PRACTICAL PHARMACOLOGY
for the
DENTAL HYGIENIST

STEVEN C. MONROTUS, B.A., D.M.D.

General Dental Practitioner;
Dental Staff, Deaconess Hospital,
Saint Louis, Missouri;
Dental Staff, Lutheran Medical Center,
Saint Louis, Missouri;
Instructor Dental Pharmacology,
Saint Louis Community College,
Saint Louis, Missouri.

1980 W. B. SAUNDERS COMPANY / Philadelphia / London / Toronto

W. B. Saunders Company: West Washington Square
Philadelphia, Pa. 19105

1 St. Anne's Road
Eastbourne, East Sussex BN21 3UN, England

1 Goldthorne Avenue
Toronto, Ontario M8Z 5T9, Canada

Library of Congress Cataloging in Publication Data

Monrotus, Steven C.
   Practical pharmacology for the dental hygienist.

   Bibliography: p.
   Includes indexes.   1. Dental pharmacology   2. Dental hygiene.
I.   Title.   RK701.M56   615′.1′0245176   79-67793   ISBN 0-7216-6434-4

Practical Pharmacology for the Dental Hygienist   ISBN 0-7216-6434-2

Last digit is the print number: 9 8 7 6 5 4 3 2 1

Dedicated to

KARL K. WEBBER, D.D.S.
my good friend and teacher
and to
STEVIE, JIMMIE, and DANNY

who made it all worthwhile

PREFACE

Since the turn of the last century the separate fields of medicine and dentistry have grown closer, and this trend has placed greater responsibility for treatment of the total patient on dental auxiliaries. Recent advances made in our understanding of the complexities of human function and treatment of disease require the expanded-function dental hygienist to prepare for this responsibility partially in the area of pharmacology. Ironically, the currently marketed textbooks of dental pharmacology for hygienists are either written or edited by researchers or periodontists who do not engage in general dental practice, do not assume the primary responsibility for delivery of dental care to the public, and do not represent a majority of the practitioners who could engage the services of a hygienist. While such textbooks are excellent works for the authors' peers, they obviously fall short of providing students a level of instruction that would prepare them to adequately manage clinical situations involving drugs and drug-related techniques encountered in a general dental practice; the difficulty students have extracting pertinent information from such references has been repeatedly demonstrated by the low scores generally seen in this area on the National Board Examination.

The dental hygienist is a clinician, not a researcher. Although theoretical aspects have been included here to clarify matters of clinical importance, no attempt has been made to improve on the many theoretical works available. An exhaustive presentation has been abandoned in favor of providing a clinically relevant base from which subsequent study may be made as the hygiene student learns to assimilate and recall details in a way analogous to that of the dental student. The design of this approach has been to produce another well-informed clinician who can interact harmoniously with the general dentist or dental specialist as dental diagnostic problems are tackled every day and solved.

The focus of this book was not on producing another typical tour de force on drugs but on serving the dual purpose of aiding the student during instruction on a rigorous subject and in passing the National Board Examination, and on training the graduate hygienist whose background in this area may be weak or poorly correlated with practice. To limit the textbook to a manageable size for classroom use, space was not wasted on definitions of terms found in medical dictionaries or on explanations of certain basic concepts of mathematics, chemistry, anatomy, or physiology unless the material was critically important. Students unfamiliar with such terms or concepts are referred to standard references for further information.

Curriculum Essentials for Dental Hygiene Education, published by the American

Dental Hygienist's Association, was used as a guide for content, and topics were organized for incorporation into a sixteen-week semester allowing time for examinations. The order of presentation of topics has been based on results of actual classroom testing, in which higher examination scores were made using the present format. New material is based only on previous material or pertinent material within the chapter and is cross-referenced. As the need arises, the beginning student is given more than one exposure to certain basic and critical information.

Certain related topics in the areas of nutrition, dental public health, patient evaluation, medical emergencies, and dental surgery and anesthesia were included in this book in the interests of completeness. Since the mechanism of action of the autonomic drugs is theoretical, the cardiovascular agents were presented ahead of them to emphasize the fact that many drugs with cardiovascular or pulmonary effects exert these effects outside the realm of autonomic receptor theory. The choices of morphine, nalorphine, and aspirin were arbitrarily made as standards of comparison to assess relative potency of similar drugs, but other analgesics could also have been used. A separate generic drug index was prepared to encourage learning of generic rather than trade names and to assist in reviewing for examinations.

Special thanks are given to Dr. Ira Shannon for his cooperation with the section on fluorides, to Paul D. Nelson for his years of encouragement, proofreading, and preparing the illustrations and indexes, and to the editors for their patience and suggestions. The students at St. Louis Community College deserve special mention for displaying an interest that became the inspiration for this textbook and without which the project would never have been begun and completed.

S. C. Monrotus, B.A., D.M.D.
St. Louis, 1980

CONTENTS

1

GENERAL PHARMACOLOGY

SECTION 1: GENERAL PRINCIPLES OF DRUG ACTION

Drug-Related Fields

There are no sharp lines of demarcation separating the various drug-related fields, but the following are useful definitions:

Pharmacology — the study of drugs.

Pharmacy — the science dealing with the procurement, preparation, and dispensing of drugs.

Pharmacodynamics — the science dealing with the mode of action and with the metabolism of drugs.

Pharmacotherapeutics — the science dealing with the use of drugs in the treatment of disease.

Pharmacognosy — the science dealing with the identification of naturally occurring drugs.

Posology — the study of drug dosage.

Toxicology — the study of poisons.

A drug is loosely defined as any chemical substance capable of affecting a biological system. Over 7500 such drugs affecting man have been described, and about 325 (4.3 per cent) of these are clinically important to the dental hygienist.

Periodic Literature

There are several sources for obtaining information on drugs and their uses.

The **United States Pharmacopeia** (USP) is issued every five years and it sets manufacturing standards related to strength and purity. The initials USP on a bottle label following the name of a drug insure that it has been manufactured with the greatest care.

The **British Pharmacopeia** (BP) is the English equivalent of the USP and is official in Canada and Great Britain.

The **National Formulary** (NF) is issued every five years and describes standards for drugs that are widely used or that have high therapeutic value.

The **AMA Drug Evaluations** (ADE) contains information on drugs introduced in the United States during the preceding ten years and on all drugs in current medical use.

The **Physician's Desk Reference** (PDR) is issued every year by some 200 drug manufacturers and contains product descriptions and a product identification section showing about 1300 tablets and capsules in full color and at actual size for easy comparison. It does not describe all drugs currently in use, but it is cross-indexed to include generic and trade names, and it describes about 2500 drug products.

Accepted Dental Therapeutics (ADT) is issued every two years by the **Council on Dental Therapeutics** of the ADA. It is designed to assist the dental practitioner in the selection of drugs for treatment of oral disease.

Facts and Comparisons (FC) is a loose-leaf listing of over 6000 drugs in current use, and it summarizes pertinent prescribing information. It is continuously updated with monthly supplements and is the most complete and up-to-date source available for rapid reference in a dental office. No dental office should be without one.

Drug Nomenclature

The **naming of drugs** becomes confusing to the student because the same drug may have several names.

The **chemical name** of a drug conveys the chemical structure and is first used when the drug is tested experimentally.

When the drug is found to be therapeutically useful the **United States Adopted Name Council** (USAN) gives it a generic name that will not conflict with other drug names. The company marketing the drug also gives the drug a **trade name** (proprietary name) which is, for promotional purposes, generally short and easy to remember.

Because the generic name is the official name of a drug and is the one used in the

USP and NF, it is preferred over the trade name(s). When the generic name of a drug is learned, it is unnecessary to learn a large number of trade names.

To illustrate the various names of a single drug we will use lidocaine as an example:

Chemical name: 2-diethyl-amino-2'6',-aceto-xylidide
Generic name: lidocaine
Trade names: Xylocaine
                Octocaine
                Doricaine
                ProLido

In all subsequent discussions we will use the generic name followed by a common trade name in parentheses, for example, lidocaine (Xylocaine).

Routes of Administration

The following are the various avenues by which drugs may be introduced into the human body:

1. Enteral Routes

a. Oral Route. The simplest way to introduce a drug into the body is by mouth, and this is the method most often used.

Advantages: Absorbing area of the intestine is large.

                  Patients are usually cooperative.

                  In overdosage most of drug can be retrieved by pumping the stomach.

Disadvantages: Some drugs are deactivated by hepatic-portal circulation.

                  Blood levels are less predictable.

                  Onset is delayed by slower absorption.

                  Gastric irritation is possible and may result in nausea.

b. Rectal Route. Drug suppositories are often placed in the rectum when the oral route is impractical or impossible.

Advantages: Patient cooperation is unnecessary.

                  The GI tract is not irritated.

                  Administration is not prevented by nausea or unconsciousness.

Disadvantages: Absorption is decreased compared to that of upper intestine.

                  Absorption is irregular and incomplete.   *Absorpth. ↓ - irreglr. + incomplete*

2. Parenteral Routes

a. Intravenous Route (I.V.). Drugs may be given through the superficial veins of the forearm, the dorsal veins of the hand, or the veins of the ankle.

Advantages: It is the most rapid method of eliciting a drug response.

The drug response is the most predictable.

Constant plasma levels are most easily obtained by this method.

This route accommodates the largest volume of drug solution.

Disadvantages: Drug injected cannot be retrieved.

Rapid injection produces undesirable effects.

Needle trauma may result in bruising.

Conscious patient is placed under stress.

b. Intramuscular Route (I.M.). Drugs may be given by injection into muscle, such as the deltoid, the lateral head of the triceps, or the gluteus medius.

Advantages: Absorption is rapid (anterior quadriceps absorbs most rapidly and is often used for hypodermoclysis).

Irritating drugs are well tolerated.

Large amounts of solution can be accommodated.

Disadvantages: Repetitive drug administration is inconvenient.

Conscious patient is placed under stress.

c. Subcutaneous Route (Sub-Q). Drugs may be injected below the dermis of the skin.

Advantages: Absorption is slow, a requirement for certain drugs, such as insulin.

Rate of absorption can be controlled with ice packs or topical epinephrine.

Disadvantages: Irritating drugs result in painful injection in conscious patient (conscious patient is placed under stress).

Only a small amount of drug solution is accommodated.

Other less frequently used parenteral routes are:

d. Intradermal Route. Drugs may be injected into the dermis of the skin (usually small amounts of local anesthetic are injected first, after which longer needles may be passed painlessly for deeper injections).

e. Intrathecal Route. Drugs may be injected into the spinal subarachnoid space (usually drugs needed to treat certain infections of the meginges).

f. Intraperitoneal Route. Drugs may be injected into the peritoneal cavity and absorbed via the mesenteric veins. This route has fallen into disuse because of the hazards of infection and adhesions.

g. Inhalation Route. Drugs in solution can be atomized and the aerosols can be inhaled, with absorption occurring via the mucous membranes of the respiratory tract. This route is often used when the agents are volatile or gaseous.

h. Topical Route. Drugs in solution may be applied anywhere on the skin or at epithelial surfaces of the eye, ear, nose, vagina, or urethra. This route is often used in the oral cavity for treatment of certain infections and administration of topical anesthetics.

Factors Influencing Drug Absorption "*SCPR*"

Solubility
Conc.
Phys. State
Route

There are several factors that influence the rapidity and degree of absorption of drugs into the body.

(4) **Route of Administration.** By far the most important factor is the route of administration. In general the parenteral routes offer more rapid and complete absorption than do the enteral routes.

(3) **Physical State.** The physical state in which the drug is administered will also affect its absorption. In general, drugs in solution are more rapidly and completely absorbed than are drugs in tablet or capsule form.

(1) **Solubility.** The solubility of a drug will also affect its rate of absorption. In general, water-soluble drugs are more rapidly and completely absorbed than are those that are fat-soluble.

(2) **Concentration.** The concentration of the drug presented to the absorbing surface will affect its absorption. In general, food or water taken before, with, or after a drug is administered orally will decrease the amount of drug absorbed and the rate of absorption. Drugs given parenterally in high concentration may result in chemical irritation with reduced absorption.

Drug Diffusion and Transportation

In order for drugs to exert their effects after administration they must first traverse cell membranes. The **cell membrane** has been described as a lipid bilayer covered on both sides by protein, and it is approximately 100 angstroms wide (1 **angstrom** = 10^{-10} meter). Special openings in the membrane called **pores** are scattered randomly on its surface, and are about 8 angstroms wide, except for **capillary pores,** which are about 30 angstroms wide. The pores are lined with positive charges and are capable of regulating the passage of small molecules and ions in and out of the cell. Drugs with molecular weights of 200 or less may pass through all membrane pores, but drugs with molecular weights *as high as 60,000* may pass through capillary pores. This process is known as **filtration.**

Extensions of the lipid bilayer also protrude through the protein covering of most membranes to the surface and in an unknown way enable lipid-soluble substances to move across the lipoprotein membrane by the process of **simple diffusion** from an area of higher concentration to an area of lower concentration. The amount of drug that diffuses is proportional to its **lipid solubility** and the concentration gradient. Therefore, whenever a drug is present outside a cell, the cell membrane becomes a barrier that exhibits a selective permeability depending on the drug's molecular size, valence (charge), and lipid solubility.

The passage of certain substances, such as glucose, across membranes is mediated by specific carrier substances within the membranes that are as yet unidentified. A drug bound to a carrier substance may pass through a membrane and be released on the other side of the membrane along its own concentration gradient by the process known as **facilitated diffusion.**

Specialized cells, such as those of nerves and muscle, are capable of transporting a substance through their membranes against an electrochemical or concentration gradient, a process which is termed **active transport**. This requires an energy expenditure, and more energy is needed to actively transport a charged particle than a neutral one.

When drugs enter the plasma they commonly undergo a reversible binding to a high molecular weight protein, **albumin.** Since only the unbound portion of the drug is active, the bound portion does not contribute to the intensity of drug action. The bound and unbound forms are in equilibrium with each other, and as more of the unbound form is used the equilibrium shifts to release more of the bound form from storage, and drug activity is prolonged. Standard doses of drugs that are highly bound may become toxic when followed by drugs that displace them from their binding sites on plasma albumin.

If all the albumin binding sites have been occupied, a drug may begin to saturate the globulin fraction of plasma as well. Certain drugs may undergo initial binding to the globulins rather than to albumin.

Sites of Drug Elimination

Drugs are removed from the body at certain sites which are classified as either major or minor in importance:

MAJOR SITES

Liver. The liver is the prime organ of drug detoxification and elimination and concentrates unmetabolized drugs and their altered metabolites in the bile or metabolizes and degrades drugs in the circulation for eventual removal by the kidney. Drugs eliminated in the bile are stored in the gall bladder and during reflex stimulation are deposited into the lumen of the small intestine, where they are eventually removed in the feces by the colon.

Kidney. The rate and extent of excretion of drugs in the urine depends upon glomerular filtration and tubular secretion acting to remove drugs from plasma and eliminate them in the urine and upon active and passive tubular reabsorption, which transports some of the filtered substances back into the plasma.

Colon. The colon eliminates drugs that are not completely absorbed after oral administration and those that are not well absorbed after biliary excretion. Drugs excreted in bile that are reabsorbed by the intestines find their way back to all other sites of elimination.

Lung. The rates of elimination of gaseous end products of metabolism depend on the partial pressures of gases in the inspired air, alveolar air, and pulmonary capillaries, the solubility of the drug in plasma, the blood flow in the tissues, and the presence of other gases.

MINOR SITES

Mammary Gland. Unless proven otherwise any drug taken by a pregnant woman should be expected to appear in the breast milk. Women receiving medication during their pregnancies should be advised not to nurse their children.

Sweat Gland. Certain drugs may appear in perspiration shortly after administration.

Lacrimal Gland. Drugs excreted into tears may be discharged to the external environment or swallowed and ultimately removed by the kidney or colon.

Salivary Gland. Drugs excreted into saliva are largely swallowed and also ultimately removed by the kidney or colon.

Non-Glandular Structures (Placenta, Epidermal Structures, and Teeth). To the extent that the fetus is a drug depot apart from the mother the placenta is considered an excretory organ for drug elimination. Slow removal of minute quantities of drugs is also possible in shed epidermis, trimmed hair and nails, and extracted teeth.

Categories of Group Drug Actions

Drugs can modify the action of cells by (1) initiating a cellular response, causing cells to produce certain materials; (2) stimulating or depressing cellular activity, causing cells to increase or decrease their functions; (3) changing the usual effect of another drug on cells, producing a different response to the drug or no response at all; and (4) exerting purely physical or chemical effects.

A **drug receptor** is a specialized cellular or tissue element with which a drug interacts to produce its biological effects; it is believed that receptors are macromolecules (proteins, lipoproteins, enzymes, or nucleic acids) that form a complex with a drug to trigger a series of chemical events. Such receptors are theoretical constructs that help to explain experimental observations and have not been demonstrated histologically; they are postulated to exist solely to explain the action of certain drugs whose actions cannot be explained otherwise, such as antihistamines (histamine H_1 and H_2 receptors), phenothiazine tranquilizers (dopamine receptors), and autonomic drugs (cholinergic and adrenergic receptors) (Chap. 5, Sec. 4; Chap. 6, Sec. 2; Chap. 7, Sec. 2). The series of chemical events triggered by the above receptors, as well as by many of the hormones (Chap. 4, Sec. 1) appears to involve the activation or inhibition of the cellular enzyme adenyl cyclase, which in turn changes the levels of cyclic AMP (adenosine monophosphate) within the target cell.

Affinity is the ability of a drug to combine with a receptor, whereas **efficacy** is the ability of a drug to induce a response subsequent to occupation of the receptor. An **agonist** is a drug that exhibits an affinity with a receptor such that combination of the drug and the receptor produces a functional change in the surrounding tissue; an **antagonist** is a drug that exhibits zero efficacy at a given receptor. Agonists therefore possess both receptor affinity and efficacy. Antagonists have affinity but lack efficacy.

Effects of Multiple Drug Administration

Whenever two different drugs are introduced into the body simultaneously they will either (1) enhance each other, (2) antagonize each other, or (3) have no effect on each other.

Enhancement of effect may come about through (1) **addition**, whereby the effect of single doses of two drugs acting in the same direction is greater than that expected for one of the drugs acting alone; (2) **summation**, whereby the combined effect of single doses of two drugs acting in the same direction is exactly equal to the algebraic sum of the individual responses; (3) **synergism**, whereby the effect of single doses of each of two drugs is greater than the algebraic sum of the individual effect when each drug is administered alone; and (4) **potentiation**, whereby the administration of a drug with no effect on a given receptor causes an exaggerated response to the administration of another drug. In some instances potentiation is used as a synonym for synergism and is broad in its meaning.

Antagonism may take the form of (1) physiological antagonism, whereby two drugs acting normally may oppose each other by acting in opposite directions; (2) chemical antagonism, whereby an active drug combines chemically with another, its antagonist, to form a compound with either no activity or less activity than the original drug; and (3) specific antagonism (competitive inhibition), whereby a drug interferes with the combination of another drug with a response system through competition for receptor sites for which both agents have a particular affinity.

No drug is so precisely specific for receptors in all patients that it is effective in exactly the desired manner, nor is any absolutely free of producing unsought reactions in some patients. Therapeutic effects primarily sought are desired drug actions, whereas additional effects not primarily sought are termed **drug reactions, or adverse drug actions**.

Whenever several drugs are administered to a patient concurrently the incidence of drug reactions increases as the number of drugs taken increases. Table 1-1 illustrates drug reaction frequency as a function of the number of drugs administered at one time.

Drug Susceptibility

Patients responding to substandard doses of a drug are considered to be **hypersusceptible** to that drug and all other chemically similar drugs. In practice, these patients are usually identified as those who complain of having a system that is sensitive to medicine of any kind and who usually refuse drug therapy.

Patients responding only to suprastandard doses of a drug are considered to be **hyposusceptible** to that drug and all other chemically similar drugs. In practice, these patients are usually identified as those who claim to have a system that is resistant to most medicine and who are usually reluctant to comply with drug therapy.

When patients are hyper- or hyposusceptible to certain drugs, they often extend their feelings of apprehension to drug therapy of any kind, including local anesthesia for root planing. Such patients would rather suffer quietly during a subgingival debridement than allow the operator to administer a dental injection to relieve their discomfort. In such cases it is best not to force treatment on a patient and in a friendly confident way complete the dental prophylaxis with respect for the patient's wishes.

Factors Affecting Patient Response

There are several factors that can affect response to drug administration:

Table 1-1. DRUG REACTION FREQUENCY*

Number of Drugs Administered	Reaction Rate
5	4.2%
6-10	7.4%
11-15	24.2%
16-20	40.0%
21 or more	45.0%

*From Martin, E. W., Hazards of Medication, 2nd ed., J. B. Lippincott, 1978, reprinted with permission.

Handwritten margin notes (top):
Age of Pt.
Age of Prescriptn.
Presence of other drugs
" of Disease
Body Temp.
The Placebo Eff.
Time of Administratn.
Variatns is Animal Species

FacTORS Eff. Pt. Response : (8)

Handwritten margin notes (right):
1 A - P
2 A - P
3 A - P
4 O - P
5 T - A
6 V - A.S.
7 B - T
8 PLA - Ef.

Variations in Animal Species. In veterinary science qualitative and quantitative differences in the response of animals to different drugs are observed. Certain drugs producing a given effect in certain animals may have the opposite effect in man or may require dosage changes based on mg/kg body weight.

Age of Patient. Standard adult doses of drugs assume that the dose is administered to a patient between 12 and 60 years of age. Infants, children, and geriatric patients require reduced doses because children have a smaller body surface area and hence a smaller body mass for drug distribution, and the elderly have a reduced metabolic rate and fail to degrade and eliminate drugs as rapidly as younger people.

Presence of Other Drugs. Although some drug combinations produce no interactions whatsoever, antagonism or enhancement of effect may occur and produce respectively no response to a given drug or an exaggerated response.

Body Temperature. Elevated body temperature in febrile states may alter the rate at which a drug is metabolized by increasing the metabolic rate, and high blood levels of a drug are more difficult to maintain over several hours. Control of high fever in infants, for example, often requires more than one antipyretic drug administered simultaneously.

Presence of Disease. Certain drugs will exert their therapeutic effects only in the presence of disease and will cause no response in the normal patient. Antipyretic drugs, for example, have no effect on normal body temperature.

Certain diseases may also affect drug susceptibility. Hyperthyroid patients, for example, are unusually sensitive to epinephrine.

Time of Administration. Some drugs are poorly absorbed when taken orally at mealtime and may require that the patient take them between meals in order to obtain the proper blood levels of the drug.

The Placebo Effect. Placebos ("sugar pills") are inert substances whose value lies in their function as symbols of the doctor's healing power. Doctors themselves are capable of affecting a patient's response by transmitting to the patient their knowledge of the potency of the drug. The positive therapeutic response of a patient to an inert substance prescribed by a doctor is called "the placebo effect" and has been shown to be a powerful tool.

The strength of the placebo effect increases with that of the medication to which it is compared. In double-blind experiments on pain relief, placebos have been reported to be 55 per cent as effective as both mild and strong analgesics. Other studies suggest that at least 50 per cent of the short-term effect of any drug that affects subjective states (pain, anxiety, and so forth) are attributable to the placebo effect.

States of mind may affect the course of cancer in some patients, and spectacular remissions in response to the administration of a placebo have been reported by several investigators. This is believed to be the result of developing in the patient's mind a very strong anticipation of cure. Such treatment, often called the "psychological approach" should be considered only in patients who are willing to expend considerable effort and to endure psychic pain, in patients who are surgically inoperable, in patients who no longer respond to radiation, and in patients for whom conventional chemotherapy is contraindicated. With these limitations in mind, the psychological approach to cancer treatment is necessarily very restricted and should be viewed only as a last resort.

Age of Prescription (Stability of Drug Preparation). Medicine of any kind that was prescribed prior to the current illness or for someone else should be disposed of by flushing down a toilet. There are many drugs that will cause patients to become violently ill if taken after their shelf-life has expired, such as minocycline (Minocin) (Chap. 2).

Different salts of the same drug may be more or less stable in solution due to decreased or increased water solubility, with resulting changes in potency as the time from manufacturing increases, as occurs with propoxyphene (Chap. 8, Sec. 2).

Dose Response Curve and Therapeutic Index

The first step in evaluating the toxicity of any drug before it is marketed is to determine its lethality in experimental animals. A large number of animals are given a test dose of the drug, and the number of deaths is plotted as a function of the dose administered. When this is done a sigmoid (S-shaped) curve is obtained, and the **lethal dose** required to kill 50 per cent of the animals so treated is defined as the LD_{50} and is expressed in units of mg/kg body weight.

In a similar way the **effective dose** required to elicit the desired response in 50 per cent of the animals tested is defined as the ED_{50} and is always less than LD_{50}.

Since all drugs are toxic at some dose, the LD_{50} is meaningless unless the ED_{50} is also known. The ratio of $LD_{50}:ED_{50}$ is known as the therapeutic ratio, or therapeutic index of the drug. The higher the therapeutic index (TI) of a drug, the less chance there will be of a toxic reaction upon its administration and the greater its use in therapy. (See Fig. 1-1.)

↑ Therapeutic index = ↓ chance of toxic reactn.

SECTION 2: ADVERSE DRUG ACTIONS

Untoward Reactions

Untoward, or undesirable reactions to drugs may take place in the body in addition to the desired responses.

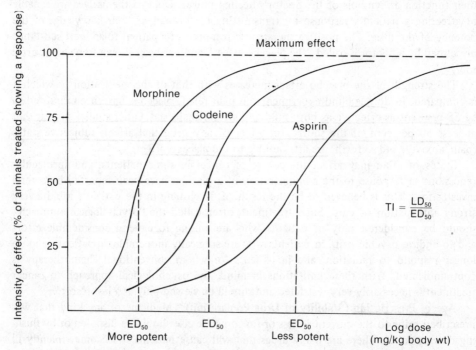

Figure 1-1. Dose response curves of three analgesic drugs comparing dosage and effectiveness.

Side Effects. In addition to a drug's main effect there are usually side effects that are observed at standard doses. These are actions of a drug other than that specifically desired. Codeine, for example, in providing analgesia for moderate pain will also stimulate the chemotherapeutic trigger zone (CTZ) of the medulla, which may initiate vomiting.

Toxic Reactions. Actions of a drug that result from overdosage are termed **toxic reactions**. **Barbiturate** intoxication, for example, which results from overdose of barbiturates, may produce respiratory arrest and death.

Hypo- or Hypersusceptibility. Inadequate or exaggerated responses not seen with a majority of patients may occur at standard doses of a drug. A dose of meperidine, for example, which is sufficient for relief of moderate pain in an average adult patient, may not produce analgesia at all in a hyposusceptible patient and may produce relief of chronic intractable pain in a hypersusceptible patient.

Allergic Hypersensitivity. Some patients react to initial contact with a drug by forming antibodies against it. Subsequent exposure to the same drug may precipitate an antigen-antibody reaction, causing a sudden violent release of histamine and widespread cellular dysfunction. There are a growing number of patients who have a history of allergy to certain drugs, for example, penicillin.

Idiosyncratic Reactions. When there has been no known previous contact of the patient with a certain drug and the drug is administered, the drug may elicit a response that is different from that which is usually observed. An idiosyncratic reaction to diazepam, for example, which is a preoperative sedative and muscle relaxant, may manifest itself with symptoms of extreme agitation and increased muscle tonus.

Allergic Reactions

Allergic reactions, or allergic hypersensitivity, is divided into two broad categories:

Contact Allergy. This form of allergy is precipitated at a mucosal surface or part of the skin in contact with the environment. Contact dermatitis, for example, may result from prior exposure to dental disclosing solution.

Intrinsic Allergy. This form of allergy is precipitated by injection, inhalation, or ingestion of a food, drug, or air-borne particle. Most allergic responses, for example, penicillin allergy, fall into this category.

Oral lesions resulting from contact allergy are termed **stomatitis venenata**, whereas oral lesions that result from the absorption of drugs are termed **stomatitis medicamentosa**.

Because allergic reactions during drug therapy may be more serious than the initial disease, it is important that the operator be aware of the potential allergic state of the patient before treatment is begun, the various side effects of any agents administered, and the correct treatment for any complications that may arise as a result of drug therapy.

The exact mechanism of an allergic reaction is at present unknown but the following is the currently accepted theory.

Whenever drugs or other foreign substances enter the circulation they may cause some cells of the reticuloendothelial (RE) system to produce antibodies against them. These antibodies are believed to be altered serum globulin molecules produced in the bone marrow, spleen, lymph nodes, and Kupffer's cells of the liver, and once formed they pass into the blood, lymph, and tissue fluid and become attached to cells.

When the patient is exposed to a second dose of the offending antigen, either it is neutralized in the bloodstream by circulating antibodies or it reaches the tissues and reacts with fixed antibodies if there are insufficient circulating antibodies in the serum.

The reaction between the drug (antigen) and the antibodies fixed to cells causes the liberation of histamine and histamine-like substances, resulting in vasodilation, increased capillary permeability, and smooth muscle spasm (Chap. 5, Sec. 4).

The two drugs used in a dental office that are most likely to produce allergic reactions are local anesthetics and penicillins (Chap. 12, Sec. 1).

Anaphylactic Reactions

Anaphylactic, or anaphylactoid, reactions are an extremely rare form of allergy characterized by a sudden complete loss of vasomotor tonus, marked hypotension progressing into respiratory and cardiac arrest, and loss of consciousness. The patient rapidly becomes cyanotic and death appears imminent.

The suddenness of this emergency can be terrifying, and prompt treatment must be provided if the patient's life is to be saved. There is no time to debate the diagnosis or plan the treatment (Chap. 12, Sec. 1).

Patients presenting with a history of such a reaction to any drug should be given antihistamines pre- and postoperatively when dental treatment is attempted (Chap. 5, Sec. 4). Patients with a history of asthma or hay fever have a greater chance of having anaphylactic reactions; if any patient is unsure about an allergy to local anesthetics, treatment should be delayed until the patient is tested by an allergist. Local anesthesia is contraindicated in patients proved sensitive or when such testing is impossible. Patients in pain requiring emergency treatment before testing can be done should be given analgesics (see Chapter 8) and, if swelling is present, antibiotics (see Chapter 2) after consultation with the patient's physician.

Urticaria (MALE VIP)

Urticaria is a disorder often associated with allergic and anaphylactic reactions and is characterized by skin lesions (rashes), myocardial and respiratory distress, visual and abdominal disturbances, itching, and often edema of the tongue. The condition is often caused by the release of histamine or a histamine-like substance. Allergic mechanisms involve antigens that may be derived from a variety of sources:

1. Inhalants, such as dust, dander, or pollen.

2. Injectants, such as drugs, vaccines, or hormones.

3. Ingestants, such as drugs or foods.

4. Contactants, such as metal filings or cosmetics.

5. Infections in teeth, gingiva, tonsils, or sinuses.

Non-allergic mechanisms may also give rise to urticaria in response to the following agents:

1. Drugs.

2. Diseases, such as carcinoma, leukemia, rheumatoid states or hormone disturbances.

3. Physical agents, such as heat, cold, trauma, or pressure.

Treatment for this condition is directed at blocking the action of histamine and maintaining the patient's "vital signs" within normal limits (Chap. 12, Sec. 1).

The important drugs which may cause urticaria in dental practice are shown in Table 1–2.

Tolerance

Tolerance is the phenomenon characterized by diminishing patient response to the administration of successive equal doses of a drug. Patients who have been taking a certain drug for some time may have acquired a tolerance to it such that higher than average doses are necessary to produce the required effect. When the drug is discontinued it may take several days to several months after the last dose for tolerance to disappear.

When a patient develops tolerance to one drug, cross-tolerance to all other drugs with a similar chemical structure is exhibited. A patient having a tolerance to codeine, for example, will also be cross-tolerant to morphine and other naturally occurring and synthetic opiates.

Orally administered preoperative medication may induce no response at all in patients who are tolerant to similar drugs — particularly sedatives, tranquilizers, central nervous system (CNS) depressants, and analgesics — and who have been taking them for a long time. Patients claiming to be tolerant to a certain group of drugs and requesting higher doses should be given only average doses consistent with their needs, and their responses should be verified.

Habituation and Addiction

Drug habituation is a condition that results from repeated consumption of a drug by the patient and is characterized by the following:

Table 1–2. DRUGS WHICH MAY CAUSE URTICARIA

Drug Groups	Member Drugs
Antiseptics and disinfectants	Iodides
Antibiotics	Penicillins Tetracyclines Sulfonamides Erythromycin
Hormones	Insulin
Analgesics	Opiates Meperidine Salicylates Propoxyphene
Sedative-Hypnotics	Barbiturates
Tranquilizers	Meprobamate
CNS depressants	Hydantoins
Enzymes	Hyaluronidase
Antineoplastics	Thiouracil

1. A desire, but not a compulsion, to continue taking the drug for the improved well being it engenders.

2. Little or no tolerance.

3. Some psychic dependence on the effects of the drug, no physical dependence.

4. Detrimental effects involving only the user.

Millions of Americans are habituated to alcohol and tobacco, as well as to certain prescription drugs, such as diazepam (Valium) or flurazepam (Dalmane).

Drug addiction is a condition that results from repeated consumption of a drug by the patient and is characterized by the following:

1. A compulsion to continue taking the drug and to obtain it by any means (Chap. 11, Sec. 2).

2. Development of tolerance.

3. Psychic and physical dependence on the effects of the drug.

4. Detrimental effects involving both the user and society.

Transmission Across Placenta

Whether or not a drug will cross the placental barrier depends upon several factors:

Stage of Pregnancy. The stage of placental development will influence transmission of drugs in either direction in that the more highly developed placenta found in later pregnancy will allow more rapid and complete diffusion of substances due to its richer vascularity.

Placental Selectivity. The placenta has a higher permeability to certain substances, for example Vitamin C, than to others. This appears to be related to the occurrence of carrier-mediated diffusion (facilitated diffusion) in the placental membranes, but this is currently hypothetical.

Molecular Weight of Drug. Drugs with a molecular weight higher than 1000 are usually unable to cross the placenta. Very few drugs have molecular weights in excess of 1000; therefore, all drugs should be assumed to cross the placenta until proved otherwise. Exceptions to this rule are rare.

Assuming adequate nutrition, there is no evidence that pregnancy itself exerts deleterious effects on the teeth of the mother. Contrary to the old wives' tale, a woman does not lose a tooth with every pregnancy.

The drugs of importance in dentistry that cross the placenta and may endanger a developing fetus are listed in Table 1–3.

Oral Effects of Certain Drugs

The following are the substances which frequently give rise to stomatitis medicamentosa:

Heavy Metals. In heavy metal toxicosis the salivary glands attempt to excrete in the saliva excess heavy metals, which can then precipitate on the teeth and gingiva and cause discolorations. The discolorations are heaviest opposite the orifices of the glands, namely, on the buccal surface of maxillary molars and the lingual surface of the mandibular

Table 1-3. DRUGS WHICH CROSS THE PLACENTA

Drugs	Effect on Fetus
Narcotics Barbiturates Nitrous Oxide	Fetal respiratory depression
Tetracyclines	Discolored teeth, inhibited bone growth
Coumarins	Intrauterine hemorrhage, fetal death
Salicylates	Neonatal bleeding tendencies
Mepivacaine	Fetal bradycardia
Cortisone	Cleft palate
Amethopterin	Cleft palate, other anomalies, abortion
Cyclophosphamide	Stunting, defects of extremities, fetal death
Thiouracil	Hypothyroidism, neonatal goiter, mental retardation

incisors. The two metals most often implicated are lead and mercury, which produce blue and blue-red discolorations respectively.

Antibiotics. Almost all antibiotics, including penicillins and tetracyclines, can be incriminated in alterations of the oral soft tissues. These changes may include a burning painful stomatitis, painful tongue, black hairy tongue, and secondary fungal infections.

Sedative-Hypnotics. Barbiturates may cause oral lesions. It is estimated that 3 to 5 per cent of patients taking barbiturates develop skin lesions, but the incidence of oral lesions is much lower.

Tranquilizers. Intraoral eruptions have been linked with meprobamate and have been described as a blistering of the lips and oral mucosa, tongue, and gingiva, with severe itching and burning.

Salicylates. Aspirin, phenacetin, and Empirin Compound may produce oral lesions in sensitized patients, resulting in painful ulcerations or burning stomatitis.

The following substances frequently give rise to stomatitis venenata:

1. Topical antibiotics.

2. Topical iodine-containing preparations.

3. Acrylic denture base materials.

4. Vulcanite denture base materials.

5. Alloys in partial denture frameworks.

6. Silver amalgam.

7. Dentifrices.

8. Mouthwashes.

9. Denture adhesives and cleaning creams.

10. Lipsticks and cosmetics.

Diphenylhydantoin (Dilantin) is well known for its production of gingival hyperplasia secondary to its use as an anticonvulsant. Many of the antineoplastic agents used in the treatment of cancer produce such oral side effects as **ulcerative stomatitis** and gingival bleeding. Oxyphenbutazone (Tandearil) therapy occasionally results in salivary gland enlargement accompanying the analgesic effect. Painful ulcerations of the oral mucosa occur when chemical burns are produced from acids and alkalies. For this reason patients should be advised never to allow an aspirin tablet to dissolve in the mucobuccal fold adjacent to a painful tooth. **Gingival hyperplasia** has also resulted from long-term use of oral contraceptives.

SECTION 3: PRESCRIPTION WRITING

Drug Schedules

The Federal Controlled Substances Act of 1970 requires every person who manufactures, distributes, prescribes, administers, or dispenses any controlled substance and who is not specifically exempted, to register annually with the Attorney General. This registration is the function of the Bureau of Narcotics and Dangerous Drugs (BNDD) of the Drug Enforcement Administration (DEA). This Act established five schedules, or groups, for restricted drugs:

Schedule I. Schedule I includes hallucinogenic substances and some opiates which have no accepted medical use and the highest potential for abuse. Examples from this group are diacetylmorphine (heroin), lysergic acid diethylamide (LSD), marijuana, and peyote.

Schedule II. Schedule II contains drugs with acceptable medical use and high potential for abuse which, if abused, may lead to severe psychological or physical dependence. Included in this group are the Class "A" narcotics, certain stimulants, and certain short- and intermediate-acting barbiturates. Examples are morphine, codeine, meperidine (Demerol), Percodan, hydromorphone (Dilaudid), cocaine, amphetamines, pentobarbital (Nembutal), secobarbital (Seconal), and amobarbital (Amytal).

Schedule III. Schedule III contains drugs with acceptable medical use and lower potential for abuse than those in Schedule II which, if abused, may lead to moderate or low psychological dependence or high physical dependence. Included are the Class "B" narcotics, certain narcotic and non-narcotic combination products, and narcotic antagonists. Examples from this group are Vicodin, Phenaphen with Codein, Tylenol with Codeine, Synalgos-DC, and naloxone (Narcan).

Schedule IV. Schedule IV contains drugs with acceptable medical use and low potential for abuse relative to drugs in Schedule III which, if abused, may lead to limited physical dependence. Included in this group are other depressants and tranquilizers. Examples are diazepam (Valium), chlordiazepoxide hydrochloride (Librium), meprobamate (Equanil), and phenobarbital (Luminal).

Schedule V. Schedule V contains drugs with accepted medical use and low potential for abuse relative to those in Schedule IV which, if abused, may lead to limited physical dependence or psychological dependence. Included are Class "X" narcotics, which are exempted preparations that may be sold over the counter (otc) without a prescription. Included are opium, morphine, and codeine mixed with specific amounts of active non-narcotics:

1. Opium, 120mg/30cc

2. Morphine or any of its salts, 15mg/30cc or 15mg/30gm

3. Codeine or any of its salts, 60mg/30cc or 60mg/30gm

Schedule V also contains certain prescription drugs relatively unimportant in dentistry.

A prescription is a dentist's order to a pharmacist directing him or her to dispense a specific drug or preparation in specific amounts for a certain person at a particular time and to instruct the person in its use. Prescriptions are applicable for drugs in Schedules II, III, IV, and some in Schedule V.

Prescriptions are legal documents for which the prescriber and pharmacist are equally responsible. Telephone prescriptions are not executed for Schedule II amphetamines or barbiturates under any circumstances, and no drug listed in Schedule II may be dispensed without a valid written prescription. In dire emergencies oral authorization for a lawful prescriber is sufficient for dispensing Schedule II narcotics, but the amount dispensed must be limited to the amount adequate to treat the patient during the emergency period only. Within 72 hours after such authorization the prescriber must submit to the pharmacist a written prescription for the amount dispensed. The pharmacist is required to notify the State Division of Health if such a prescription has not been received within the designated 72 hours. Many pharmacists make it a rule to refuse under any circumstances to dispense Schedule II products with authorization given by phone.

Controlled substances stored in a dental office must be kept in a locked cabinet or safe. Criminal violations of this law are punishable by fines, prison terms, or both.

Individual states' criteria for the various schedule categories sometimes differ from the Federal ones; when the Federal and State restrictions differ, the more stringent requirements prevail with respect to refilling prescriptions and to the records which must be kept.

Parts of a Written Prescription

The modern prescription retains six basic components:

The Heading. At the top of the prescription appears the heading which includes the dentist's name, office address, and phone number, the patient's name and address, and the date. Occasionally the age of the patient is also included.

The Superscription. The superscription appears below the heading on the left side of the script (prescription blank). It is represented by the symbol "Rx.," an abbreviation for the Latin word *recipe* ("take thou"). It is believed to stand for the sign of Jupiter, father of the Roman gods, whose help the ancient prescriber wished to invoke to make the medicine effective. When a prescription is written on a blank slip of paper the symbol "Rx" should appear to identify the document. In most offices script pads are printed with the heading and superscription printed on them to save time in writing.

The Inscription. The inscription states the name(s) and concentration(s) of the prescribed ingredients. In prescribing certain commercial preparations the name only is sufficient, for example, Percodan.

The Subscription. The subscription contains the dosage form desired (tablets, capsules, pediatric suspensions, and so forth) and the number of such doses to be dispensed. If the medication is a special recipe of the dentist this part of the prescription should also contain specific directions to the pharmacist for compounding the ingredients.

The Signature (*Signatura, Signa*). The signature comprises instructions for the patient's use, that is, how much medicine to take, how to take it, and how often to repeat it. Although prescriptions are written today in English certain Latin abbreviations are still in common use (Table 1–4). This part of the prescription always begins with the abbreviation "Sig." to identify that these are the instructions to the patient.

The Dentist's Signature. The prescriber signs his or her name at the bottom of the prescription authorizing the dispensing of the medication. If the medication is a controlled substance, the prescriber's DEA number (BNDD number) is written immediately below the signature. Every dentist is issued a different number by the Federal Government, which is checked by the pharmacist before the prescription is filled. The number always begins with the letter "A" (for America) followed by the first letter of the dentist's last name, and it ends in a seven digit number (Fig. 1–2).

It is recommended that the dentist indicate on the prescription whether or not the prescription is to be renewed and, if so, how many times. This information may be quickly designated on many scripts by filling in a small form printed on them, usually in the lower left corner. Without such information on the prescription, a patient is usually refused any refills until the pharmacy contacts the prescriber for proper authorization. If it is permissible for the pharmacist to dispense a less expensive generically equivalent drug than what is listed in the inscription, the prescriber signs his or her name to the left of the bottom line above the words "substitution permitted;" when this is not permissi-

Table 1–4. COMMONLY USED LATIN ABBREVIATIONS

Latin Phrase	Abbreviation	Meaning
signa	Sig.	label, "take"
statim	stat.	immediately
numero	no.	number
qua tres hora	q.3h.	every 3 hours
qua quattour hora	q.4h.	every 4 hours
qua sex hora	q.6h.	every 6 hours
bis in die	b.i.d.	twice a day
ter in die	t.i.d.	three times a day
quater in die	q.i.d.	four times a day
hora somni	H.s.	at bedtime
per os	P.O.	by mouth
non per os	n.P.O.	nothing by mouth
pro re nata	p.r.n.	as needed
ante cibum	a.c.	before meals
post cibum	p.c.	after meals
recipe	Rx.	"take thou"
non repitatur	non rep.	do not repeat

Handwritten annotations: every (next to q.3h./q.4h./q.6h. rows); q o d - every other day; h = hour; q = every; Ex. q6h; p̄ - after; ā - line; c̄ - with; s̄ - w/o

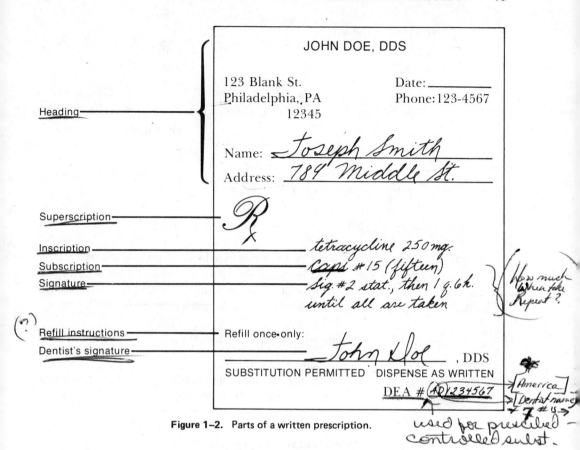

Figure 1–2. Parts of a written prescription.

ble, the prescriber signs his or her name to the right of the bottom line above the words "dispense as written."

Commonly Used Conversion Factors

In the metric system the three fundamental units of length, weight, and time are expressed as meters, grams, and seconds, respectively. The following prefixes are used to denote magnitude:

pico	10^{-12}	trillionth
	10^{-11}	
	10^{-10}	
nano	10^{-9}	billionth
	10^{-8}	
	10^{-7}	
micro(μ) . .	10^{-6}	millionth
	10^{-5}	
	10^{-4}	
milli(m) . .	10^{-3}	thousandth
centi	10^{-2}	hundredth
deci	10^{-1}	tenth

(UNITS)   ($10^0 = 1$)

deka . . . . 10^1		tenfold
hecto . . . . 10^2		hundredfold
kilo . . . . . 10^3		thousandfold
10^4		
10^5		
mega . . . . 10^6		millionfold
10^7		
10^8		
giga . . . . . 10^9		billionfold
10^{10}		
10^{11}		
tera . . . . . 10^{12}		trillionfold

In determining drug dosage, weight is expressed in milligrams, micrograms, and grains. Volume is expressed as cubic centimeters and fluid ounces. Concentration is expressed as weight per unit volume, percent solution, or as a ratio of weight:volume. Relationships of the units of weight, volume, and concentration are as follows:

Weight relationships (mg, μg, gr)

$$1 \text{ g (gram)} = 15 \text{ gr (grains)}$$
$$= 10^3 \text{ mg (milligrams)}$$
$$= 10^6 \text{ } \mu\text{g (micrograms)}$$
$$1 \text{ gr} = 60 \text{ mg}$$

Volume relationships (cc, fl oz)

1 tsp (teaspoon)	= 5 cc (cubic centimeters)
	= 5 ml (milliliters)
	(1 cc = 1 ml)
1 tbsp (tablespoon)	= 15 cc
	= 3 tsp
	= 1/2 fl. oz.
1 fl oz (fluid ounce)	= 30 cc
	= 2 tbsp
	= 6 tsp

Concentration (weight-volume) relationships (mg/cc, μg/cc)

1 per cent solution = 1 g/100 cc = 10^3 mg/10^2 cc = 10 mg/cc
2 per cent solution = 2 g/100 cc = 2 × 10^3 mg/10^2 cc = 20 mg/cc, etc.
1:1000 = 1 g/10^3 cc = 10^3 mg/10^3 cc = 1 mg/cc
1:100,000 = 1 g/10^5 cc = 10^6 μg/10^5 cc = 10 μg/cc, etc.

A gram of weight is defined as the gravitational force at sea level exerted upon 1 cc of water (H_2O) at its temperature of maximum density (4°C).

Children's Dose Calculation

Calculation of children's dosage presents special problems because dose is based on body weight, which is proportional to body surface area, and body weight is variable with age. Several formulas have been developed for this purpose:

1. Infants (up to age 1)

   a. Clark's Rule:

$$\text{Infant dose (ID)} = \frac{\text{Wt (lbs)} \times \text{Adult dose}}{150}$$

   b. Fried's Rule:

$$\text{ID} = \frac{\text{Age (mos)} \times \text{Adult dose}}{150}$$

2. Children (ages 1 to 12)

   c. Young's Rule:

$$\text{Child dose (CD)} = \frac{\text{Age (yrs)} \times \text{Adult dose}}{\text{Age (yrs)} + 12}$$

   d. Cowling's Rule:

$$\text{CD} = \frac{\text{Age (at next birthday)} \times \text{Adult dose}}{24}$$

The weakness in the above formulae is that body weight is variable with age and in many cases the dose based on age is underestimated. A more accurate formula bases the dose on body surface area:

$$\text{CD} = \frac{\text{Body surface area (m}^2) \times \text{Adult dose}}{2.00}$$

This formula is based on the assumption that the average adult male patient has a body surface area of 2.00 m^2.

For any given height and weight, tables in reference books and Figure 1–3 may be consulted to determine body surface area. By drawing a straight line between the height and weight scales of Figure 1–3 and determining the point of intersection on the middle scale, accurate determination of child dose can be made. (See Fig. 1–3.)

The relationship between body surface area and per cent adult dose is roughly linear; i.e., for every 0.2m^2 increase in body surface area, the per cent adult dose increases approximately 11 per cent.

It is generally agreed that a child at age eight should be able to tolerate one half the adult dose of any given drug, and a child at age 12 can safely be given a full adult dose without fear of overdosage.

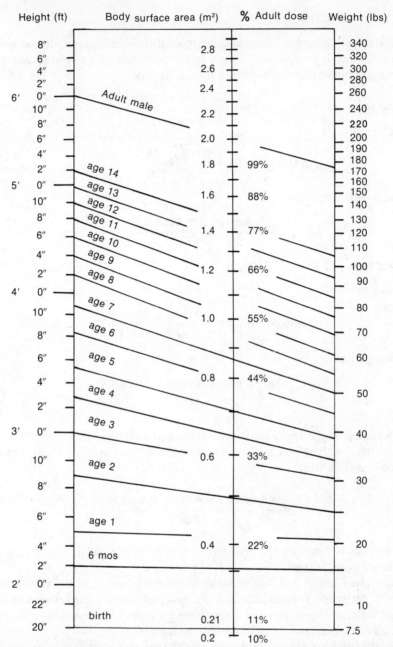

Figure 1–3. Dubois body surface chart. (Modified from information prepared by Boothby and Sandiford of the Mayo Clinic.)

Patient Compliance

It is generally assumed that the more a patient knows about the medicine he is taking the more likely he will be to take the medicine on schedule. The personal observation of the author in writing thousands of prescriptions for dental patients in the course of private practice has been that this assumption seems correct for some patients, while with others more errors are seen in the medication schedule as the patient's knowledge about his medicine increases.

Lengthy discussions with the patient concerning the actions of the medicine and the reasons the doctor has prescribed it should be avoided. A good rule to follow is "the less said, the better," except in those circumstances when the patient is a member of a health profession and less likely to become confused with a technical explanation. Even under these circumstances it is the doctor, not the hygienist, who is best capable of leading the discussion; when the doctor prefers not to answer any questions patients may have concerning the actions of a drug, the hygienist should not attempt to answer them either.

It sometimes seems that the incidence of postoperative complications in dentistry is proportional to patient inability to follow postoperative instructions. Therefore, the dental hygienist should realize that as an extension of his or her dentist employer, choice of words used with a patient can be as much a part of the treatment as the medicine itself.

TEST QUESTIONS

1. All of the following are drug-related fields EXCEPT:
   - (a) posology
   - (b) pharmacodynamics
   - (c) pharmacotherapeutics
   - (d) pharmacy
   - (e) necrology
   - (f) toxicology
2. The most complete source that is used for obtaining information about drugs in current use and that is updated with monthly supplements is:
   - (a) Physician's Desk Reference
   - (b) United States Pharmacopeia
   - (c) Facts and Comparisons
   - (d) National Formulary
   - (e) AMA Drug Evaluations
   - (f) Accepted Dental Therapeutics
3. Generic names should be learned in favor of other drug names because a generic name:
   - (a) will not conflict with other drug names
   - (b) is the official name listed in the U.S.P. and N.F.
   - (c) when learned makes the learning of a large number of trade names unnecessary
   - (d) conveys the chemical structure
   - (e) is short and easy to remember for promotional purposes
   - (f) a, b, and c
   - (g) b, c, and d
   - (h) c, d, and e
   - (i) all of the above
4. All of the following are parenteral routes of administration EXCEPT:
   - (a) subcutaneous
   - (b) inhalation
   - (c) topical
   - (d) rectal
   - (e) intramuscular
   - (f) intravenous
5. Injection at the most rapidly absorbing intramuscular site in the body is used to elicit as rapid a drug response as possible when an intravenous route is impractical or impossible, and this site is located in the:
   - (a) gluteus medius
   - (b) anterior quadriceps
   - (c) gastrocnemius
   - (d) lateral head of the triceps
   - (e) deltoid
   - (f) none of the above

6. A disadvantage of using the intravenous route is that:
   (a) drugs once injected cannot be recalled
   (b) it accommodates only a small volume of solution
   (c) it is NOT the most rapid method of eliciting a drug response
   (d) constant plasma levels of a drug cannot be easily obtained
   (e) drug response is more unpredictable than with other routes
   (f) none of the above

7. Drug absorption is influenced by all of the following EXCEPT:
   (a) route of administration
   (b) physical state
   (c) solubility
   (d) concentration
   (e) molecular weight
   (f) none of the above

8. Specialized excitable cells, such as nerve, muscle, and odontoblasts, are capable of transporting a drug across their cell membranes against an electrochemical or concentration gradient by a process that is termed:
   (a) filtration
   (b) simple diffusion
   (c) facilitated diffusion
   (d) active transport

9. All of the following are sites of drug elimination EXCEPT:
   (a) liver
   (b) kidney
   (c) colon
   (d) lung
   (e) mammary gland
   (f) pancreas

10. Drugs can modify the action of cells by:
    (a) initiating a cell response
    (b) stimulating or depressing existing cell activity
    (c) changing the usual effect of another drug on cells
    (d) exerting physical or chemical effects
    (e) all of the above
    (f) none of the above

11. A specialized cellular or tissue element with which a drug interacts to produce its biological effects and which is postulated to exist solely to explain the actions of certain drugs whose actions cannot be explained otherwise is a:
    (a) unit membrane
    (b) receptor
    (c) synergist
    (d) binding site on albumin

12. A drug that exhibits zero efficacy at a given receptor is a(n):
    (a) synergist
    (b) potentiator
    (c) agonist
    (d) antagonist

13. When two different drugs are introduced to the body simultaneously, enhancement of effect may come about through:
    (a) addition
    (b) summation
    (c) synergism
    (d) potentiation
    (e) all of the above
    (f) none of the above

14. A clinical response to a substandard dose of a drug is termed:
    (a) hyposusceptibility
    (b) hypersusceptibility
    (c) tolerance
    (d) toxic reaction

15. All of the following are factors affecting patient response to drugs EXCEPT:
    (a) variations in animal species
    (b) age of patient
    (c) molecular weight of drug
    (d) presence of other drugs
    (e) presence of disease
    (f) body temperature
    (g) time of administration
    (h) placebo effect
    (i) age of prescription

16. The therapeutic ratio or index is expressed as:
    (a) $LD_{50}:ED_{50}$
    (b) $ED_{50}:LD_{50}$
    (c) mg/kg
    (d) a positive number greater than one
    (e) a and d
    (f) b and d

17. All of the following are untoward reactions to drugs EXCEPT:
    (a) side-effects
    (b) toxic reactions
    (c) hypersusceptibility
    (d) allergic hypersensitivity
    (e) habituation
    (f) idiosyncratic reactions

18. The drugs most likely to precipitate allergic reactions in dental treatment are:
    (a) penicillins
    (b) local anesthetics
    (c) narcotics
    (d) a and b
    (e) b and c
    (f) a and c

19. A rare form of allergy characterized by sudden loss of vasomotor tonus, marked hypotension, and loss of consciousness progressing into cardiac and respiratory arrest is a(n):
    (a) toxic reaction
    (b) idiosyncratic reaction
    (c) anaphylactic reaction
    (d) urticaria episode
    (e) heart attack
    (f) none of the above

20. A disorder which is characterized by skin lesions, myocardial and respiratory distress, itching, visual and abdominal disturbances, and tongue edema and which often results from the release of histamine or a histamine-like substance is:
    (a) a toxic reaction
    (b) an idosyncratic reaction
    (c) an anaphylactic reaction
    (d) urticaria
    (e) a heart attack
    (f) none of the above

21. A diminishing response to successive equal doses of a drug is termed:
    (a) potentiation
    (b) tolerance
    (c) placebo effect
    (d) hyposusceptibility

22. Drug habituation in comparison with drug addiction is characterized by:
    (a) little or no tolerance developed
    (b) both psychic and physical dependence on the effects of the drug
    (c) detrimental effects involving both the user and society
    (d) none of the above

23. Whether or not a drug crosses the placenta depends upon:
    (a) the molecular weight of the drug
    (b) the stage of pregnancy
    (c) placental selectivity for the drug
    (d) all of the above

24. Stomatitis medicamentosa may be caused by any of the following EXCEPT:
    (a) heavy metals
    (b) antibiotics
    (c) sedative-hypnotics
    (d) tranquilizers
    (e) vitamins
    (f) salicylates

25. According to the Federal Controlled Substances Act of 1970, drugs that have acceptable medical use and high potential for abuse and that, if abused, may lead to severe psychological or physical dependence would be in Schedule:
    (a) I
    (b) II
    (c) III
    (d) IV
    (e) V

26. The Latin phrase "pro re nata," abbreviated p.r.n., means:
    (a) immediately
    (b) four times daily
    (c) as needed
    (d) by mouth

27. The portion of a written prescription containing the instructions to the patient for taking the medicine is the:
    (a) heading
    (b) superscription
    (c) inscription
    (d) subscription
    (e) signature

28. In determinations of drug dosage, concentration is expressed as:
    (a) weight per unit volume
    (b) per cent solution
    (c) as a ratio of weight:volume
    (d) a and b
    (e) b and c
    (f) all of the above

29. An acetaminophen elixir contains 120 mg/cc; if you want a child to take 300 mg you would give:
    (a) ½ teaspoon
    (b) 1 teaspoon
    (c) 1½ teaspoons
    (d) 2 teaspoons

30. A phenobarbital elixir contains 20 mg/5 cc; if you want a child to take 60 mg you would give:
    (a) 1 teaspoon
    (b) 2 teaspoons
    (c) 1 tablespoon
    (d) 2 tablespoons

31. Intravenous influsion of 50 cc of dextrose 5 per cent solution would result in administration of:
    (a) 2.5 mg
    (b) 25 mg
    (c) 250 mg
    (d) 2500 mg

32. A dental hygienist administers one full carpule (1.8 cc) of lidocaine 2 per cent with epinephrine 1:100,000 for mucosal anesthesia during root planing. The patient has received _(1)_ of lidocaine and _(2)_ of epinephrine.
    (a) (1) 36 mg and (2) 18 µg
    (b) (1) 36 mg and (2) 180 µg
    (c) (1) 36 µg and (2) 18 µg
    (d) (1) 36 µg and (2) 180 µg

33. Epinephrine 1:1000 solution for emergency use contains:
    (a) 10 µg/cc
    (b) 100 µg/cc
    (c) 1 mg/cc
    (d) 10 mg/cc
    (e) 100 mg/cc
    (f) 1 g/cc

34. One teaspoon of 0.4 per cent stannous fluoride solution contains:
    (a) 10 mg
    (b) 20 mg
    (c) 30 mg
    (d) 40 mg

35. According to body surface charting, a child at age _____ should be able to tolerate ½ the adult dose of any given drug.
    (a) 2
    (b) 4
    (c) 6
    (d) 8

2

ANTISEPTICS, DISINFECTANTS, AND ANTIBACTERIAL AGENTS

SECTION 1: ANTISEPTICS AND DISINFECTANTS

Definitions

An **antiseptic** is a drug that inhibits but does not necessarily destroy microorganisms, whereas a **germicide** is a drug capable of destroying microorganisms. Germicides that are lethal for pathogenic (disease-producing) microorganisms are termed **disinfectants**.

The most common use for these agents in dental hygiene practice is in cold treatment of contaminated surfaces of certain non-penetrating dental instruments, such as handpieces and prophylactis angles. However, these drugs also find use as pre-injection and pre-incision wipedowns, as surgical scrubs, in root canal irrigation, and as ingredients in intra-alveolar and periodontal packs, as well as in topical agents.

For all of the above uses the drugs are dissolved in solution prior to administration to thoroughly wet the contaminated surface upon application.

Limitations

Antiseptics and disinfectants cannot be relied upon to kill *Mycobacterium tuberculosis*, hepatitis virus B, or spores, and the use of these agents should be reserved for treatment of accessible infections in the oral cavity and for disinfection of certain non-penetrating instruments. Although some manufacturers claim that their germicides will kill all pathogens, the use of these products is not a sovereign remedy for a lack of sterilization equipment. There are a growing number of dentists who are illogically using only cold chemical disinfection for treatment of their penetrating instruments between patients, and those who employ hygienists should be persuaded to obtain the necessary equipment before hiring one.

The term **sterilization** implies the complete destruction of all microorganisms, whether pathogenic or non-pathogenic. All penetrating instruments, such as forceps, elevators, curettes, and scalers, should be either steam sterilized in an autoclave at 121°C at 15 lbs pressure for 15 minutes, or dry heat sterilized at 160°C for 1 hour.

Loose surgical instruments may be sterilized in the operating suites of most modern hospitals by subjecting them to steam in an autoclave at 270°C for three minutes; wrapped instruments will be sterilized at the same temperature after seven minutes in the autoclave. This process is termed "high speed" sterilization.

Common Uses

Dental hygienists will commonly encounter the following agents in a dental office:

70 per cent **isopropyl alcohol** finds use as a pre-injection skin wipedown and an intraoral solvent for temporary crown and bridge cements.

Eugenol (clove oil) is one of dentistry's oldest medicines and is both an antiseptic and an anodyne having a sedative effect on exposed irritated dentin. The oil is mixed with zinc oxide powder to form zinc oxide eugenol (ZOE) The final product(s) of the reaction are as yet unknown, but the reaction may be accelerated by the addition of zinc acetate (to form modified ZOE). This agent finds use as an ingredient in temporary fillings and cements, periodontal and intra-alveolar packs, and pressure-indicating paste.

Five per cent **sodium hypochlorite** (Clorox) is used by some dentists in a diluted form to irrigate and disinfect the main root canals of teeth.

Formocresol finds use in endodontic therapy and may be used to disinfect and mummify remnants of pulp tissue following pulp removal and prior to canal debridement.

Three per cent **hexachlorophene** (pHisoHex) is used in oral surgery or subgingival curretage as a surgical scrub prior to gloving.

Four per cent **Chlorhexidine gluconate** (Hibiclens liquid) is also used as a surgical scrub prior to surgical procedures.

Benzalkonium chloride (Zephiran) may be used to disinfect skin pre-operatively and for sterile storage of instruments and hospital utensils. To protect metal instruments stored in solution from rust, four Anti-Rust tablets per quart should be added to the solution, and the solution changed at least once a week. Since anionic detergents and soaps reduce the antibacterial activity of the solution, all instruments should be thoroughly rinsed before storage.

Two per cent **glutaraldehyde** (Cidex) is said to kill *M. tuberculosis*, spores, and viruses on penetrating instruments after a ten hour soak and is ideally suited for disinfection of endodontic files or other instruments likely to rust when heated. It is not deactivated by soap, blood, or mucus.

Three per cent **hydrogen peroxide** is used by some dentists during cavity preparation to disinfect dentinal surfaces prior to filling. The release of oxygen provides the antiseptic action.

Ten per cent **carbamide peroxide** (Gly-Oxide, Cank-Aid) also releases oxygen on contact with mouth tissues, reduces inflammation, inhibits odor-forming bacteria, and relieves pain of periodontal pockets, aphthous ulcers, denture sores, and various other oral lesions.

Several **mercury compounds** are available for external use as general antiseptics. Among these are **thimerosal** (Merthiolate), **merbromin** (Mercurochrome), **phenylmercuric nitrate** (Phe-Mer-Nite), and **mercocresols** (Mercresin).

There are likewise several **iodine compounds** that can be used as antiseptic solutions and surgical scrubs. Anhydrous copper sulfate may be mixed with glyceryl zinc iodide to form **Gray's astringent**, which can be used intraorally to disinfect periodontal pockets, gingival infections, and surgical wounds following electrosurgery. Two per cent **iodine in alcohol** (iodine tincture) may be applied to skin wounds, but to avoid irritation the area should not be bandaged, and the skin will be stained. **Povidone-iodine** (Betadine, Pharmadine, ACU-dyne, Isodine, Mallisol, Polydine) retains the germicidal property of iodine without irritation to skin and mucous membranes and is non-staining. Treated areas may be taped or bandaged. **Poloxamer-iodine** (Prepodyne, SeptoDyne), also a water-soluble iodine complex, releases iodine at a determined rate, resulting in prolonged action.

In addition to the agents just discussed there are many over-the-counter (otc) throat lozenges, troches, mouthwashes, and sprays that can be used for minor mouth irritations. These supply antiseptic and analgesic effects and usually contain combinations of **hexylresorcinol, cetylpyridinium chloride**, or **phenol** in a flavored base with **benzocaine**.

Negatol (Negatan) 45 per cent solution, although used primarily as a styptic, has germicidal properties in dilutions up to 1:100 and can be applied full strength to oral lesions (Chap. 5, Sec. 3).

Direct and Indirect Pulp Capping

Dental caries, or dental decay, is an infection of the teeth and is treated by means of surgical removal of the diseased portion of the tooth and placement of disinfectants and antiseptic fillings when the disease encroaches on the pulp, or nerve, of the tooth. When decay is deep there are two popular methods of treatment: (1) the indirect pulp cap, and (2) the direct pulp cap.

When decay is examined microscopically, it can be seen divided into various zones depending on depth. There is a zone of hard decay that has not yet decalcified between the zone of soft decay which has decalcified and is radiographically visible and the sound portion of the tooth. If a pulp exposure, or nerve exposure, is suspected pre-operative to complete caries removal, an indirect pulp cap may be performed. In this procedure all decay is removed except a small portion of hard decay close to the pulp, and the tooth is lightly dampened with a sponge, or cotton pledget, and filled with a zinc oxide eugenol temporary filling. It is then hoped that the antiseptic properties of the filling will arrest any further growth of the cavity to give the pulp time to migrate away from the area. As the pulp tissue retreats centripetally it lays down secondary dentin at the rate of about 4 microns per day. Since zinc oxide eugenol is hygroscopic (water-attracting), if the tooth is not dampened with water before insertion of the filling, the material will attract water from the dentin and sensitize it. For this reason zinc oxide eugenol is never placed in a bone-dry tooth unless the pulp has already been removed. After a minimum of four to six weeks the tooth is completely excavated and a sound floor of paper-thin dentin separates the pulp from the cavity preparation, thus avoiding a pulp exposure.

If the operator elects to do complete caries removal and a small pulp exposure is encountered (less than 0.5 mm in diameter), a "base" may be applied to the exposure site, and the tooth may be closed for four to six weeks with a temporary filling. This is termed a direct pulp cap. The base material most often used in permanent teeth is calcium hydroxide (Dycal), and that used in primary teeth, **zinc oxide eugenol** (Cavitec). There is increasing evidence that any chemically pure substance placed on the exposed pulp tissue will stimulate the formation of a secondary calcific bridge in dentinogenesis; however, it has been shown that placement of calcium hydroxide (Dycal) on pulp exposures of primary teeth will cause internal root resorption.

When a pulp exposure is greater than 0.5 mm in diameter, pulpectomy and endodontic therapy is indicated, and the entire pulp is removed down to the root apex.

The pulp is not healthy in any carious tooth (Chap. 4, Sec. 2) but it should respond favorably to an indirect or direct pulp cap, provided that the tooth is diagnosed as vital before treatment. Many failures are due to attempting treatment on non-vital, gangrenous teeth or to errors in diagnosis. The presence of hemorrhage at the exposure site indicates vitality. Recent studies indicate that a solution containing **9-aminoacridine** 0.2 per cent and **benzalkonium chloride** 0.1 per cent has greater antibacterial activity and is less irritating than eugenol when applied directly to pulp exposures of any size.

The greatest criticism most general dentists have of pulp capping procedures is the unpredictable incidence of postoperative sensitivity that can result in the patient's blaming the dentist for improper technique. Because dentists also consider that healing is unpredictable and that the pulp may become non-vital in spite of treatment, as well as that modern endodontic therapy is relatively simple, pulp capping procedures have been slow to establish a foothold in many dental practices.

Pulpotomy and Pulpectomy

It is generally agreed that the more cellular a tissue the greater is its healing potential. When primary and permanent tooth pulps are examined microscopically, a histological difference is seen between the two; i.e., the primary **tooth pulp** is cellular throughout, whereas the permanent tooth pulp is relatively acellular, except in the area of the pulp chamber. When the pulp of a primary tooth is vital (alive), it should therefore be possible to remove only the most severely infected portion of the pulp from the pulp chamber below the cavity and to expect the remaining pulp tissue to remain vital. A **pulpotomy** is a procedure that results in the removal of the coronal third of a vital primary tooth pulp, disinfection of the remaining pulp stumps, and temporary closure of the tooth. If the tooth pulp is non-vital (gangrenous), and the tooth can be saved, the entire pulp tissue is removed down to the root apices, and the tooth is disinfected and temporarily closed in a procedure called a **pulpectomy**. Pulpotomies are not performed on permanent teeth because removal of pulp tissue from the pulp chamber will be followed by rapid degeneration of the remaining pulp tissue in the main root canals due to the decreased cellularity; this can lead to further infection and possible pain. Neither are pulpotomies performed on gangrenous (non-vital) teeth when pulpectomy is indicated.

The main agent used to disinfect pulp stumps during pulpotomies is formocresol; this drug has an extremely disagreeable odor, and it will burn any soft tissue that it contacts. Dry sponges (cotton pellets) used to transfer formocresol from the jar to the tooth should be only lightly dampened with the solution, and the top should be closed on the jar immediately after use to avoid the escape of noxious vapors.

Other less widely used disinfectants and anti-inflammatory compounds that have been used for pulpotomies include hydrocortisone 2.5 per cent solution and solutions of

9-aminoacridine 0.2 per cent and benzalkonium chloride (Zephiran) 0.1 per cent.

According to Sargenti the apical third of a vital infected pulp is sterile and will not undergo degeneration when endodontic therapy is completed in one sitting using the N2-RC2B sealant (Chap. 13, Sec. 2).

Some evidence suggests that potent agents such as formocresol should not be used to disinfect pulp stumps of primary teeth because these drugs can leak into the bone and damage the enamel-forming cells (ameloblasts) of the permanent tooth buds, resulting in enamel hypoplasia of the permanent tooth. Since the enamel of the permanent incisors, cuspids, and bicuspids should be completed by age six the incidence of enamel hypoplasia secondary to iatrogenic use of formocresol is almost non-existent in children having a mixed dentition; when pulpotomies are indicated in children aged two to five, and the operator is concerned about the possibility of **enamel hypoplasia, hydrocortisone** 2.5 per cent solution may be substituted for formocresol, or pulpectomy may be performed as an acceptable alternative.

Treatment Planning

In producing a "treatment plan" for a patient it should be borne in mind that a cavity is always larger in the mouth than it appears on a dental radiograph, because the zone of soft decay is the only part that has decalcified. Whenever a radiograph shows a moderate sized cavity in a young tooth with a large pulp, or a relatively "small" shadow indicating leakage underneath an old crown or filling, the patient should be informed preoperatively, at the consultation appointment, that the possibility exists that the nerve of the tooth may be infected and need to be treated. The phrase "root canal" should be avoided in beginning discussions with the patient because this may be frightening.

Teeth that have large open holes in them should be lightly dried with dry sponges and temporary zinc oxide eugenol fillings should be placed in them without drilling and before dental prophylaxis. It is not wise to disturb such teeth with a spoon excavator in attempts to remove some of the "leathery dentin;" this may result in a pulp exposure. It is also not wise to dry the tooth lightly with a blast of air; this will irritate the pulp and can result in pain when the tooth was previously asymptomatic. If a patient's teeth bother him or her more after they have been cleaned, he or she will be inclined to blame the dentist and the hygienist, even when a lifetime of neglect is the cause of the disease.

SECTION 2: ANTIBACTERIAL AGENTS

General Uses and Gram's Staining

In dental practice whenever a patient presents with both pain and swelling it is almost always because of an infection, and antibiotics are usually indicated. An antibiotic is a substance either produced by an organism or made synthetically that exerts an antagonistic effect on another organism. When the offending pathogen is known, an antibiotic may be selected that will be effective against that pathogen; the pathogens most often implicated in dental infections are bacteria and fungi.

Antibiotics are not so specific that they "hit" only the offending pathogen; the clinician should keep in mind that antibiotic therapy can disrupt microbial equilibria and allow microorganisms normally held in check to overgrow, resulting in **superinfection.**

Superinfection is defined as a proliferation of microorganisms that are different from those causing the original infection. To avoid the possibilities of superinfections and untoward reactions (Chap. 1, Sec. 2), antibiotics should not be routinely prescribed for minor infections unless a definite need for them exists. All infections do not require antibiotic coverage, and many respond to local disinfection and to building the general resistance of the body to disease by administration of therapeutic vitamins and minerals (Chap. 3, Sec. 1).

If a patient discontinues an antibiotic without taking the entire amount prescribed those organisms that have only been weakened will develop into resistant strains that will be harder to kill later with the same drug. This results in a situation worse than that of giving no drug at all, because another drug must be used that is usually not the drug of choice. Dental patients should therefore be advised to take all of the drug prescribed.

Bacteria are classified according to the Gram's method of staining:

1. A smear is made on a microscope slide.

2. The smear is then stained with crystal violet for one minute, washed in water, stained with Gram's iodine for one minute, and washed in water again.

3. The smear is decolorized in acetone-alcohol and washed in water.

4. The smear is counterstained with safranin for 20 seconds, washed, and allowed to dry.

Organisms that retain the violet stain and do not decolorize are termed gram-positive, whereas those that decolorize and pick up the pink safranin stain are termed gram-negative.

Oral infections may involve maxillary and mandibular bone or overlying soft tissue and fascial spaces, or both. Most often they are caused by gram-positive organisms, although there are an increasing number of gram-negative oral infections. Antibiotics effective against both gram-positive and gram-negative organisms are termed "broad spectrum," or "extended spectrum" drugs.

All antibiotics are bacteriostatic at low doses; i.e., at low doses they will inhibit the growth of bacteria. As the dose is increased some antibiotics become bactericidal, or lethal to bacteria.

There is no other phase of dental hygiene practice that may justifiably arouse more fear and anxiety on the part of the patient and dentist then management of acute infections of the head and neck. A patient may present with a seemingly minor gingival infection that may turn on him like a violent monster within 24 hours, requiring several weeks of hospitalization before it is resolved. For this reason dental infections of any kind should be treated early and aggressively.

Penicillins

In dental practice the most important antibiotics effective against gram-positive organisms are the penicillins. These are the drugs of choice for most oral infections and for prophylaxis against subacute bacterial endocarditis (Chap. 13, Sec. 1) secondary to bacteremia resulting from dental procedures in a patient with a heart prosthesis or a history of rheumatic or congenital heart disease.

One "unit" of penicillin has the activity of 0.6 μg of penicillin G (1 mg penicillin G = 1667 units); therefore, the usual adult dose of 250 mg q.i.d contains 400,000 units per dose. Pediatric suspensions of various penicillins are available at concentrations of 125, 250, and 500 mg/tsp. Large doses of penicillins may be used even in children because penicillins have an almost non-existent toxicity.

Some bacteria can manufacture a substance (penicillinase) that can break the penicillin molecule into a by-product that has no antibiotic activity. This ability serves to classify the penicillins into two main groups: (1) penicillinase-sensitive penicillins, including penicillin G salts, penicillin V, and the broad spectrum penicillins; and (2) penicillinase-resistant penicillins (see Table 2–1). Drugs in the latter group are more toxic than those in the former, cause more side effects, are less effective against organisms that do not produce penicillinase, and are therefore indicated only for infections resistant to penicillin G and caused by penicillinase-producing staphylococci. All the penicillins exert their effects by interfering with the synthesis of the bacterial cell wall.

Sensitivity Reaction to Penicillins

Penicillins are, together with local anesthetics, the most likely group of drugs to cause allergic reactions in dentistry. This tendency to elicit allergic reactions is the most serious drawback to the widespread use of penicillins for infections.

It is estimated that 2.5 million people in the United States are allergic to penicillin, and allergic reactions occur in about 8 per cent of those patients receiving the drug. Any history of allergy to penicillin should be carefully noted on the patient's medical history form, but a negative history is no assurance that penicillin allergy does not exist. Patients with other allergies are more likely to be allergic to penicillin than patients who are not allergic to anything.

Skin tests have been devised to determine whether or not a patient will show an allergic response to administration of penicillin, but the tests are not completely reliable,

Table 2–1. THE PENICILLINS

Penicillinase-Sensitive Penicillins	
	Broad Spectrum Penicillins
Penicillin G sodium	Ampicillin (Amcill, Polycillin, Pensyn, Principen, Totacillin, Omnipen)
Penicillin G potassium (Pentids, Pfizerpen G, Sugracillin)	Hetacillin (Versapen)
Penicillin G procaine (Crysticillin, Duracillin, Wycillin)	Amoxicillin (Amoxil, Larotid, Polymox, Trimox)
Penicillin G benzathine (Bicillin, Permapen)	Carbenicillin disodium (Geopen, Pyopen)
PenicillinV (phenoxymethyl penicillin)	Carbenicillin indanyl disodium (Geocillin)
Penicillin V potassium (Penicillin VK, Pen-Vee K, V-Cillin K, Robicillin VK)	Ticarcillin disodium (Ticar)
Phenethicillin potassium (Maxipen)	

Penicillinase-Resistant Penicillins
Methicillin sodium (Azapen, Celbenin, Staphcillin)
Nafcillin sodium (Nafcil, Unipen)
Oxacillin sodium (Prostaphlin, Bactocill)
Cloxacillin sodium (Tegopen, Cloxapen)
Dicloxacillin sodium (Dynapen, Pathocil, Veracillin, Dycill)

and they could precipitate an anaphylactic reaction (Chap. 1, Sec. 2). Such testing should not be done in a dental office unless it is performed by trained people, with emergency drugs and equipment available.

Minor reactions to penicillin may be followed by more serious reactions after a second exposure, and any history of reaction to penicillin is sufficient justification for employing another drug.

When broad spectrum penicillins are indicated for treatment of upper respiratory infections and otitis media, many physicians are now prescribing amoxicillin rather than ampicillin because the frequency and severity of skin reactions with amoxicillin is reduced. Skin reactions to ampicillin in particular have become a common pediatric problem.

Erythromycin, Streptomycin, and Vancomycin

For those patients allergic to penicillin the antibiotic of choice is **erythromycin**, a bacteriostatic drug that is bactericidal for the staphylococci and hemolytic streptococci often involved in dental infections. It is effective against essentially the same microorganisms as the penicillins and is believed to act by interfering with bacterial protein synthesis. As with the penicillins the usual adult dose is 250 mg q.i.d, but the pediatric suspensions are available in concentrations of 125, 200, 250, and 400 mg/tsp. The following are the available preparations:

1. Erythromycin (E-Mycin, Ilotycin, Robimycin)

2. Erythromycin stearate (Bristamycin, Wintrocin, Erypar)

3. Erythromycin estolate (Ilosone)

4. Erythromycin ethylsuccinate (Pediamycin, E.E.S.)

5. Erythromycin gluceptate (Ilotycin gluceptate)

6. Erythromycin lactobionate (Erythrocin lactobionate)

The **aminoglycosides** are a group of bactericidal antibiotics used in the treatment of certain gram-negative infections. Although they are broad spectrum agents, they are associated with significant renal and neurological toxicity and even neuromuscular blockade and respiratory paralysis when given with or soon after muscle relaxants or general anesthetics. Bacterial resistance to aminoglycosides, except for streptomycin sulfate, develops slowly. **Streptomycin sulfate** is usually reserved for acute fulminating infections, such as pneumonia, meningitis, acute gonorrhea, brucellosis, chancroid, plague, and tuberculosis, and is marketed only in injection form in 1 and 5 gram vials; the usual adult dose is 1 gram I.M., followed by a schedule of between 1 and 4 grams daily in divided doses until the infection disappears or until signs of ototoxicity appear.

Vancomycin (Vancocin) is a glycopeptide antibiotic that is also associated with significant nephro- and neurotoxicity; it is indicated for treatment of potentially life-threatening infections in patients who have not responded to penicillins or cephalosporins, or of such staphylococcal infections as osteomyelitis, pneumonia, or soft-tissue infections. It is available in injection form as 500 mg in a 10 cc vial and as a powder for oral use against staphylococcal enterocolitis, marketed as 10 grams in a screw-capped container. The usual adult dose is 500 mg q.6h. or 1 gram q.12h. I.V.

The prevention and treatment of staphylococcal endocarditis (Chap. 13, Sec. 1) involve the use of penicillins, erythromycin, penicillins plus streptomycin, or erythromycin plus vancomycin, depending on the route of administration desired and the allergic status of the patient.

Tetracyclines

Another alternative in cases of penicillin allergy is treatment with **tetracyclines**, a group of broad spectrum bacteriostatic antibiotics. The usual adult dose of a tetracycline is 250 mg q.i.d, except for doxycycline and minocycline (100 mg b.i.d) and demeclocycline and methacycline (150 mg q.i.d). The pediatric suspensions contain in 2 tsps. exactly the same doses as the adult preparations.

Care must be exercised not to prescribe any of the tetracycline pediatric suspensions to children under the age of 16 (during the period of enamel development) to avoid enamel hypoplasia and permanent discoloration of the primary and permanent teeth. The following are the available preparations:

1. Tetracycline (Achromycin V, Panmycin, Robitet, Tetracyn, Cyclopar, Sumycin, Bristacycline)

2. Tetracycline phosphate complex (Tetrex)

3. Chlortetracycline HCl (Aureomycin)

4. Oxytetracycline (Terramycin, Oxlopar)

5. Doxycycline (Vibramycin, Doxychel)

6. Demeclocycline HCl (Declomycin)

7. Minocycline (Minocin, Vectrin)

8. Methacycline (Rondomycin)

As with erythromycin, the tetracyclines are believed to act by interfering with bacterial protein synthesis, but they are notably ineffective for prophylaxis against subacute bacterial endocarditis (Chap. 13, Sec. 1).

Lincomycin and Clindamycin

Lincomycin and clindamycin are chemically dissimilar to any other antibiotics; adult doses are 500 mg q.i.d and between 150 and 300 mg q.i.d respectively, and the pediatric suspensions contain 250 mg/tsp and 75 mg/tsp respectively.

Lincomycin is essentially a bacteriostatic drug that interferes with bacterial protein synthesis and that is bactericidal to some organisms. It has been used successfully against staphylococci that are resistant to penicillin, but it is not effective against gram-negative organisms. It should receive consideration in cases of actinomycosis and osteomyelitis.

Clindamycin is a bactericidal drug with the same mechanism of action as lincomycin but a slightly broader spectrum of activity. Compared to lincomycin, clindamycin causes less gastrointestinal upset, is better absorbed orally, and has a greater margin of safety in patients with renal insufficiency. It is the drug of choice for osteomyelitis secondary to alveolar osteitis (dry socket) (Chap. 13, Sec. 2).

A serious and sometimes fatal episode of colitis may appear concurrent with lincomycin or clindamycin therapy or several weeks after cessation of therapy. Patients taking either drug should be advised to discontinue the drug immediately at the first sign of diarrhea during treatment and to report passage of blood or mucus in the stool during or after treatment to their physician.

Lincomycin (Lincocin) is available as 250 and 500 mg capsules, and clindamycin (Cleocin) is available as 75 and 150 mg capsules. Both are also available in injection form.

Cephalosporins

The **cephalosporins** are a group of broad spectrum, antibiotics structurally related to the penicillins that, like the penicillins, exert their effects by interfering with the synthesis of the bacterial cell wall. They may be either bacteriostatic or bactericidal, depending on the dose, organism susceptibility, the tissue concentration of the drug, and the rate at which the organisms are multiplying. These drugs are available for oral dosage as 250 and 500 mg capsules and in pediatric suspensions of 125 and 250 mg/tsp.

The cephalosporins may be considered in severe oral infections when better-known agents cannot be used or will be ineffective, but they should be used with caution, if at all, in patients who are allergic to penicillin. While generally less effective against gram-positive organisms than penicillins, they are valuable secondary agents for use against gram-negative organisms and penicillinase-producing staphylococci. Inhibition of gram-negative organisms requires higher doses than does inhibition of gram-positive organisms.

The following are the available preparations:

1. Cephalothin sodium (Keflin Neutral)

2. Cephaloridine (Loridine)

3. Cephalexin (Keflex)

4. Cephaloglycin (Kafocin)

5. Cefazolin sodium (Kefzol)

6. Cephradine (Velosef)

7. Cephapirin sodium (Cefadyl)

The usual therapeutic dose varies from 250 to 1000 mg q.i.d, depending on the severity of the infection. Cephalexin and cephradine are particularly useful to dentists in treatment of oral infections and to the physician in treating upper respiratory infections and infections of the paranasal sinuses.

Sulfonamides

The **sulfonamides** are broad spectrum bacteriostatic agents chemically similar to para-aminobenzoic acid (PABA). They may be used rarely against oral infections when better-known agents cannot be used or will be ineffective.

Folic acid is a nutrient essential to bacterial function, but some bacteria cannot utilize pre-formed folic acid; they must manufacture their own. PABA is an essential ingredient for folic acid synthesis. Since the sulfonamides are chemically similar to PABA, they may be mistakenly incorporated into folic acid synthesis by the bacteria, thus competitively inhibiting folic acid production and therefore impeding bacterial functioning. The sulfonamides are not effective against bacteria that can utilize preformed folic acid.

Certain local anesthetics are also chemically similar to PABA and may interfere with the sulfonamides when administered concurrently (Chap. 9, Sec. 1).

The sulfonamides (sulfa drugs) may be grouped as follows:

1. Systemic, short- and intermediate-acting

   a. Sulfadiazine
   b. Sulfacytine (Renoquid)
   c. Sulfamerazine
   d. Sulfisoxazole (Gantrisin)
   e. Sulfamethoxazole (Gantanol)
   f. Sulfachlorpyridazine (Sonilyn)
   g. Sulfamethizole (Thiosulfil)

2. Systemic, long-acting

   a. Sulfamethoxypyridazine (Midicel)
   b. Sulfameter (Sulla)

3. Miscellaneous

   a. Phthalylsulfathiazole (Sulfathalidine)
   b. Sulfasalazine (Azulfidine)
   c. Sulfapyridine

Sulfonamides are available as 250, 325, and 500 mg tablets and in pediatric suspensions of 250 and 500 mg/tsp. Several multiple sulfonamide products are also available:

1. Triple sulfa (Terfonyl, Neotrizine)

   167 mg Sulfadiazine
   167 mg Sulfamerazine   } per tablet or tsp
   167 mg Sulfamethazine

2. Sulfonamides Duplex

   250 mg Sulfadiazine
   250 mg Sulfamerazine   } per tsp

3. Sul-V

   100 mg Sulfadiazine
   100 mg Sulfamerazine
   100 mg Sulfamethazine   } per tablet or tsp
   100 mg Sulfacetamide
   100 mg Sulfamethizole

Sulfonamides are generally administered in a 2 to 4 grams loading dose followed by maintenance doses of between 1 and 2 grams q.i.d, except for sulfacytine (500 mg, then 250 mg q.i.d), sulfamethizole (between 0.5 and 1.0 gram t.i.d or q.i.d), and sulfapyridine (500 mg q.i.d).

Antifungal Agents

The **antifungal agents** are used primarily to treat systemic and localized fungal infections and to prevent fungal superinfections resulting from therapy with broad spectrum antibiotics.

Nystatin (Nilstat, Mycostatin) acts by binding to fungal cell membranes and allowing leakage of intracellular components, and it is indicated for systemic fungal infections caused by *Candida (Monilia) albicans* and related species. It is supplied in tablets of 500,000 units and usual adult doses are between 500,000 and 1,000,000 units t.i.d. for at least 48 hours after clinical cure to prevent relapse. There are several nystatin-tetracycline combinations available (Declostatin, Achrostatin V, Tetrastatin, Terrastatin, Comycin). Nystatin oral suspension (100,000 units/cc) is indicated for treatment of fungal infections of the oral cavity, and the dose for adults and children is between 400,000 and 600,000 units q.i.d (one half of dose in each side of mouth, retaining the drug as long as possible before swallowing). The dose for infants is 200,000 units q.i.d. Local treatment should also be continued at least 48 hours after perioral symptoms have disappeared.

Other less important fungicidal drugs include flucytosine (Ancobon), amphotericin B (Fungizone), and griseofulvin (Grisactin, Grifulvin V). These are alternate drugs used to treat systemic fungal infections when nystatin would be inappropriate due to its selective topical action.

Postoperative Infectious Complications

Many patients who present for routine subgingival débridement and dental prophylaxis have neglected their dentition for years and are forced into seeking dental care because of pain or swelling in the mouth. When the pre-operative diagnosis is an oral infection, it is sometimes advisable to defer cleaning the teeth of such a patient, even though there may be massive calculus deposits, until certain teeth are extracted or certain soft-tissue infections are brought under control by means of curettage, irrigation, local disinfection, or antibiotic therapy.

Postoperative infectious complications associated with elective oral surgery, particularly extraction of impacted teeth, may pose drug-related problems, such as (1) selection of an appropriate antibiotic in patients who claim to be allergic to many drugs, (2) treatment of persistent infections that have not resolved in spite of antibiotic therapy, or (3) treatment of untoward reactions (Chap. 1, Sec. 2).

Patients with a medical history of allergy to many drugs, including antibiotics, will usually, but not always, develop allergy to a newly administered antibiotic within 48 hours after the first dose. Since patients are most commonly allergic to penicillin, if any antibiotics are to be given, a tetracycline or erythromycin should be chosen. If the patient continues to show allergic reactions, lincomycin or clindamycin can be tried. A sulfonamide would be the next choice, and last on the list would be agents chemically similar to penicillins (cephalosporins). The aminoglycosides streptomycin and vancomycin are generally not considered for the long-term outpatient therapy necessary for persistent oral infections because of the risks of nephro- and neurotoxicity.

The veins of the brain and face have no valves to prevent backward flow of blood, and the tissue pressures resulting from facial swelling can cause the normal gravitational channels to become blocked, resulting in venous flow that backs up along alternate routes to the cavernous sinus, brain, and meninges. Such backward venous flow is increased by muscular movement, and infections of the face superior to the horizontal plane running through the corners of the mouth are potentially life-threatening in that serious complications may develop if treatment is delayed (brain abscess, meningitis, or cavernous sinus thrombosis). Treatment of severe odontogenic infections of the face involves administration of antibiotics for prolonged periods (ten days or more), but if an oral infection is still raging out of control after five days of treatment using a single antibiotic, it is safe to conclude that the organisms causing the infection are resistant to that particular agent and that another should be substituted. "Shotgun therapy" using oral antibiotics to treat vaguely localized dental pains is contraindicated and may lead to superinfections.

The most common untoward reactions to antibiotics are side-effects involving the gastrointestinal tract (diarrhea, cramping, and similar reactions) and allergic hypersensitivity (macular rashes usually limited to the skin of the trunk of the body). Mild allergic reactions are best treated with the diphenylmethane tranquilizer and antihistamine diphenhydramine (Benadryl) 50 mg q.4h. as needed (Chap. 7, Sec. 2). Diarrhea is best treated with cholestyramine (Questran) 9 grams t.i.d. before meals; this drug is a bile-acid-sequestering resin that combines with bile in the intestine to form an insoluble complex in the feces and that induces constipation.

The extraction of maxillary cuspids, bicuspids, or molars with periapical abscess (Chap. 13, Sec. 2) and roots in intimate relation with the floor of the maxillary sinus may result in direct spreading of infection into the sinus, if the sinus floor has been perforated by disease. The purulent discharge from the nose or tooth socket that is produced by acute maxillary sinusitis can be cultured and Gram stained (Chap. 2, Sec. 2). Treatment consists of administration of antibiotics that are deemed effective against the organisms cultured and that the patient is not allergic to, antihistamine-decongestants to bring early relief to the nasal obstruction, mild analgesics to control pain, and additional surgery can be performed if needed. When the organisms cultured are gram-positive, the antibiotics given usually include methicillin I.V. between 8 and 12 grams daily, cloxacillin P.O. between 1 and 2 grams daily, and penicillin V P.O. between 1 and 2 grams daily. If the patient is allergic to penicillin the agents usually chosen are erythromycin P.O. between 1 and 2 grams daily, tetracycline P.O. between 1 and 2 grams daily, or clindamycin I.V. between 1.2 and 2.4 grams daily or P.O. between 0.6 and 1.2 grams daily. When gram-negative organisms are also cultured in significant numbers the antibiotics usually chosen are ampicillin I.V. or I.M. between 4 and 6 grams daily, cephalosporins I.V. between 6 and 8 grams daily or P.O. between 2 and 4 grams daily, or tetracycline P.O. between 1 and 2 grams daily. When patients with infections of these organisms are also allergic to penicillins, the treatment is often limited to administration of tetracycline P.O. between 1 and 2 grams daily or sulfonamides P.O. 2 and 4 grams daily. Opportunistic fungal infections of the sinus by **Candida** or related species can be managed with repeated antral lavages with nystatin or by giving amphotericin BI.V.

The majority of hospitalized patients who receive antibiotic therapy are treated prophylactically during the postsurgical phase, usually by administration of penicillins or cephalosporins, and these patients have no evidence of infection. Prophylactic antibiotic therapy following dental surgery is generally discontinued after five days.

TEST QUESTIONS

1. A drug that inhibits but does not necessarily destroy microorganisms is termed a(n):
   (a) antiseptic
   (b) germicide
   (c) disinfectant
   (d) styptic

2. Disinfectants cannot be relied upon to consistently kill:
   (a) *Mycobacterium tuberculosis*
   (b) hepatitis B virus
   (c) spores
   (d) all of the above

3. All of the following are common dental office antiseptics and disinfectants EXCEPT:
   (a) isopropyl alcohol
   (b) eugenol
   (c) formocresol
   (d) glutaraldehyde
   (e) carbamide peroxide
   (f) negatol
   (g) glyceryl zinc iodide
   (h) zinc oxide
   (i) povidine-iodine

4. Direct pulp capping of primary teeth using calcium hydroxide is contraindicated in order to preclude the possibility of:
   (a) enamel hypoplasia
   (b) internal root resorption
   (c) external root resorption
   (d) root caries

5. Pulpotomies on permanent teeth are contraindicated because:
   (a) dental caries is not completely removed
   (b) calcium hydroxide results in enamel hypoplasia
   (c) the remaining pulp tissue will rapidly degenerate
   (d) formocresol results in internal root resorption

6. Enamel hypoplasia of permanent teeth secondary to use of prescribed potent agents during primary tooth pulpotomies can only be produced at ages:
   (a) 2 to 5
   (b) 4 to 8
   (c) 6 to 10
   (d) 8 to 12

7. Zinc oxide eugenol is NEVER placed into a bone-dry tooth unless endodontic therapy has been performed previously because:
   (a) thermal shock will produce pain
   (b) the material attracts water from the dentin and sensitizes it
   (c) the material is irritating to pulp tissue
   (d) the material requires moisture to inhibit recurrent caries

8. The microorganisms most commonly implicated in dental infections are:
   (a) viruses
   (b) bacteria
   (c) fungi
   (d) rickettsiae
   (e) a and b
   (f) b and c
   (g) c and d
   (h) all of the above

9. Microorganisms that do not decolorize and that do not retain the violet stain are termed:
   (a) gram-positive
   (b) gram-negative
   (c) both a and b
   (d) neither a nor b

10. Antibiotics that are lethal to microorganisms when given in high doses are termed:
    (a) broad spectrum
    (b) bacteriostatic
    (c) bactericidal
    (d) parenteral anti-infectives

11. 400,000 units of penicillin is approximately equal to:
    (a) 150 mg
    (b) 250 mg
    (c) 500 mg
    (d) 1000 mg

12. When a patient presents with allergy to penicillins, which of the following are used cautiously, if at all?
    (a) tetracyclines   (c) sulfonamides
    (b) cephalosporins   (d) antifungal agents

13. The drug of choice for dental infections in patients allergic to penicillins is:
    (a) minocycline   (d) erythromycin
    (b) streptomycin   (e) clindamycin
    (c) vancomycin   (f) cephalexin

14. The prevention and treatment of staphylococcal endocarditis may involve the use of:
    (a) penicillins   (d) vancomycin
    (b) erythromycin   (e) all of the above
    (c) streptomycin   (f) none of the above

15. Tetracycline pediatric suspensions are contraindicated for treatment of dental infections to preclude the development of:
    (a) dizziness and staggering   (c) internal root resorption
    (b) enamel hypoplasia   (d) nausea and vomiting

16. Patients taking lincomycin or clindamycin should be carefully watched for signs of:
    (a) headache   (d) diarrhea and colitis
    (b) nausea and vomiting   (e) visual disturbances
    (c) dizziness   (f) tinnitus

17. The cephalosporins are structurally related to:
    (a) tetracyclines   (c) aminoglycosides
    (b) penicillins   (d) sulfonamides

18. Antibiotics which competitively inhibit folic acid synthesis in microorganisms are the:
    (a) penicillins   (c) aminoglycosides
    (b) tetracyclines   (d) sulfonamides

19. In order for nystatin to be an effective antifungal agent it must be administered by the:
    (a) intravenous route   (c) oral route
    (b) intramuscular route   (d) topical route

20. All of the following potentially fatal complications may result from neglect of infections of the head and neck EXCEPT:
    (a) brain abscess   (c) trismus
    (b) meningitis   (d) cavernous sinus thrombosis

21. Dental patients should not receive antibiotic therapy with single drugs for longer than:
    (a) three days   (c) seven days
    (b) five days   (d) nine days

22. The most common side-effects of antibiotic therapy are:
    (a) dizziness   (e) a and b
    (b) diarrhea   (f) b and c
    (c) allergic reactions   (g) c and d
    (d) drowsiness   (h) all of the above

3

VITAMINS
AND
FLUORIDES

[handwritten notes:]
Vitms — Stored | not Stored | Min'ls. | Trace Min'ls
fat-solb. A,D,E,+ K | H₂O solb. B complex | Na,K,Ca | Fe, I, Cu, Mn,
H₂O solb. B₁₂ | + C | + Mg | Zn, Co, Mb,
 | | | Se, Cr, Sn, V,
 | | | F, Si, Ni

SECTION 1: VITAMINS

Vitamins and certain mineral elements are essential for health, have catalytic properties, are consumed in food in amounts less than 1 gram/day, and are usually absorbed unchanged. Vitamins may be stored in the body (fat-soluble A, D, E group, K, and water-soluble B_{12}) or may not be stored and require daily intake (water-soluble B complex and C). Minerals having biological importance may be grouped as the major minerals (Na, K, Ca, and Mg) or as minor (trace) minerals comprising less than 0.005 per cent of body weight (Fe, I, Cu, Mn, Zn, Co, Mb, Se, Cr, Sn, V, F, Si, and Ni).

The Food and Nutrition Board of the National Academy of Sciences, National Research Council publishes **Recommended Dietary Allowances** (RDAs) to provide standards of nutrition for different age groups. These RDA values are not requirements but recommended daily intakes that apply only to healthy persons and are not intended to cover nutritional requirements in disease states (Table 3–1).

Retinol (Vitamin A)

[handwritten: (nietolopia) night blindness]

Retinol (vitamin A) is needed for the proper maintenance of normal epithelial tissue and for the formation of the photoreceptor pigments in the retina involved in night, day, and color vision. One international unit (IU) of vitamin A is equal to 0.3 µg of retinol, and the RDA is 4000 IU for women and 5000 IU for men.

Symptoms of vitamin A deficiency include night blindness and xeropthalmia, and the usual therapeutic dosage is between 25,000 and 50,000 IU/day. Vitamin A tablets sold for the prevention and relief of sunburn have induced acute hypervitaminosis A even when taken according to the manufacturer's directions. Chronic toxicity usually results from taking doses above 100,000 IU for several months. Symptoms of overdosage include headache, irritability, and vomiting.

It is rare for the dental hygienist to encounter a patient with vitamin A deficiency, except in developing countries, where the staple food may be deficient in this nutrient, and patients display an increased susceptibility to infections. However, when a therapeutic multi-vitamin mineral is given in conjunction with other dental treatment the

Table 3-1 RECOMMENDED DIETARY ALLOWANCES FOR DIFFERENT AGE GROUPS*

Age (yrs)	Children			Adult Males					Adult Females						
	1-3	4-6	7-10	11-14	15-18	19-22	23-50†	51+	11-14	15-18	19-22	23-50†	51+	P††	L§
Vitamin A (IU)	2000	2500	3300	5000					4000					5000	6000
Vitamin B_1 (mg)	0.7	0.9	1.2	1.4	1.5		1.4	1.2	1.2	1.1		1.0	1.1	+0.3	+0.5
Vitamin B_2 (mg)	0.8	1.1	1.2	1.5	1.8		1.6	1.5	1.3	1.4		1.2		+0.3	+0.5
Vitamin B_3 (mg)	9	12	16	18	20		18	16	16	14		13	12	+2	+4
Vitamin B_5 (mg)	10?			10?					10?						
Vitamin B_6 (mg)	0.6	0.9	1.2	1.6	2.0				1.6	2.0				2.5	
Vitamin B_9 (µg)	100	200	300	400					400					800	600
Vitamin B_{12} (µg)	1.0	1.5	2.0	3.0					3.0					4.0	
Vitamin C (mg)	40			45					45					60	80
Vitamin D (IU)	400			400					400						
Vitamin E (IU)	7	9	10	12	15				12					15	
Vitamin K (mg)	2?			2?					2?						

*Adapted from *Recommended Daily Dietary Allowances*, revised 1974, Food and Nutrition Board, National Academy of Sciences, National Research Council.
†Reference male or reference female
††Pregnant
§Lactating

amount of vitamin A taken in a daily dose must be carefully noted. When the capsule contains 10,000 IU of vitamin A, a daily dose of 5 capsules should not be exceeded.

Vitamin A is available in various concentrations in over-the-counter multi-vitamin–mineral combinations (Myadec, Theragran-M, Therapax-10 with minerals, Multicebrin), as well as in tablet and capsule form in doses of 5, 10, 25, and 50,000 IU.

Vitamin B Complex

All of the components of the vitamin B complex are considered as a whole because the effect of one of them on the body is usually related to the presence of the others in sufficient concentration. They have a sedative effect on the nervous system in saturation doses and with the mineral magnesium (Mg) are termed "nature's tranquilizers." This group includes thiamine (vitamin B_1), riboflavin (vitamin B_2), niacin (nicotinic acid, niacinamide, vitamin B_3), pantothenate (vitamin B_5), pyridoxine (vitamin B_6), folate (folic acid, folacin, vitamin B_9), and cobalamine (vitamin B_{12}). The controversial laetrile (amygdalin, vitamin B_{17}) has no useful purpose and is not part of the vitamin B complex. Symptoms of overdosage of vitamin B complex have not yet been described, but the dental hygienist may be the first to suspect symptoms of deficiency.

The RDA for thiamine (vitamin B_1) is listed in Table 3–1 along with the RDAs for other nutrients. It is needed for proper myocardial function and neuronal function and in the metabolism of carbohydrates. Deficiency results in beriberi, a condition of fatigue, pre-cordial pain, nervousness, abdominal discomfort, anorexia, and constipation. It may arise from (1) increased B_1 requirements, as in pregnancy, fever, or hyperthyroidism; (2) impaired absorption of B_1 from long-term diarrhea; or (3) impaired absorption secondary to alcoholism or liver disease. Treatment consists of administration of vitamin B complex containing between 5 and 30 mg B_1/day.

Riboflavin (vitamin B_2) is needed for proper maintenance of mucous membranes and in energy and protein metabolism. Deficiency results in angular stomatitis (cheilosis) a condition of maceration of the mucosa at the corners of the mouth and vermilion surface of the lips, which may become secondarily infected with fungi (*Candida albicans*) to produce grey-white lesions termed "perlèche." The tongue usually has a deep purplish-red color. Diagnosis depends on laboratory tests, therapeutic trials, and elimination of other causes, because cheilosis and glossitis may also be caused by B_6 deficiency, edentia, or ill-fitting dentures. Treatment consists of administration of vitamin B complex containing between 10 and 30 mg B_2/day.

Niacin (nicotinic acid, niacinamide, vitamin B_3) is involved in oxidation-reduction reactions and in carbohydrate and tryptophan metabolism. Deficiency results in pellagra, a condition characterized by glossitis and stomatitis beginning in the area of Stensen's duct and followed by progression throughout the mouth, skin lesions, and further nervous and gastrointestinal involvement. Since niacin therapy may cause flushing, itching, burning, or tingling sensations, and niacinamide does not, treatment consists of administration of vitamin B complex containing between 100 and 1000 mg niacinamide/day.

Pantothenate (vitamin B_5) is associated with release of energy by carbohydrate metabolism and is needed for synthesis and degradation of fatty acids and steroid hormones. The RDA is not known, but 10 mg/day is probably adequate to satisfy human requirements. The central reflex that leads to bruxism can be controlled in some cases with oral saturation doses of calcium pantothenate, 100 mg/day for several days.

Pyridoxine (vitamin B_6) is needed for proper amino acid and fatty acid metabolism and deficiency may result in angular stomatitis (cheilosis) indistinguishable from B_2 deficiency, skin lesions, and anemia. The tongue is usually inflamed. Treatment consists of administration of vitamin B complex containing between 25 and 100 mg B_6/day.

Folate (folic acid, folacin, vitamin B_9) is needed for proper formation of red blood corpuscles, and deficiency may cause megaloblastic anemia, stomatitis, or glossitis. Treatment consists of administration of vitamin B complex containing 1 mg B_9/day.

Cobalamine (vitamin B_{12}) is essential to cell growth and reproduction, to formation of blood cells, and in synthesis of nucleoprotein and myelin, and it is necessary to prevent pernicious anemia and some psychiatric disorders. Symptoms of deficiency are very similar to B_6 deficiency (cheilosis, skin lesions, and anemia). Treatment consists of administration of vitamin B complex containing between 5 and 20 μg B_{12}/day and in pernicious anemia between 1 and 2 μg B_{12}/day I.M. to maintain remissions.

The clinical use of the vitamin B complex extends beyond mere treatment of cheilosis or glossitis, owing to the sedative effect of these vitamins on the nervous system. They are often given in capsule form pre-operatively, with magnesium, zinc, and vitamin C (Vicon-C), to diabetics, patients who are slow to heal, patients needing multiple extractions, the elderly or debilitated, and to those who cannot take antibiotics. This vitamin complex helps patients to better cope with the stress encountered as the result of extensive subgingival débridement or subgingival curettage.

Ascorbate (Vitamin C)

Ascorbic acid (ascorbate) is not a true vitamin but a mammalian liver metabolite needed for the proper formation of collagen in connective tissue, proper maturation of white blood cells, and improvement of the uptake of oxygen in cellular respiration. It has been nicknamed "the surgeon's vitamin" because it aids cellular respiration during general anesthesia, it inhibits hemorrhage along suture lines, and it's deficiencies are associated with the inability of wounds to heal.

Humans are prone to develop deficiencies of ascorbate because (1) the human liver has lost its ability to manufacture ascorbate from other substances, necessitating dietary intake; and (2) the tabular maximum (T_m), or active tubular secretion capacity, for ascorbate going from the proximal tubule into the peritubular capillaries and thus back to the plasma is very low (only 1.77 mg/min) in comparison with other substances such as glucose (T_m = 320 mg/min). Unless ascorbate is given in time-release form, maintaining a saturation level in the tissues of 120 mg over several hours to avoid rapid spilling into the urine, the body will rid itself of a dose of any size within 95 min after ingestion.

There is increasing evidence to suggest that the daily requirement of ascorbate for the average adult is 3000 mg, rather than the current RDA of 45 mg, which represents the amount required to prevent deficiency symptoms (scurvy). Between what is needed to prevent scurvy and what humans need for optimum health is a vast "grey zone" into which most patients fall. Inflammatory diseases and surgical operations increase the body's requirement of this nutrient.

In patients with scurvy, the gums become swollen, purple, spongy, and friable and bleed easily when air is blown on them (scorbutic gingivitis). Left untreated, the teeth will eventually loosen, old scars will break down, and spontaneous hemorrhages may occur in any part of the body. Ascorbic acid 250 mg q.i.d. should be given until signs of deficiency have disappeared, followed by maintenance doses of between 300 and 500 mg/day in divided doses for several months. Response is most rapid when superimposed infections are treated and calculus removal is accomplished.

Since every member of the dental staff is exposed to upper respiratory infections every day, a daily regimen of vitamin C 1000 mg t.i.d. in time-release form will offer good protection against air-borne viruses, which can be inhaled during dental procedures. Patients who require extensive surgery, who have healed slowly previously, or who have a history of diabetes should be given vitamin C, vitamin B complex, magnesium, and zinc (Vicon-C) pre-operatively. Female patients sometimes complain of irritation around the external opening of the urethra when they are taking 1000 mg or more of vitamin C daily when it is not in time-release form, because of the effect of vitamin C in acidifying the urine. These patients should be advised to increase their water intake, to avoid salty food and drink, and to take the non–time-release pills farther apart.

Because acidification of the urine can result in precipitation of calcium stones in the renal pelvis, the ureters, or the urinary bladder in some patients, vitamin C therapy should be used cautiously in patients with a history of kidney or bladder stones and only with the physician's consent.

Vitamin C is available in tablet doses of 25, 50, 100, 250, 500, and 1000 mg in non–time-release form and in doses of 250, 500, and 1000 mg in time-release form, and it is also an ingredient in many over-the-counter multi-vitamins with minerals and in combination products.

It is currently believed that megascorbic therapy (daily intake of vitamin C greater than 1000 mg) helps in detoxification of heavy metals, such as mercury (Hg), that have accumulated in the body because of long-term exposure. In the case of mercury, which is combined with silver alloys to make dental fillings, the maximum exposure written into law by Congress and specified by the Public Health Service is 0.01 parts mercury vapor per million parts of air (0.1 mg Hg/m^3 air). The vapor pressure above mercury stored in jars without lids or above discarded amalgam scraps can be 100 times this amount. Toxic concentrations can accumulate gradually even with careful technique, and hazardous levels can be reached without a large spill. Mercury can vaporize at a very low temperature ($10°$ F) and can be rapidly absorbed into the bloodstream; although mercury absorption poses little problem for patients, continual exposure of dental personnel can result in a buildup that can affect the nervous system, red blood corpuscles, liver, and kidneys. The net result can be erethism (abnormal irritability), hand tremors, or kidney, eye, and skin disorders. Recent surveys have shown potentially toxic mercury levels in between 10 and 15 per cent of dental offices surveyed, with an additional 40 per cent having serious problems associated with the handling of mercury and amalgam; this represents half of all dental offices in which the hygienist may be working. A daily regimen of vitamin C 1000 mg in time-release form will offer dental personnel a somewhat wider margin of safety in dealing with occupational mercury contamination, in conjunction with other safety measures (use of mercury vapor sniffers, pre-measured amalgam capsules, or powdered sulfur scattered along walls).

There appears to be a relationship between dietary sodium ascorbate and phenytoin (diphenylhydantoin, Dilantin) in the treatment of epileptic seizures; epileptic animals given phenytoin but deprived of ascorbate have recurrent seizures that disappear when a diet containing ascorbate is resumed (Chap. 7, Sec. 3).

The incidence of viral hepatitis B in transfused patients is about 7 per cent in those who receive little or no vitamin C following blood transfusion, compared to 0.2 per cent in those who receive 2 grams of vitamin C or more daily, indicating that it has a prophylactic effect against post-transfusion hepatitis (Chap. 5, Sec. 3).

Vitamin D group

Ergocalciferol (vitamin D_2) or **cholecalciferol** (vitamin D_3), or both, are needed for proper absorption of calcium and phosphorus, for renal tubular reabsorption of phosphorus, for calcification of bone, and for magnesium metabolism. One μg of vitamin D equals 40 IU, and the RDA is 10 μg (400 IU). Cholecalciferol (vitamin D_3) is formed in human skin by exposure to sunlight or ultraviolet radiation, which has led to the nickname "the sunshine vitamin." Daily requirements for this nutrient are extremely variable, depending on the amount of ultraviolet radiation to the skin and the efficiency of calcium and phosphorus metabolism.

If the supply of vitamin D is inadequate, if its metabolism is abnormal, or if tissues are resistant to its action, a metabolic bone disease called rickets (in children) or osteomalacia (in adults) may ensue. This may ordinarily be cured by administration of 1600 IU vitamin D per day. Adults receiving 100,000 IU daily for several months may show signs of toxicity (hypervitaminosis D) with symptoms of nausea, vomiting, and weakness. Treatment includes placing the patient on a low calcium diet and discontinuing the vitamin.

Vitamin D is available in tablet and capsule form in doses of 25 and 50,000 IU. Whenever vitamin D therapy is instituted, an adequate dietary intake of calcium is necessary for clinical response.

Vitamin E group

The vitamin E group includes the alpha, beta, gamma, and delta tocopherols, with alpha the most active biologically. **Alpha-tocopherol** is an intracellular antioxidant involved in the stability of membranes and having close metabolic relationships with selenium (Se). Deficiency of vitamin E in humans results in rupture of red blood corpuscles and is thought to be related to infant "crib death syndrome." Administration of this vitamin has been used as an adjunct in the treatment of thrombophlebitis and is thought to aid is the dissolution of fresh blood clots (Chap. 5, Sec. 1). Skin burns heal more rapidly when topical vitamin E is applied to the affected area, supplemented with 1200 units daily orally. The vitamin also opens up collateral circulation and has been successfully used as a part of treatment of angina pectoris and intermittent claudication.

The RDA for vitamin E is unknown but is believed to be between 12 and 15 mg/day. The potencies of the various forms of vitamin E vary, and dosage is based on activity and is standardized as international units (IU). Therefore, 1 mg of vitamin E may contain from 0.89 to 1.49 IU, depending on the chemical form it is in.

Dentists and dental hygienists are often victims of inadequate leg circulation and should consider vitamin E supplementation in daily doses of 400 IU. There is no evidence that administration of vitamin E will beneficially alter the course of periodontal disease, but there are very few chronic degenerative diseases that fail to respond to vitamins C and E combined.

Vitamin E should not be taken by hypertensive persons because in one third of these it will elevate blood pressure, in another one third it will decrease blood pressure, and in the remaining one third the blood pressure will remain the same. The hygienist cannot predict with certainty whether or not any given hypertensive patient will fall into a specific response category.

Recent evidence has shown that mice with vitamin E deficient diets will develop lung disease when exposed to 13 ppm nitrous oxide for long periods of time. Those given high doses of vitamin E do not experience any adverse effects from exposure to nitrous oxide. It is known that nitrous oxide interferes with the production of prostaglandin E_2, a hormone regulating blood production in the lungs, and vitamin E seems to have the scavenger effect of removing free radicals from the polluted air before they can interfere with prostaglandin synthesis. Dentists and hygienists exposed to nitrous oxide are also advised to take between 200 and 400 IU vitamin E daily.

Vitamin E capsules are available in doses of 30, 50, 100, 200, 400, 600, 800, and 1000 IU, mainly as *dl*-alpha-tocopheryl acetate.

Vitamin K group

Vitamin K is necessary for proper liver formation of certain blood coagulation factors (prothrombin factor II, proconvertin factor VII, plasma thromboplastin component factor IX, and the Stuart-Prower factor X) that are required for clotting (Chap. 5, Sec. 1). Deficiency of phytonadione (vitamin K_1), menadione (vitamin K_3), or menadiol sodium diphosphate (vitamin K_4) results in uncontrolled hemorrhage. Intestinal bacteria are capable of manufacturing vitamin K for the use of the host but are essentially absent from the intestine of the newborn during the first three to five days of life. Infants are especially prone to hemorrhages, especially breast-fed infants, since breast milk is a poor source of Vitamin K.

Phytonadione (vitamin K_1) should be given in doses of 1 to 2 mg I.M. to every newborn to prevent intracranial hemorrhage incidental to birth trauma, and should be given preoperatively to hemophiliacs (Chap. 5, Sec. 3) whenever oral surgery is contemplated.

Vitamin K is available in 5 mg tablet form and in various doses for injection.

Diet Evaluation

Studies indicate that health exists only in a state of homeostasis, or physiological equilibrium, produced by a balance of functions and chemical composition within an organism. The body is designed to operate within a very narrow range of fluctuation, and both increases and decreases in body functions or chemical constituents may signify the development of disease. Dr. Albert Szent Gyorgi the co-discoverer of vitamin C has said, "Full health is the state in which we feel best, work best, and have the greatest resistance to disease." Research has shown that when the body is in perfect health, i.e., in homeostasis, it is more difficult for disease to take hold, if indeed disease can begin at all in such a theoretically healthy body.

Studies have also shown that the human body is composed of roughly 100 trillion cells, each of which performs about 1200 separate chemical reactions every day to keep the body homeostatic, or free of disease. About 3000 chemicals are used in the reactions, and all of them must come from the air we breathe, the water we drink, and the food we eat. Of these chemicals, 2998 (oxygen and water are excepted) are supplied only in the diet.

According to estimates, the modern human body is basically the same as in the primitive human, having the same methods of digestion and assimilation, the same enzymes and hormones. Studies indicate that the early human was primarily a meat eater and that nutrients necessary to support life came from freshly killed raw meat and to a lesser extent, in times of game scarcity, from raw plant food. This situation was altered when humans began cultivation and the incidence of plant food in their diet increased. As members of a health profession we should not advocate a return to raw meat, nor cave dwelling, but we must understand what makes the body's physiological mechanisms operate at their optimal level. The closer we can come to our natural diet of animal protein and raw or slightly cooked plant food, the more we can expect to be free of disease.

Body chemistry imbalances may be brought about by many factors operating over a long period of time, some of which we are powerless to control, e.g., our genetic predisposition to disease and the stress of living. But if we add to this other factors we can control, such as an inadequate diet, a diet high in refined food, sugar, and caffeine, inadequate oral hygiene, inadequate rest, and habits such as smoking, at some point the body will begin to break down. This breakdown is first apparent in the mouth but eventually involves all the body systems. It is a slow insidious process that goes on for years without the patient's knowledge, until finally symptoms of chronic degenerative diseases appear (dental decay and gum disease, arthritis, diabetes, hardening of the arteries, and coronary heart disease). By then it is too late to be concerned about prevention, and crisis care is needed (Fig. 3–1).

Every cell is meant to be bathed in a fluid that is only so high or low in blood sugar and that acts like a miniature sugar carburetor; if we feed the cell too much sugar it will physiologically sputter, and if the mixture is too lean the cell will physiologically choke. Basic to all other forms of dental treatment are recommendations aimed at maintaining the blood sugar within normal limits so that cells in the teeth and gums cannot be overcome by disease.

Our American technology has grown faster than our knowledge of nutrition, and advertisers in their zeal to sell a product are presumably not aware that the public believes

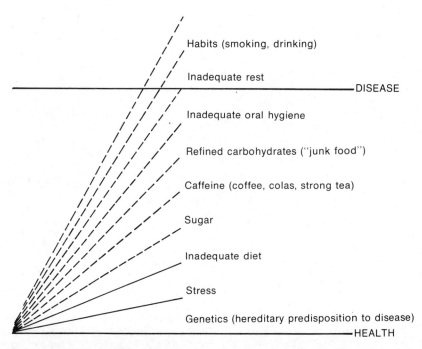

Figure 3–1. Additive factors in the production of chronic degenerative disease. Uncontrollable factors are in solid lines. By controlling the other factors the entire stack will fall down below the level at which the body breaks down.

the advertising at face value. Colas and other sweetened drinks have become a substitute for water. The sugar and caffeine in colas, which taken once in a while would not do excessive harm, are today taken in such quantities that the body's normal functions are impaired, allowing the body to deteriorate. The same can be said for routine consumption of other refined carbohydrates (cold box cereal, snack food, junk food, white bread, soda, gum, candy, pastries, table sugar, and commercial ice cream and additional abusable substances such as coffee, tobacco, and alcohol (Fig. 3–2).

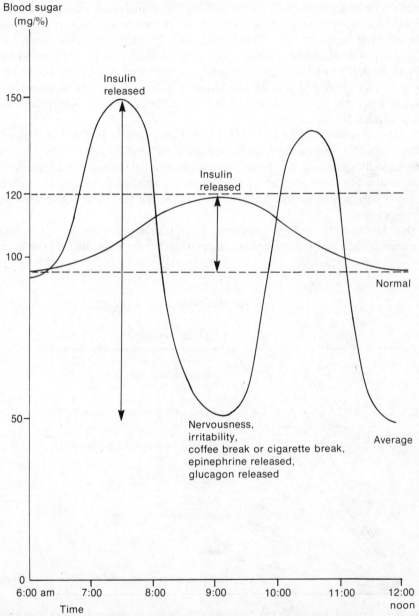

Figure 3–2. Blood sugar curves of normal (high protein) and average (high refined carbohydrate) diets

Americans may have the best health care delivery system in the world, but in this country alone (1) 30 per cent of the population is afflicted with some symptoms of arthritis; (2) there are more than 20 million diabetics, diagnosed and undiagnosed; (3) 50 per cent of all adult males have symptoms of arterial or heart disease; (4) seven out of eight have some difficulty in metabolizing carbohydrates; (5) three out of five adults have lost all their teeth in one or more dental arches; and (6) there are over 100 million unfilled cavities in the mouths of Americans, with the decay rate almost doubling, resulting in enough repair work to keep every dentist busy 24 hours a day for the next 50 years.

To maintain our health we must have a basically natural diet and avoid those things that tend to upset our blood sugar. There is just no other way that results in long-range success. The success of any dental treatment will depend on how closely the patient follows the hygienist's recommendations for changes in diet. With patient's with advanced oral disease, it is usually necessary for them to consider taking many nutrients in pill form to add to their diet that which is removed in processing.

When it has been determined that a patient's oral disease is of sufficient magnitude to warrant investigation into its cause, the hygienist should request and analyze a seven-day diet diary of everything the patient is eating and drinking except water and at what time during the day or night each thing is consumed. The total number of food choices during the week is divided into the number of animal protein, whole carbohydrate, and refined carbohydrate food choices and multiplied by 100 to obtain the percentage of each type of food in the diet.

In general no more than one third (33 per cent) of the diet should consist of refined carbohydrates, with a goal of reducing this to 10 per cent if possible. The remainder of the diet should be evenly balanced between animal protein (meat, fish, fowl, eggs, and cheese) and whole carbohydrates (raw and slightly cooked plant food).

Patients with severe oral disease will probably have diets high in refined carbohydrates and low in animal protein and should be advised accordingly. There is no need to limit the number of eggs per week due to alarm about excessive cholesterol, since only 20 per cent of the body's cholesterol is drawn directly from the diet. Eighty per cent of the body's cholesterol is made in the liver from acetate radicals found in refined carbohydrates, and the amount of cholesterol in the diet is not a significant factor in the development of atherosclerosis in the vast majority of people. Furthermore, eggs are particularly rich in lecithin, which has been shown to be cholesterol-lowering, and eliminating cholesterol totally from the diet encourages the body to manufacture excess amounts.

Deaths of dieters using liquid protein appear to result from excessively low levels of such essential nutrients as calcium, magnesium, phosphorus, iron, zinc, and copper, not from toxic components.

SECTION 2: FLUORIDES

Fate of Ingested Fluoride

Virtually every food contains trace amounts of fluoride, but larger quantities are found in some foods, such as tea and certain types of fish. Once absorbed from the gastrointestinal tract or lungs, fluoride is distributed to the extracellular fluid, and the major portion is deposited in bone and teeth as fluorapatite. Ameloblasts concentrate ten times more fluorapatite in the outer layers of tooth enamel than along the inner layers near the dentinoenamel junction. Ingested fluoride has no effect on previously formed enamel and is only beneficial when it can be locked into the developing enamel rod structure, i.e., during the critical years of enamel formation (up to age 16). Fluorapatite is more resistant to acid dissolution than is apatite and will therefore be less likely to initiate decay.

Excretion of fluoride is rapid and takes place almost entirely in the kidney.

Effects of High and Low Fluoride Intake

The optimal fluoride level in a food and water supply will produce maximal protection against dental caries without adverse effects, and this level has been determined to be 1 mg/day and 1 ppm (part per million). There is currently no evidence to show that fluoride is essential to nutrition in humans or animals, and no ill effects have been correlated with excessively low fluoride intake.

When the fluoride level rises to 1.5 ppm, white spots and flecking on the enamel is observed, and at higher concentrations severe pitting and staining occurs, which is termed chronic endemic dental fluorosis (mottled enamel). Although this enamel is unsightly, it is very resistant to acid dissolution. Fluorosis is most evident in permanent teeth, and deciduous teeth are affected only at high levels of fluoride intake. Bony changes are usually seen only after prolonged high intake in adults.

It is generally accepted that maximal protection from dental decay can be accomplished by ingestion of drinking water containing 1 ppm fluoride and food containing 1 mg/day of fluoride, in conjunction with other preventive measures.

When excessive fluoride vapor is inhaled, the results are intense nasal and eye irritation, headache, a sense of suffocation, bronchitis, and glottal and pulmonary edema. The human toxicity threshold for inhaled fluoride vapor is unknown, but exposure of industrial workers to air containing 3.6 mg fluoride/m^3 for several years produced radiographic findings consistent with fluorosis, but no clinical disability. Treatment consists of respiratory support, oxygen under positive pressure, and prednisone P.O. between 30 and 80 mg/day in divided doses for adults.

Accidental ingestion of excessive fluoride results in a salty or soapy taste in the mouth, tremors, convulsions, shock, and, possibly, in renal failure. The toxic dose ranges from two to five grams for adults, but it is less for children and is approximately 600 mg at age three (Chap. 1, Sec. 3). Treatment consists of inducing emesis (with syrup of ipecac or mustard water), followed by having the patient drink large quantities of milk and having him transported to the emergency room of the nearest hospital, whereupon 10 cc of calcium gluconate 10 per cent should be administered I.V.; these measures are directed at attempting to form insoluble calcium fluoride (CaF_2). Large doses of vitamin C given I.V. have been shown to increase survival time and prevent marked weight loss in animals given toxic levels of fluoride. No evidence of toxicity was noted in adult cancer patients treated with sodium fluoride 80 mg q.i.d. for six months, with equivalent findings for children taking between 20 and 50 mg q.i.d. No apparent signs of toxicity were observed in an adult cancer patient treated with 5600 mg of sodium fluoride given in 400 and 500 mg doses over a nine day period.

Fluoride Supplements

It is generally agreed that water supplies with less than 0.3 ppm (parts per million) of fluoride require supplementation of 0.5 mg/day for children under three and 1 mg/day for children over 3; water supplies with between 0.3 and 0.7 ppm require supplementation of 0.25 mg/day for children under three and 0.5 mg/day for children over three (see discussion later in this chapter). Because of increased use of fluoridated water in food processing, fluoride supplements have their greatest use in treating breast-fed babies in non-fluoridated communities. Extensive use of commercial formulas and foods will provide more than 1 mg/day, whereas an intake of greater than 0.5 mg/day at age six months may cause mottled enamel.

Since all the available fluoride supplements utilize sodium fluoride, they are contraindicated in patients on low-sodium or sodium-free diets or in patients being treated with a diuretic (Chap. 8, Sec. 1). Fluoride supplementation may cause skin reactions, such as eczema, atopic dermatitis, or urticaria, which disappear upon discontinuing therapy.

Sodium fluoride tablets are available in concentrations of 0.55 mg (Luride 0.25 mg Lozi-Tabs), 1.1 mg (Luride 0.5 mg Lozi-Tabs), and 2.21 mg (Luride 1.0 mg Lozi-Tabs, Karidium, Phos-Flur). Each of these supplies fluoride in concentrations of 0.25, 0.5, and 1.0 mg respectively, and each is chewable (except Karidium). Infant drops are available in concentrations of 0.125 mg/drop (Karidium), 0.1 mg/drop (Luride), 0.25 mg/drop (Fluoritab, Flura-Drops), and 0.5 mg/cc (Pediaflor).

The effect of prenatal fluoride supplements on caries was studied in 771 children whose mothers had during pregnancy either drunk fluoridated water only, taken a vitamin-fluoride tablet daily, or taken a 2.2 mg sodium fluoride tablet daily. In each of the groups the number of caries-free children was 25, 69, and 97 per cent respectively. The children whose mothers had taken the sodium fluoride tablets had no evidence of fluorosis. Based on these findings a 2.2 mg sodium fluoride tablet should be taken by a pregnant woman daily from the third to the ninth month of pregnancy, but at the present time prenatal fluoride supplements are not recommended because of the lack of a sufficient number of clinical studies.

Fluoride dietary supplements are unnecessary when the drinking water contains fluoride in a concentration of 0.7 ppm or more.

Water Fluoridation

Antifluoridationists have three main arguments against fluoridation of public drinking water, namely, that (1) fluoridation is too expensive and gives city taxpayers inadequate returns for tax dollars invested in the program, (2) fluoride may be a carcinogen, and (3) forcing fluoridation on the public without voter referendum constitutes a flagrant violation of the right of citizens to choose for themselves.

In 1978 it cost the taxpayer living in St. Louis, Missouri about 11 cents per person to gain this additional protection against dental decay (Table 3–2). This is less than the cost of a single local phone call and gives one of the best returns of any investment so small in size. It is reasonable to assume that similar data could be obtained from other American cities with similar populations; therefore, the argument that water fluoridation gives inadequate returns for the dollars invested is unsupported by facts. It has been

Table 3–2. COST OF FLUORIDATION OF DRINKING WATER
IN ST. LOUIS IN 1978

Approximate population of St. Louis, Missouri (1978)	505,000
Total 1978 operating budget for the city of St. Louis, Missouri	$ 214,785,025
Cost of sodium fluoride added to St. Louis water supply, adjusted to 1 ppm (900 tons at $59.70 per ton) per year in 1978	$ 53,730 (1/40th of 1 per cent of total budget)

shown by Ast, Cons, Pollard, and Garfinkel in 1970 that the average initial complete dental care cost for a poor child living in a fluoridated city ($16.93) was less than the same cost of care for a poor child living in a non-fluoridated city ($40.78). Supplemental incremental care also was reported to cost less in the fluoridated city. The difference ($23.85) is significantly more than the cost of turning a large non-fluoridated city such as St. Louis, Missouri, into a fluoridated one (11 cents).

In 1975 a study conducted by Burk and Yiamouyiannis compared cancer mortality rates among residents of fluoridated and non-fluoridated American cities; the methodology and conclusions of that study have been questioned by scientists and health organizations throughout America, including the National Cancer Institute and the American Dental Association. Many courts today are ordering the discontinuance of water fluoridation based only on the findings of this study, although this authority had previously been placed in the hands of the State Department of Environmental Resources by the State Supreme Courts. At the time this chapter is being written there is no evidence directly linking excess fluoride in the body to malignancy; even if fluoride has an extremely long latent period in carcinogenesis a significant number of animals subjected to experimentally induced fluoride toxicosis in recent years should have developed cancer if fluoride were carcinogenic. Since the incidence of cancer is 25 per cent in the overall population and since there are so many suspected carcinogenic agents, the isolation of any single one of them in any study on cancer mortality, which involves holding the levels of the others constant, is virtually impossible. Any substance foreign to the body may be a carcinogen when administered to an absorbing surface in a concentration that is high enough, but many scientists are arguing whether fluoride is truly foreign to the body or whether it is necessary in trace amounts. While the issue is debated, dental decay continues to be the most prevalent disease in the world. The statistically high degree of correlation between fluoridation of drinking water and decreased incidence of dental decay in regions where the water is naturally low in fluoride has been repeatedly verified, whereas the correlation with cancer mortality has not.

The benefits of fluoridation are best realized during the critical years of enamel formation (up to age 16), as the fluoride is deposited in the developing layers of enamel in this period. However, this portion of the population is not registered to vote and cannot legally exercise a freedom of choice. Compared to its benefits to non-voters fluoridation is not meant to greatly benefit the voting public; therefore, a referendum banning water fluoridation, if passed, would not only discriminate against non-voting children but would also open up a Pandora's box of dental disease, resulting in suffering that could have been prevented by the adult voting population.

Topical Fluoride Treatments

Frequent application of fluoride to exposed tooth surfaces has been shown to inhibit caries, and the surface layers of cementum and dentin have a markedly greater affinity for fluoride than does enamel. There is no convincing evidence that any type of infrequent fluoride application has any major impact on the control of dental microbial plaque diseases. Daily use of a fluoridated dentifrice and occasional use of a fluoride gel at home to supplement office fluoride treatments will greatly reduce the incidence of dental caries, but fluoride therapy alone should not be considered a sovereign remedy for control of odontolysis.

There are three types of office fluoride solutions: (1) sodium fluoride (NaF), (2) stannous fluoride (SnF_2), and (3) acidulated phosphate fluoride (APF). The properties of sodium fluoride are very similar to APF. In comparison with sodium fluoride, SnF_2 is simpler to use, more beneficial in reducing caries in fluoridated areas, more effective in adults, and capable of arresting existing caries. However, it has an unpleasant taste, it is unstable in solution, and it will stain teeth slightly.

In a series of experiments Dr. Ira Shannon has shown that reduction of enamel solubility is greatest with sequential APF and SnF_2 treatments, less with combined APF and SnF_2, still less with SnF_2 alone, and least with APF alone (Table 3–3).

Sodium fluoride rinses are marketed in concentrations of 0.05 per cent (Fluorigard Dental Rinse, Fluorinse, Kari-Rinse, Sodium Fluoride Home Rinse) and 0.2 per cent (Fluorinse, Point-Two Dental Rinse); the gel is available only in a concentration of 1.1 per cent (Kari-Gel). Stannous fluoride rinses and gels are available only in concentrations of 0.4 per cent (Gel-Kam, Iradicav Stannous Fluoride). Acidulated phosphate fluoride rinse is marketed as Iradicav Acidulated Phosphate Home Fluoride 0.02 per cent and the gel as Fluoride 0.5 per cent.

There is evidence that topical application of 8 per cent stannous fluoride solution to cavity preparations reduces the incidence of recurrent caries underneath restorations. Contraindications to this preventive procedure include (1) anterior restorations, which may appear stained underneath and unsightly esthetically, and (2) acid-etched restorations, which may not be as retentive because of reduced enamel solubility induced by fluoride.

Topical fluoride treatments should be individualized for each patient in consultation with the dentist. Using an office mouth rinse, such as Gel-Kam, is easier than utilizing fluoride trays; the patient simply rinses the fluoride solution in his mouth for 60 seconds, expectorates, repeats the procedure for another 60 seconds and is instructed not to rinse his mouth for two hours. The procedure is rapidly accomplished with no gagging or excessive salivation, but it requires full control of the swallowing reflex, which is not mature prior to age six. A 1.23 per cent APF gel is recommended for tray application, and is mandatory between ages three and six. A thixotropic gel (Gel II) is desirable for developmentally disabled patients (those with mental retardation, genetic syndromes, autism, cerebral palsy, epilepsy, and so forth) or for children who intensely dislike topical fluoride because it tends to liquefy within the tray at mouth temperature. Nursing bottle caries is best treated with topical application of 0.5 per cent APF gel once daily after thorough deplaquing to arrest active decay until the teeth can be restored or ex-

Table 3–3. ENAMEL SOLUBILITY REDUCTION (ESR) WITH DIFFERENT OFFICE FLUORIDE SOLUTIONS*

	ESR with Acidulated Phosphate Fluoride (APF)	ESR with APF Plus Stannous Flouride 0.4%	ESR with Stannous Fluoride 0.4%
Initial Protection	71.1%	95.7%	74.6%
Durability of Protection Following:			
Acid Etching #1	72.9%	93.6%	94.1%
Acid Etching #2	41.5%	92.2%	60.0%
Acid Etching #3	19.0%	87.6%	34.9%
Acid Etching #4	5.5%	75.3%	12.4%

Comparison of ESR Following:

	ESR with APF (0.62%)	ESR with Stannous Flouride 0.4%	ESR with APF Followed by Stannous Flouride	ESR with APF Plus Stannous Flouride Mixture
Single and Multiple Fluoride Applications	79.5%	81.1%	95.8%	92.8%

*References:
Shannon, I.L., Edmonds, E.J., Madsen, K.O.: Single, double and sequential methods for fluoride applications. J. Dent. Child, 41:35, 1974.
Shannon, I.L., Edmonds, E.J.: Chemical alterations of enamel surfaces by single and sequential treatments with fluorides. J. Am. Dent. Assoc., 19:135, 1973.
Shannon, I.L., Paoloski, S.B., Wescott, W.B.: Laboratory fluoride experiments in dental hygiene curriculum. J. Dent. Educ., 39:28, 1974.

tracted; extremely small amounts of the gel on the tops of cotton swabs are all that is needed, and no more than 30 cc of the gel should be prescribed at any one time. Stannous fluoride is marketed as 10 mg effervescent tablets that are to be dissolved in 10 cc of tap water to produce a 0.1 per cent solution for mouth rinsing (Stan-Care); this product appears to have less likelihood of accidental overdosage than mouth rinses marketed in glass containers that resemble soda bottles, and it would not counteract diuretic therapy for hypertension because it contains no sodium.

The beneficial effects of topically administered fluoride to tooth structure include (1) reduction in enamel solubility, (2) surface energy reduction (decreased plaque accumulation and tenacity of deposits), and (3) inhibition of microbial enzyme systems. General recommendations for a sound preventive program include (1) professionally applied topical fluoride treatment at each dental recall visit, (2) use of an ADA-approved fluoride-containing dentifrice (Crest, Colgate, Aim, Maclean's, or Aqua-Fresh) at least twice daily, and (3) fluoride supplements (drops, tablets) up to age six in communities with suboptimal fluoride levels in the central water supply. Mouth rinses should not replace fluoride supplements until age six because the swallowing reflex is not sufficiently mature prior to that time. The potency of fluoride should not be underestimated and it should be used with the same caution as any other prescription drug. Only commercial preparations should be used; concentrated solutions should not be added to pumice ad libitum in order to devise a special fluoride concoction.

TEST QUESTIONS

1. All of the following are minor (trace) minerals needed for optimum health EXCEPT:
   (a) iron
   (b) copper
   (c) zinc
   (d) mercury
   (e) cobalt
   (f) chromium

2. All of the following vitamins are stored in the body EXCEPT:
   (a) A
   (b) B complex, excluding B_{12}
   (c) C
   (d) D group
   (e) E group
   (f) K group
   (g) B_{12}
   (h) a and c
   (i) b and c
   (j) c and g
   (k) d and e
   (l) e and f
   (m) e and g

3. A drug needed for the proper maintenance of epithelial tissue and for the formation of the retinal photoreceptor pigments involved in day, night, and color vision is:
   (a) retinol
   (b) thiamine
   (c) riboflavin
   (d) niacin
   (e) pyridoxine
   (f) ascorbate

4. All of the following are components of the vitamin B complex EXCEPT:
   (a) thiamine
   (b) riboflavin
   (c) niacin
   (d) pantothenate
   (e) pyridoxine
   (f) folate
   (g) cobalamine
   (h) amygdalin

5. Beriberi results from deficiency of:
   - (a) retinol
   - (b) thiamine
   - (c) riboflavin
   - (d) niacin
   - (e) pyridoxine
   - (f) folate
   - (g) cobalamine
   - (h) ascorbate

6. Pellagra results from deficiency of:
   - (a) thiamine
   - (b) riboflavin
   - (c) niacin
   - (d) pyridoxine
   - (e) folate
   - (f) cobalamine
   - (g) ascorbate
   - (h) retinol

7. Pernicious anemia results from deficiency of:
   - (a) retinol
   - (b) thiamine
   - (c) riboflavin
   - (d) niacin
   - (e) pyridoxine
   - (f) folate
   - (g) cobalamine
   - (h) ascorbate

8. Scurvy results from deficiency of:
   - (a) retinol
   - (b) thiamine
   - (c) riboflavin
   - (d) niacin
   - (e) pyridoxine
   - (f) folate
   - (g) cobalamine
   - (h) ascorbate

9. Stomatitis and glossitis may result from deficiency of:
   - (a) retinol
   - (b) thiamine
   - (c) riboflavin
   - (d) niacin
   - (e) panthothenate
   - (f) pyridoxine
   - (g) folate
   - (h) cobalamine
   - (i) ascorbate
   - (j) a, b, e, and i
   - (k) c, d, f, g, and h
   - (l) a through i

10. A mammalian liver metabolite involved in proper maturation of white blood cells, formation of collagen in connective tissue, uptake of oxygen during general anesthesia, and microhemorrhage along suture lines is:
    - (a) glucagon
    - (b) ascorbate
    - (c) alpha-tocopherol
    - (d) niacin
    - (e) pantothenate
    - (f) cholecalciferol

11. Time release vitamin C is preferable to non–time-release vitamin C because within _____ after ingestion of a large non–time-release dose the body rids itself of this nutrient completely.
    - (a) 35 min
    - (b) 65 min
    - (c) 95 min
    - (d) 125 min

12. The body tissues of the average adult are saturated with vitamin C at a level of:
    - (a) 45 mg
    - (b) 90 mg
    - (c) 120 mg
    - (d) none of the above

13. The body is prone to develop deficiencies of ascorbate because:
    - (a) it is not stored in the human body
    - (b) it is not manufactured in the human liver
    - (c) the human tubular maximum for ascorbate is very low
    - (d) all of the above

14. The incidence of post-transfusion hepatitis may be reduced with _____ in a daily dose of 2 grams or more
   (a) vitamin B complex
   (b) ascorbate
   (c) cholecalciferol
   (d) alpha-tocopherol
   (e) phytonadione
   (f) retinol

15. Toxic reactions to excessively high doses of vitamins (hypervitaminosis) may occur with administration of:
   (a) vitamin A
   (b) vitamin B complex
   (c) vitamin C
   (d) vitamin D group
   (e) vitamin E group
   (f) vitamin K group
   (g) a and d
   (h) b and e
   (i) c and f
   (j) all of the above
   (k) none of the above

16. An intracellular antioxidant concerned with the stability of membranes, dissolution of fresh blood clots, improvement of collateral circulation, and having close metabolic relationships with selenium is:
   (a) retinol
   (b) ascorbate
   (c) cobalamine
   (d) alpha-tocopherol
   (e) cholecalciferol
   (f) phytonadione

17. Vitamin E supplementation should NOT be considered for hypertensives because:
   (a) in one third of all hypertensives it will elevate blood pressure
   (b) it may act as a physiologic antagonist to antihypertensive drugs the patient may be taking
   (c) the clinical response cannot be predicted with certainty
   (d) all of the above

18. A substance that is necessary for the hepatic synthesis of certain blood coagulation factors and that should be administered to hemophiliacs prior to dental procedures that will result in significant hemorrhage is:
   (a) alpha tocopherol
   (b) ascorbate
   (c) phytonadione
   (d) pyridoxine
   (e) cholecalciferol
   (f) folate

19. Uncontrollable factors that contribute additively to the production of chronic degenerative disease include:
   (a) inadequate oral hygiene, poor diet, and insufficient rest
   (b) genetics and stress
   (c) diets high in sugar, caffeine, and refined carbohydrates
   (d) habits (consumption of tobacco and alcohol)

20. The amount of cholesterol in the diet is NOT a significant factor in the production of atherosclerosis in the vast majority of patients because:
   (a) most of the cholesterol in the body is made in the liver from refined carbohydrates
   (b) some cholesterol is needed in the diet to discourage the body from manufacturing excessive amounts
   (c) both a and b
   (d) neither a nor b

21. The optimum fluoride level in a daily food supply is ___(1)___, whereas the optimum level in a central water supply is ___(2)___.
    - (a) *(1)* 1 ppm and *(2)* 1 mg
    - (b) *(1)* 1 mg and *(2)* 1 ppm
    - (c) *(1)* 10 ppm and *(2)* 10 mg
    - (d) *(1)* 10 mg and *(2)* 10 ppm

22. A mother phones a dental office stating that her three year old child has just swallowed about 2 ounces of Fluorigard Dental Rinse (0.05 per cent sodium fluoride) and is nauseated. The child has ingested ___(1)___ of sodium fluoride and treatment consists of ___(2)___.
    - (a) *(1)* 30 mg and *(2)* inducing emesis, ingesting milk, and I.V. calcium
    - (b) *(1)* 30 mg and *(2)* inducing emesis, ingesting water, and I.V. sodium
    - (c) *(1)* 100 mg and *(2)* inducing emesis, ingesting milk, and I.V. calcium
    - (d) *(1)* 100 mg and *(2)* inducing emesis, ingesting water, and I.V. sodium

23. Fluoride dietary supplements are unnecessary when the drinking water contains fluoride in a concentration of at least:
    - (a) 0.3 ppm
    - (b) 0.5 ppm
    - (c) 0.7 ppm
    - (d) none of the above

24. The highest enamel solubility reduction occurs with administration of:
    - (a) 1.64 per cent stannous fluoride
    - (b) 0.62 per cent acidulated phosphate fluoride
    - (c) combined b and a
    - (d) b, then a

25. Recommendations for a sound preventive program would include all of the following EXCEPT:
    - (a) topical fluoride treatment at each recall visit
    - (b) use of an ADA-approved fluoride dentifrice
    - (c) use of mouth rinses prior to age six
    - (d) use of fluoride supplements in communities with suboptimal fluoride in the central water supply

26. The beneficial effects of fluoride to tooth structure include all of the following EXCEPT:
    - (a) enamel solubility reduction
    - (b) increase in enamel hardness
    - (c) surface energy reduction
    - (d) inhibition of microbial enzyme systems

4

HORMONES

SECTION 1: ENDOCRINOLOGY

Thyroid and Parathyroid Hormones

A **hormone** is a chemical substance that is manufactured and secreted into the body fluids by one or more cells, and that, by its action, exerts an effect on other cells of the body. All hormones are drugs by definition.

Hormones are divided into two groups according to the location of their points of secretion relative to that of their target tissues: (1) local hormones exert their effects in the vicinity where they are secreted, whereas (2) general hormones are transported by the blood to distant sites where they exert their effects. Exocrine glands discharge their secretion into ducts, while endocrine glands discharge their secretion directly into the blood. This chapter will focus on those endocrine hormones of interest in clinical dentistry.

The thyroid gland is located in the neck just inferior to the larynx and is wrapped around the lateral and anterior surfaces of the trachea (Fig. 4–1). This gland contains two types of secretory cells: (1) follicular and (2) parafollicular.

The follicular cells concentrate iodine in four closely related iodinated hormones, which are abbreviated as follows:

T_1 = monoidotyrosine	= 1 iodine atom per molecule
T_2 = diiodotyrosine	= 2 iodine atoms per molecule
T_3 = triiodothyronine	= 3 iodine atoms per molecule
T_4 = tetraiodothyronine (thyroxine)	= 4 iodine atoms per molecule

The effect of these thyroid hormones is to increase the metabolic rate of the body by increasing heart and respiratory rate, cardiac output, blood volume, and enzyme activity. T_3 is synthesized by the combination of T_1 and T_2, and T_4 may be synthesized by the addition of T_1 to T_3 or by the addition of T_2 to T_2.

T_4 represents about 95 per cent of the circulating thyroid hormone, T_3 about 5 per cent, and T_1 and T_2 are only found in trace amounts. There is evidence to suggest that body tissues convert T_4 to T_3 before any physiological effect is observed, and T_3 is about five times as potent as T_4. Dental patients present with normal thyroid function are termed euthyroid.

The parafollicular cells manufacture calcitonin, a polypeptide that works in an unknown way to allow serum calcium to attach to binding sites in calcifying structures. It is thought to have a possible role in tooth development, as well as in maintenance of the inorganic phase of bone.

Hypothyroidism, or depressed thyroid activity, when present in infancy results in a characteristic mental and physical retardation termed cretinism. The adult form of the disease is termed "myxedema," and when it occurs in childhood, "juvenile myxedema." The consistent oral findings with the disease are malocclusion, delayed tooth eruption, and increased tendency to develop periodontal disease. The gingival tissue is often inflamed, and when non-inflamed, it may be pale and enlarged. The teeth are usually poorly shaped and carious. The cretin, or thyroid dwarf, is often uncooperative owing to the mental retardation; general anesthesia may be indicated even for diagnostic radiographs and routine dental prophylaxis. Severe hypothyroids cannot withstand stress easily and are unusually sensitive to narcotics (Chap. 8, Sect. 1) and barbiturates (Chap. 7, Sec. 1).

The following preparations are used to treat hypothyroidism:

Desiccated Thyroid (Thyroid USP, Thyrocrine, Thyro-Teric, Thyroid Strong, Thyrar, S-P-T) contains the hormones T_4 and T_3 in their natural state and ratio (19:1 by weight).

Liotrix (Euthroid, Thyrolar) is a mixture of the hormones T_4 and T_3 in a 4:1 ratio by weight and may be used when more T_3 is desirable.

Levothyronine sodium (Synthroid, Levoid, Letter, Cytolen, Ro-Thyroxine) contains T_4 and is absorbed better than the extract of desiccated thyroid.

Liothyronine sodium (Cytomel, Ro-Thyronine) is used with hypothyroids who are allergic to thyroid extract, and it contains T_3.

Calcitonin (Calcimar) is available only in injection form and is administered I.M. or Sub-Q.

Hyperthyroidism, or increased thyroid activity, is associated with a lump in the anterior neck, called a goiter, or enlarged thyroid gland. The retro-orbital tissue is also hypertrophied, and this results in exophthalmos, or "pop-eyes". Oral examination reveals accelerated tooth eruption and a marked loss of the alveolar processes. Radiographic findings show a diffuse demineralization of the jawbone and rapidly progressing periodontal destruction. Oral surgery or any extensive and painful operations should be avoided with these patients, and their dental appointments should be short and simple. Epinephrine is contraindicated (Chap. 6, Sec. 2), and general anesthesia is advisable to minimize the endogenous release of epinephrine that may occur during administration of a local anesthetic. Patients receiving antithyroid agents such as **Propylthiouracil** or **methimazole** (Tapazole) over a prolonged period may have agranulocytosis and be susceptible to oral infections. No treatment of any kind should be begun by the hygienist on any patient presenting with a visible goiter, exophthalmos, or a history of taking an antithyroid drug, until the dentist has received approval from the patient's physician. A complete blood count (CBC) may be necessary before routine subgingival débridement and dental prophylaxis to exclude the possibility of leukopenia, and pre-medication is usually required.

The **parathyroid** glands are usually four in number and are located on the posterior surface of the thyroid. Each gland measures about 3 by 6 mm and has a thickness of about 2 mm. Occasionally there are thoracic parathyroid glands located in the anterior or posterior mediastinum. The glands secrete parathormone, a small protein which is released in response to falling serum calcium levels and which allows calcium to be mobilized from calcified structures to prevent low-calcium tetany. It also has the long-term effect of increasing calcium reabsorption and phosphate excretion by the kidneys.

Hyperparathyroidism, or increased parathyroid activity, is best treated with surgical excision of the parathyroids. **Hypoparathyroidism,** or depressed parathyroid activity, can be controlled with parathormone injections, administration of calcium and vitamin D (Chap. 3, Sec. 1), or administration of **dihydrotachysterol** (Hytakerol). The last drug given orally has the effect of mobilizing bone calcium, is faster acting than vitamin D, and will not cause tolerance if used over a long period. It also reduces the risk of hyper-calcemia because it is less persistent than is vitamin D after treatment is discontinued.

Controlled hyper- or hypoparathyroid patients can usually be satisfactorily managed in the office without hospitalization. The hypoparathyroid patient may show severe dental hypoplasia and oral candidiasis that are very resistant to treatment (Chap. 13, Sec. 2). Hyperparathyroid patients present with inflamed gingival tissues, severe alveolar breakdown, excessive tooth mobility, recurrent gingival tumors, and dental radiographs with radiolucencies unrelated to tooth apices and with a generalized loss of trabecular detail.

Pancreatic Hormones

The pancreas is an exocrine and endocrine gland situated transversely across the posterior wall of the abdomen, in the epigastric and left hypochondriac regions, and is between 12.5 and 15 cm long. It is composed of two types of tissues: (1) the acini, which secrete digestive juices into the duodenum, and (2) the islets of Langerhans, which secrete glucagon and insulin into the blood. The islets are composed of alpha cells, which manu-facture glucagon and beta cells, which manufacture insulin (Fig. 4–1).

The function of glucagon is to activate liver phosphorylase, an enzyme needed for the breakdown and release of liver glycogen into the circulation. It is secreted whenever the blood sugar falls to as low as 70 mg per cent, and 1 μg glucagon/kg body weight will elevate blood sugar 20 mg/per cent. For this reason, it has been called the "hyperglycemic factor."

The function of insulin is to accelerate glucose transport across the cell membrane and into the cells of skeletal muscle, adipose tissue, heart, and smooth muscle organs. Glucose cannot pass into cells by means of membrane pores and must rely on facilitated diffusion, which operates very poorly without insulin. Insulin also potentiates the action of pituitary growth hormone, which has almost no effect in the absence of insulin.

Prolonged elevation of blood glucose, resulting either from diets higher in sugar, caffeine, or refined carbohydrates, or from excessive levels of growth hormone, gluco-corticoids, or thyroxine, can make the beta cells of the pancreatic islets "burn out," or atrophy, from excessive demands on insulin production. The eventual result of partial or complete cessation of insulin production is diabetes mellitus. There are presently 10 million diagnosed diabetics in America alone, with an estimated 10 million cases that are undiagnosed.

The symptoms of diabetes mellitus include general weakness, weight loss, increase in appetite and in food intake (polyphagia), increased thirst (polydipsia), and increased passage of urine (polyuria). Diabetic coma and insulin shock (Chap. 13, Sec. 1) result from hyperglycemia and acidosis, and hypoglycemia, respectively. Diabetes is known to depress the activity of ascorbate (vitamin C), and the usual oral findings are red and edematous gingival tissues similar to those of scurvy, painful suppuration of the gingivae,

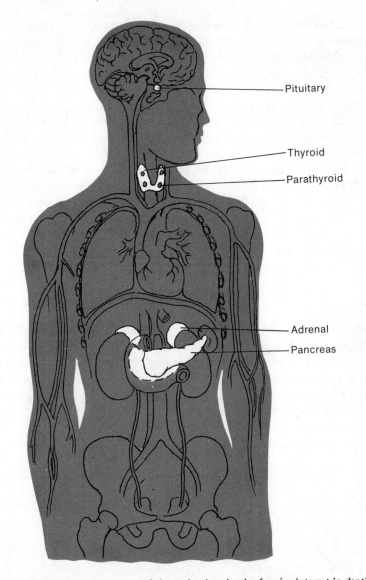

Figure 4–1. Topographical anatomy of the endocrine glands of major interest in dentistry.

recurrent periodontal abscesses, extensive periodontal breakdown, excessive tooth mobility, rapid deposition of calculus, decreased salivary flow, increased carious teeth, and arteritis of the dental pulp, which may manifest itself as an unexplained odontalgia.

Diabetics also have vascular complications that result in decreased ability to heal. Before extractions, periodontal surgery, subgingival curettage or débridement, the patient should be pre-medicated with a sedative and vitamin-mineral preparation. A prophylactic antibiotic may also be given if the patient has a severe infection or a tendency to develop alveolar osteitis ("dry socket") (Chap. 13, Sec. 2). Local anesthesia without epinephrine is preferred, since epinephrine and general anesthetics cause a rise in blood sugar. Before any dental work is begun on a diabetic, he should be questioned about what he ate at his last meal, when he ate it, and how long ago he took his insulin or antidiabetic drugs.

The following are the insulin preparations available:

1. **Insulin injection** (Regular Iletin)

2. **Insulin Zinc Suspension** (Lente Iletin, Lente Insulin)

3. **Prompt Insulin Zinc Suspension** (Semilente Iletin, Semilente Insulin)

4. **Extended Insulin Zinc Suspension** (Ultralente Iletin, Ultralente Insulin)

5. **Globin Zinc Insulin**

6. **Isophane Insulin Suspension** (NPH Iletin, Isophane Insulin)

7. **Protamine Zinc Insulin Suspension** (Protamine Zinc & Iletin, Protamine Zinc Insulin)

In some cases of diabetes mellitus the pancreas is producing insulin but cannot release it into the circulation in sufficient quantities. In these circumstances an oral hypoglycemic agent is given to stimulate the release of endogenous insulin. The sulfonylureas are derivatives of sulfonamides and have hypoglycemic effects, while being devoid of antibacterial effects (Chap. 2, Sec. 2). The following sulfonylurea preparations are available:

1. **Tolbutamide** (Orinase) 500 mg

2. **Acetohexamide** (Dymelor) 250 mg, 500 mg

3. **Tolazamide** (Tolinase) 100 mg, 250 mg, 500 mg

4. **Chlorpropamide** (Diabinese) 100 mg, 250 mg

The following are the available hyperglycemic agents:

1. **Glucagon injection**

2. **Diazoxide** (Proglycem) 50 mg 100 mg, 50 mg/cc oral suspension

Diabetics have abnormally high levels of plasma glucagon, which not only stimulates insulin release but also formation and release of cyclic AMP (adenosine monophosphate), and this activates liver and skeletal muscle phosphorylases and allows stored glycogen to be released into the circulation as glucose and thus raise blood sugar levels. Although glucagon stimulates formation and release of cyclic AMP in liver tissue in a way analogous to that of beta adrenergic stimulation (Chap. 6, Sec. 2), insulin suppresses the accumulation of cyclic AMP in fat and liver tissue. Therefore, the action of glucagon in the pancreas (insulin release) tends to oppose the action of insulin in fat and the liver (inhibition of cyclic AMP activity). This arrangement has a certain amount of survival value in that high sugar levels in the blood returning to the pancreas would release insulin at the same time that glucagon release would be suppressed and would not contribute to further insulin release, tending to dampen the wide oscillations in blood sugar, that might occur without such a mechanism.

The conclusion that stimulation of alpha adrenergic receptors inhibits pancreatic insulin release, while beta adrenergic stimulation leads to release of insulin is well supported by experimental data (Chap. 6, Sec. 2).

Periodontal Syndromes Linked With Diabetes

There are two periodontal syndromes that are related to pancreatic diabetes, or diabetes mellitus:

Acute Periodontoclasia Secondary to Diabetes. The acute form is characterized by rapid alveolar bone loss, multiple gingival abscesses, severely mobile teeth that are painful upon percussion, and generalized gingival inflammation. This form is usually seen in patients with uncontrolled diabetes or with controlled diabetes and acute dental infection.

Chronic Periodontoclasia Secondary to Diabetes. The chronic form is characterized by continued progressive bone loss around the teeth in patients with controlled diabetes, and it appears to be related to the duration of the diabetes. In spite of adequate control of the diabetes, there is radiographical evidence of continual periodontal breakdown.

Because mastication may be painful or difficult or because mucosal soreness may make it difficult to wear dentures, diabetics may turn to foods that are nutritionally poor, such as refined carbohydrates. Once periodontal health has been achieved, nutritional counseling and oral hygiene instructions are necessary to maintain the patient's health, and these duties are delegated to the dental hygienist.

Adrenocorticosteroids

The two adrenal, or suprarenal, glands are located on the superior pole of each kidney and consist of an inner medulla surrounded by an outer cortex. The adrenal medulla and cortex are anatomically close, but they are two distinct glands physiologically; the medulla manufactures the catecholamines epinephrine (85 per cent) and norepinephrine (15 per cent) (Chap. 6, Sec. 2), while the cortex manufactures glucocorticoids, mineralocorticoids, and sex hormones (male androgens and female estrogens). All of the adrenocortical hormones are termed steroids (Fig. 4–1). Control of the formation of steroid hormones is another function of cyclic AMP within both the adrenal cortex and the gonads.

Steroid hormones are associated either with glucocorticoid (anti-inflammatory) effects, mineralocorticoid (self-retaining) effects, or with both. **Glucocorticoids** act as anti-inflammatory agents, increase muscle strength, stimulate fat deposition, and promote conversion of protein into glucose (gluconeogenesis). **Mineralocorticoids** regulate blood levels of sodium (Na) and potassium (K) by acting on the kidney to increase renal tubular reabsorption of sodium and renal excretion of potassium.

The following compounds are associated with only glucocorticoid activity:

1. **Triamcinolone** (Aristocort, Kenacort, Rocinolone, Cenocort Forte, Trilone)

2. **Triamcinolone acetonide** (Kenalog)

3. **Dexamethasone** (Decadron, Hexadrol, Dexone, Gammacorten, Deksone)

4. **Methylprednisolone** (Medrol)

5. **Methylprednisolone sodium succinate** (Solu-Medrol)

6. **Methylprednisolone acetate** (Depo-Medrol, Medralone)

7. **Meprednisone** (Betapar)

8. **Paramethasone acetate** (Haldrone)

9. **Betamethasone** (Celestone)

10. **Fluprednisolone** (Alphadrol)

The only compound with pure minerolocorticoid activity is:

1. **Desoxycorticosterone acetate** (Doca Acetate, Percorten acetate)

The following compounds have both glucocorticoid and mineralocorticoid effects:

1. **Adrenal Cortical Extract** (Recortex)

2. **Cortisone** (Cortone, Adricort)

3. **Hydrocortisone** (Cortef, Solu-Cortef, Hydrocortone)

4. **Hydrocortisone acetate** (Biosone, Fernisone, Hydrocortone Acetate, Cortef Acetate, Cortril Acetate)

5. **Prednisone** (Meticorten, Orasone, Deltasone, Delta-Dome, Fernisone, Lisacort, Paracort, Ropred, Servisone, Sterapred)

6. **Prednisolone** (Delta-Cortef, Fernisolone-P, Prednis, Predoxine, Ropredione, Sterane)

7. **Prednisolone acetate** (Fernisolone, Sterane, Meticortelone acetate, Ropredlone, Dura-pred)

8. **Prednisolone sodium phosphate** (Hydeltrasol)

9. **Prednisolone sodium succinate** (Meticortelone)

10. **Fludrocortisone acetate** (Florinef Acetate)

The dental hygienist may come into contact with the use of steroid hormones in the following office situations:

1. The patient's medical history may reveal that he or she is taking a steroid for any of a wide variety of disorders or allergic states.

2. Steroids are usually stocked in the dental office emergency drug kit to aid in elevating blood pressure and to potentiate vasopressors in the treatment of shock-like hypotension.

3. Triamcinolone acetonide (Kenalog) 0.1 per cent or hydrocortone acetate 2.5 per cent ointment may be prescribed by the dentist for the treatment of pubertal gingivitis or treatment of certain oral lesions up to 1 cm in diameter.

4. Steroid-antibiotic solutions (Hydrocortone Ophthalmic Suspension) are used topically in the oral cavity on exposed pulp tissue when profound local anesthesia cannot be obtained and endodontic therapy is indicated.

5. Hydrocortisone 1.2 per cent and prednisolone 0.21 per cent are components of the root canal sealant used in the N2 (Sargenti) endodontic method practiced in many offices.

6. Dexamethasone I.M. is often administered postoperatively to dental patients recovering from general anesthesia for reduction of cerebral edema.

Hypofunction of the adrenal cortex gives rise to **Addison's disease,** producing symptoms of progressive weakness, weight loss, hypotension, and pigmentation of skin and mucous membranes. The patient may also suffer from anorexia, vomiting, diarrhea, headaches, paresthesias, irritability, or loss of memory. Pigmentation of the oral mucosa may be the first sign of the disease and appears as irregular bluish-black or brownish-gray spots. During an acute exacerbation of these symptoms (adrenal crisis), the systolic pressure may be between 50 and 80 mm Hg (Chap. 12, Sec. 1). An adrenal crisis may follow operative procedures or acute infections in patients with Addison's disease, in patients who are receiving anticoagulant therapy owing to destruction of adrenocortical tissue by spontaneous hemorrhage, or in patients on long-term steroid therapy that may give rise to depressed adrenocortical function. Such patients may not be able to react satisfactorily to a stressful situation without an increase in steroid dosage, and each patient's physician should be consulted prior to any dental procedures. Since the long-term use of steroids interferes with the body's defense mechanism, prophylactic antibiotic therapy (Chap. 2, Sec. 2) may be indicated if severe infection is present or anticipated, and hospitalization may also be indicated.

Hyperfunction of the adrenal cortex results in symptoms of hypertension, obesity, an abnormal glucose tolerance test, reduced ability to heal, reduced resistance to infection, and possible psychiatric aberrations. The complex of symptoms is known as **Cushing's syndrome** and may be produced by adrenal tumors, pituitary tumors, or administration of high levels of steroids. Treatment consists of surgical removal of tumorous tissue or gradual reduction of steroid dosage.

Patients with hyperadrenalism are poor risks for any type of dental procedures, and the hazards facing the dental profession in these patients are poor healing, susceptibility to infections, hypertensive crises, abnormal bone fractures, and possibly uncontrolled diabetes. Emergency treatment should be given with the advice of the patient's physician, and routine treatment should be deferred until the physician has had time to treat the hyperadrenalism.

Pituitary Growth Hormone

The secretion of pituitary growth hormone, or somatotropin, is controlled by the lower paraventricular area of the hypothalamus, and the hormone is manufactured in the adenohypophysis, or anterior lobe of the pituitary gland. Its function is to promote increased cell size and cell division by increasing the rate of protein synthesis of all cells, by increasing the mobilization of fats for energy, and by decreasing the rate of carbohydrate utilization throughout the body (Fig. 4–1).

Decreased secretion of all the adenohypophyseal hormones, including growth hormone, is termed panhypopituitarism. This results in pituitary dwarfism, which is a state characterized by small stature, hypothyroidism, depressed function of sexual organs, and decreased secretion of glucocorticoids by the adrenal glands. The pituitary dwarf usually is not mentally retarded, and hospitalization for dental procedures is usually not indicated. Use of pedondontic instruments may be necessary.

When the pituitary gland is excessively active prior to puberty and before the epiphyses of the long bones have become fused to the bone shafts, giantism will result. The pituitary giant is normal in every respect except for his or her tall stature and tendency to develop diabetes mellitus secondary to degeneration of the beta cells of the pancreatic islets of Langerhans due to overstimulation and overactivity. Such a person may therefore have full-blown diabetes and be unaware of it. When oral surgical procedures or sub-gingival débridement is considered in these patients, it should be approached with the same precautions as in diabetics.

If the increased pituitary activity occurs after puberty, and the bone epiphyses have fused with their bone shafts, acromegaly will result. A person with this disorder cannot grow taller, but his bones can grow in thickness, and his soft tissues can enlarge, resulting in mandibular prognathism, macroglossia, and enlargement of the nose, supraorbital ridges, vertebrae, hands, and feet. A history of separation of the teeth in an adult or growth of the mandible after age 20 should arouse suspicion of acromegaly. It may be difficult to use ordinary instruments in these patients, owing to their macroglossia. If kyphosis is present the patient may experience some discomfort in the dental chair in the supine position. Hospitalization should be considered in those patients in which a general anesthetic is indicated.

Somatotropin is only available as **Asellacrin** for injection.

The release of adenohypophyseal hormones, including TSH (thyroid stimulating hormone), ACTH (adrenocorticotrophic hormone), and growth hormone (somatotropin), in response to hypothalamic releasing factors appears to also involve cyclic AMP at certain points in the series of relays leading to the ultimate arrival of these hormones at their target cells.

Pubertal Gingivitis

During puberty there is increased androgen activity in males and increased estrogen activity in females, which may result in enlargement of the gingiva, a condition termed gingivitis of puberty. The affected areas are usually reddened and bleed easily, but there are no pathognomonic findings with this disease. The entire gingival tissue may be affected, or it may be limited to a local area. The exact mechanism leading to this abnormality is obscure, but the hormonal changes are believed to be involved. This type of hypertrophic gingivitis also occurs in pregnancy and occasionally during menstruation.

Treatment is directed at local measures, namely, subgingival débridement, restoration of faulty subgingival margins, and oral hygiene instruction. Stubborn pubertal gingivitis that does not respond to these measures may be treated with either

1. hydrocortisone acetate 2.5 per cent ointment, or

2. triamcinolone acetonide 0.1 per cent (Kenalog Orabase)

The latter drug is 20 times more potent than the former, and no serious local or systemic side effects have been reported when this agent is used for oral lesions. (Chap. 9, Sec. 1).

SECTION 2: MICROENDOCRINOLOGY

Hypothalamic-Parotid Gland Endocrine Axis

The tooth is a separate functioning organ that has an active metabolism extending from the cells of the pulp to at least as far as the dentinoenamel (DE) junction. Between five and ten minutes following intraperitoneal injection of radioactive acriflavine hydro-chloride, it has been seen to reach the odontoblastic tubules. The odontoblasts themselves are osmotic pumps that control an active transport system for movement of dentinal fluid within the hard structures of the tooth, and when this system fails, the incidence of dental caries increases.

Saliva is continually seeking to enter the tooth through the interprismatic substance of the enamel, which is composed of keratin and is maintained by the flow of nutrients from the odontoblastic tubules. Movement of dentinal fluid is usually greater than fluid flow into the tooth, and the interprismatic substance is maintained in a state of health. The rate of movement of dentinal fluid is controlled by **parotin**, an endocrine hormone secreted by the parotid salivary glands. The submandibular and sublingual glands, as well as the other minor salivary glands, do not control fluid movement in the dentin; only the parotid gland does.

It has been shown that the hypothalamus of the brain normally secretes the hypothalamic parotid-hormone releasing factor, which circulates through the blood to the parotid glands and enables stored parotin to be secreted into the circulation and thus find its way to the teeth. It has also been shown that parasympathetic stimulants encourage outward flow of dentinal fluid in animals deprived of their salivary glands. Therefore, anything that depresses function of either the parotid gland or hypothalamus will increase the incidence of dental decay by interrupting the hypothalamic-parotid endocrine axis (see Chapter 6, Section 2).

This fact has major significance in dental hygiene practice. Sugar in the diet lowers the serum phosphorus below 3.5 mg/per cent (3.5 mg per 100 cc of blood), which in turn depresses the hypothalamus. External radiation used to treat certain malignancies of the jaws and pharynx may unavoidably pass through the parotid glands, depressing their normal functions. Tumors of the parotid glands themselves may require surgical excision of the parotids. Although the formation of parotin has not been substantiated in man, and the current information is based only on animal model experiments, it would be safe to conclude that dental patients presenting with a history of radiotherapy to the mouth or jaws, parotid gland excision, or with diets high in sugar will require special consultation in order to prevent the eventual loss of all the teeth due to dental caries. Certain laboratory mammals fed diets very low in sugar (Purina laboratory chow) do not have appreciable dental decay, but when these animals are irradiated, the incidence of decay increases sharply, even when the organisms in the animals' mouths are eating nothing but Purina. When certain other laboratory animals are fed diets high in sugar and have the dentinal fluid transport mechanism in their teeth stimulated with parasympathetic stimulants, such as bethanecol, the caries incidence is often reduced by between 95 and 100 per cent, even when the organisms in the animals' mouths have a plentiful supply of sugar and the animals' parotid glands have been removed. Although the environment external to a tooth may be destructive because acid comes in contact with the tooth surface, whether or not dental decay occurs is dependent, in at least some mammals, on the physiologic activity within the host, and not the mere presence or absence of acid at the enamel surface. It is entirely possible that in humans dental decay is a local problem superimposed on a larger systemic imbalance, which represents the invisible part of the "iceberg;" this would help explain the common clinical observation of uncontrolled decay in mouths that are essentially free of local irritants or that have a high level of oral hygiene.

Balancing Body Chemistry

The body chemistry evaluation (BCE) has been developed in recent years as a therapeutic modality used to correct chronic degenerative diseases, including dental decay and peridontal disease. It is based on the findings that certain mineral profiles are routinely seen in the blood and hair samples of the patients suffering from certain diseases, that certain organ systems may have an effect on the destruction of peridontal tissues, and that food intake may affect disease states. The patient is asked to provide the dentist with the following information: (1) a completed **Cornell Medical Index** (CMI) questionnaire, (2) **seven-day diet diary** of everything the patient is eating or drinking except water, and (3) **blood and hair samples** taken every three months for a period between six and nine months long. The results of these tests are corollated and recommendations are made to the patient about diet, medications, and vitamin and mineral supplementations to bring the body chemistry back to within normal limits. If peridontal surgery is needed it is usually performed at the end of the testing, although it may be necessary to perform it prior to testing owing to the extent of the disease.

The success of this program depends on patient cooperation (proper diet, follow-up examinations, and treatment), which may be difficult to achieve. Such treatment may ultimately involve hundreds of dollars worth of dental investment, which further jeopardizes patient cooperation. In those offices where BCE is routinely practiced, the dental hygienist will be involved with calculations of total protein, whole carbohydrates, refined carbohydrates, and total food choices in the patient diet diaries, and with patient diet consultations.

Although analysis of blood gives an indication of extracellular activity, it reveals only what is *available* to cells, not what cells are *receiving*. Hair analysis gives an indication of intracellular activity with regard to trace mineral concentrations. **Trace minerals** are elements required in small amounts for normal cellular activity to take place, and those that are studied for practical application are calcium (Ca), copper (Cu), lead (Pb), iron (Fe), magnesium (Mg), manganese (Mn), potassium (K), sodium (Na), zinc (Zn), mercury (Hg), cadmium (Cd), chromium (Cr), and lithium (Li). By studying which elements activate or inhibit certain enzyme systems, one deduces why certain systems may break down in the absence of particular trace minerals.

When one knows which values are low and which values are high, supplementation with "chelated minerals" may be effective in getting high values down and low values up. **Chelation** is a type of weak chemical bond in which a metal element is attached to an amino acid or amino group ($-NH_2$) of a protein. The gastrointestinal tract is believed to be lined with negatively charged chemical groups to which positively charged minerals have a great tendency to attach themselves, being poorly absorbed as a result. By bonding to an amino acid or protein having several free negative charges, the mineral is held within the protein structure and will pass more freely into the circulation. Once absorbed and transported to the tissues, cells deficient in the element have the ability to break the weak bonds of the chelate and transport the mineral into the cell. This process is referred to as "chelating in."

Some amino acid preparations can be given I.V., and these have the ability to "chelate out" certain minerals known to be in excess in cells and to allow the resultant mineral-protein products to be easily excreted. This form of therapy is best accomplished with close monitoring of the patient in the hospital.

Some studies have suggested that the absorption of chelated minerals ranges from 50 to 85 per cent, whereas the absorption of plain mineral salts may be less than 5 per cent; other studies have suggested that chelated minerals, especially those combined with soya protein, are more poorly absorbed than are the plain mineral salts, which are almost completely absorbed. Since there is evidence for and against chelating minerals to be used as diet supplements and since chelation increases the cost of treatment, at the present time there appears to be no practical advantage to be gained by using chelated minerals instead of plain mineral salts. The results of further studies should be evaluated before definite attitudes on chelation are formulated, since it is possible that some minerals may be more completely absorbed in a chelated form and other minerals may not.

Magnesium (Mg) is the major divalent intracellular cation and is necessary for activation of 78 per cent of the body's enzyme systems. Potassium (K) is the major monovalent intracellular cation. Many of the body's inefficiencies are due to deficiencies of both magnesium and potassium. Lead (Pb), mercury (Hg), and cadmium (Cd), when present in cells, are contaminants.

TEST QUESTIONS

1. Severe hypothyroidism (cretinism, myxedema) necessitates a reduction in dosage of:
   (a) antihistamines and belladonna alkaloids
   (b) narcotics and barbiturates
   (c) tranquilizers and non-barbiturate sedatives
   (d) none of the above
2. The hygienist should not begin dental treatment on severely hyperthyroid patients presenting with _____ until the dentist obtains proper medical clearance.
   (a) a visible goiter
   (b) exophthalmos
   (c) a history of taking antithyroid drugs, such as methimazole or propylthiouracil
   (d) all of the above
3. Patients with diabetes mellitus should be pre-medicated with a _____ prior to periodontal surgery, subgingival curettage, or subgingival débridement.
   (a) sedative and vitamin-mineral combination
   (b) narcotic and antihistamine
   (c) antithyroid drug
   (d) none of the above
4. Patients with diabetes mellitus should NOT be given local anesthesia with _____ because this will cause a rise in blood sugar.
   (a) insulin   (c) enzymes
   (b) epinephrine   (d) all of the above
5. An adrenal crisis may be caused by an acute oral infection or stressful dental procedure in patients with:
   (a) Addison's disease
   (b) long-term steroid therapy
   (c) anticoagulant therapy
   (d) all of the above
6. Routine dental treatment for patients with Cushing's syndrome or other forms of hyperadrenalism should be deferred until the hyperadrenalism is medically treated in order to avoid:
   (a) uncontrolled diabetes mellitus   (d) poor healing
   (b) abnormal bone fractures   (e) infections
   (c) hypertensive episodes   (f) all of the above

7. A history of separation of the teeth of an adult or growth of the mandible after age 20 should excite suspicion toward:
   (a) hyperthyroidism
   (c) acromegaly
   (b) hyperadrenalism
   (d) myxedema
8. Pituitary giants have a great tendency to develop:
   (a) panhypopituitarism
   (c) mental retardation
   (b) diabetes mellitus
   (d) pubertal gingivitis
9. Within ten minutes after intraperitoneal injection, radioactive acriflavine hydrochloride will reach the:
   (a) enamel surface
   (c) odontoblastic tubules
   (b) interprismatic substance
   (d) none of the above
10. An endocrine hormone that influences dentinal fluid flow, that is released by a "releasing factor" from the hypothalamus, and that is depressed by excess sugar, caffeine, and refined carbohydrates in the diet is:
    (a) phosphorylase
    (d) somatotropin
    (b) triiodothyronine
    (e) parotin
    (c) glucagon
    (f) hydrocortisone
11. An endocrine hormone that accelerates the facilitated diffusion of glucose across cell membranes and in which the action depends upon sufficient quantities of pituitary growth hormone is:
    (a) phosphorylase
    (d) insulin
    (b) triiodothyronine
    (e) parotin
    (c) glucagon
    (f) hydrocortisone
12. The _(1)_ salivary glands promote dentinal fluid movement which can also be encouraged by _(2)_ stimulating drugs such as bethanecol
    (a) *(1)* parotid and *(2)* sympathetic
    (b) *(1)* parotid and *(2)* parasympathetic
    (c) *(1)* submandibular and *(2)* sympathetic
    (d) *(1)* submandibular and *(2)* parasympathetic
13. Dentinal fluid movement can be interrupted by any of the following EXCEPT:
    (a) external radiation to the mouth or jaws
    (b) surgical excision of the parotid glands
    (c) decrease in serum phosphorus below 3.5 mg/per cent
    (d) diets high in sugar, caffeine, or refined carbohydrates
    (e) depressed hypothalamic activity
    (f) injection of parasympathetic stimulating drugs
14. A body chemistry evaluation may include any of the following EXCEPT:
    (a) Cornell Medical Index questionnaire
    (b) seven-day diet diary
    (c) complete blood count and urinalysis
    (d) blood and hair samples over a period between six and nine months long

ANTICOAGULANTS AND ANTIHISTAMINES

SECTION 1: FACTORS IN THE ARREST OF HEMORRHAGE

Extrinsic and Intrinsic Thromboplastin Generation

It is absolutely essential that the practicing dental hygienist have a clear understanding of the mechanism of coagulation of blood, since a variable amount of bleeding is produced during subgingival débridement and dental prophylaxis. Teeth cannot be thoroughly cleaned without causing injury to small blood vessels in the gingival tissues, resulting in hemorrhage.

Platelets (thrombocytes) are present in whole blood in quantities between 200,000 and 400,000/mm^3 in the normal individual. **Fibrinogen,** a plasma protein, is normally present in concentrations between 0.2 and 0.4 per cent of blood plasma (whole blood minus cellular components). Hemorrhage occurring because of injury of small blood vessels is controlled by (1) platelets and injured tissues, which release substances that modify vascular permeability and smooth muscle tonus; (2) the vascular adherence and agglutination of platelets; (3) the conversion of plasma fibrinogen to a network of fibrin threads; and (4) the drawing together of the wound edges by retraction of the clot and drying of the exudate.

74

The study of blood coagulation has been simplified by using a Roman numeral system of nomenclature for the various clotting factors. These are listed in Table 5-1. All of the clotting factors have a very short duration in the circulation (half-lives are between 5 and 120 hrs), and it is possible that some coagulation goes on all the time and that the factors are continually used up. The dissolution of these fresh clots is related to the amount of alpha tocopherol (vitamin E) in the diet. Thrombophlebitis is amenable to treatment with vitamin E 400 IU daily.

Thromboplastin is an essential ingredient in the clotting process and may be generated through the extrinsic pathway or the intrinsic pathway (Fig. 5-1).

Skin and underlying vascular injury results in the release of substances including (1) histamine (Chap. 5, Sec. 4) or a histamine-like substance which triggers a "triple response," (i.e., vasodilation in the immediate area, vasodilation in the surrounding area through axon reflexes, and increased vascular permeability with coincident extravascular movement of plasma proteins, resulting in edema and vascular compression); (2) a vasoconstrictor, thought to be serotonin released from platelets, which may result in complete vascular occlusion for an interval between 20 and 120 minutes long; and (3) tissue (extrinsic) thromboplastin, a normal cellular component, which initiates the formation of a more permanent change, the fibrin clot. A measurement of these factors is the bleeding time, or the interval required for cessation of bleeding from a blotted cutaneous stab wound. The bleeding time normally ranges from three to eight minutes. Extrinsic thromboplastin is therefore released whenever there is cell damage of any kind.

Blood plasma also contains factors capable of generating intrinsic thromboplastin in the absence of cell damage by contact with a roughened or wettable surface, including factors III, IV, VIII, IX, XI, and XII. Factors that accelerate this conversion are factors V and X. Formation of intrinsic thromboplastin is thought to begin with adsorbed Hageman factor XII and to involve the recently discovered Fitzgerald and Fletcher factors, which currently have no Roman numeral designation.

It is immaterial to the body whether thromboplastin is generated extrinsically by cell damage or intrinsically by contact with a roughened or wettable surface (see Fig. 5-1). Thromboplastin may be generated during dental procedures either intrinsically or extrinsically depending on the situation. Hemorrhage secondary to most dental procedures, such as extractions, periodontal surgery, or dental prophylaxis, involves the extrinsic pathway, whereas thrombi resulting from the contact of blood with roughened vascular surfaces within intact vessels are generated intrinsically.

Table 5-1. NOMENCLATURE FOR THE BLOOD CLOTTING FACTORS

Fibrinogen factor I
Prothrombin factor II
Platelet factor III
Calcium factor IV
Accelerin factor V
Factor VI (This term is no longer used.)
Convertin factor VII
Antihemophilic globulin factor VIII
Plasma thromboplastin component factor IX
Stuart-Prower factor X
Plasma thromboplastin antecedent factor XI
Hageman factor XII
Fibrin stabilizing factor XIII

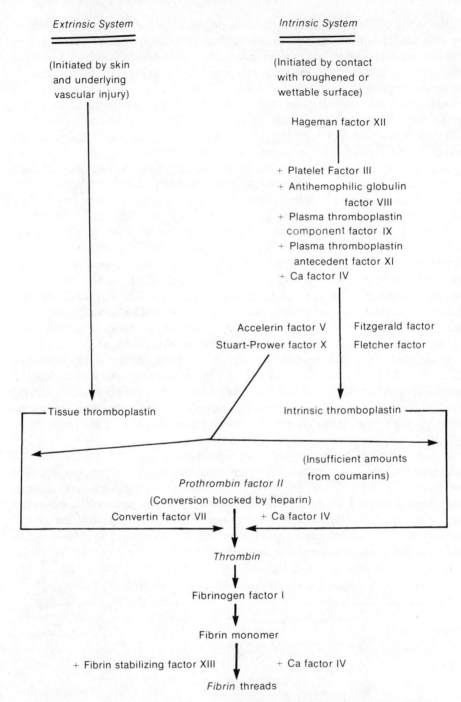

Figure 5–1. Comparison of extrinsic and intrinsic mechanisms of blood coagulation.

There are four primary screening tests to determine whether a bleeding disorder results from a vascular, platelet, or plasma coagulation abnormality. These are, for the platelet phase, (1) bleeding time (between 3 and 8 min) and (2) platelet count (between

200,000 and 400,000/mm^3), and for the coagulation phase, (3) partial thromboplastin time (between 22 and 37 sec) and (4) prothrombin time (between 10 and 14 sec, or less than 2 sec deviation from control. The coagulation time (between 6 and 17 min) is usually used to monitor heparin therapy (Chap. 5, Sec. 2) but has been replaced in many hospitals with the partial thromboplastin time.

The prothrombin time (PT) is a measure of extrinsic system activity (factors I, II, V, VII, and X), whereas the partial thromboplastin time (PTT) is a measure of intrinsic system activity (factors I, II, V, VIII, IX, X, XI, XII, Fitzgerald, and Fletcher). Routine hospital admission orders for tests for dental patients will usually include measurement of bleeding time and of PTT, since the bleeding time test reveals platelet function (both platelet factor III release and clot retraction) and since the PTT test measures the activity of a greater number of clotting factors than does the PT.

Prothrombin Conversion and Fibrin Formation

The action either of tissue (extrinsic) thromboplastin or of intrinsic thromboplastin is, in the presence of calcium ions, to catalyze the reaction that converts plasma prothrombin factor II to the active proteolytic enzyme thrombin. Three known accelerating factors in this conversion are accelerin factor V, convertin factor VII, and Stuart-Prower factor X.

Thrombin then acts on fibrinogen factor I, which comprises between 0.2 and 0.4 per cent of blood plasma, and splits off two molecular peptide groups, thereby permitting subsequent polymerization to form fibrin threads. The intertwining of fibrin threads acts as a network that holds back blood cells and prevents their escape. Fibrin stabilizing factor XIII and calcium ions are needed for polymerization to take place.

Fibrinolysis and Prevention of Intravascular Clotting

Retraction of the fibrin clot with the expression of serum (plasma minus fibrinogen) occurs by a contractile mechanism contained in the enmeshed platelets. Clot breakdown, or clot lysis, is necessary to remove old clots after they have done their job and occurs when plasma profibrinolysis (plasminogen) is converted to the active enzyme fibrinolysin (plasmin).

Intravascular disease processes or injury may result in the deposition of fibrin, platelets, and enmeshed blood cells within intact vessels. If clot lysis is impaired, the thrombus thus formed may either break loose and occlude small vessels as a thromboembolus or be invaded by connective tissue, receiving an endothelial lining and thereby reducing the size of the vessel lumen. The possibility of thrombus formation and embolic occlusion may be reduced with anticoagulant therapy, long-term use of salicylates, or vitamin E supplementation.

SECTION 2: ANTICOAGULANTS

Heparin Sodium

Heparin sodium (Hepathrom, Panheprin, Depo-Heparin) is stored naturally in granules in mast cells and circulating basophils and is made from animal tissues. It acts to inhibit the formation of fibrin clots (1) by acting as an antithromboplastin, blocking the conversion of prothrombin factor II to thrombin, (2) by inhibition of Stuart-Prower factor X, thereby retarding the rates at which intrinsic thromboplastin is generated and prothrombin factor II can be converted, and (3) by inhibition of fibrin stabilizing factor XIII, preventing the formation of a stable fibrin clot. Although clotting time is prolonged by heparin sodium, it does not significantly alter the concentrations of the clotting factors of the blood, and bleeding time is usually unaffected.

Heparin sodium is not active when given orally and must be given by I.V. or Sub-Q injection. An initial dose of 10,000 units is followed with a daily dose between 20,000 and 60,000 units. Its action appears to be associated with its large electronegative charge, which facilitates combination with a variety of proteins. This may also account for its inability to cross the placenta or failure to appear in milk after administration.

Heparin sodium is used to prevent and treat venous thrombosis, to prevent clotting in arterial and heart surgery, as an adjunct to treatment of stroke, and in the preheparinized tubes used for blood transfusions and collection of blood samples. Patients receiving heparin sodium are usually hospitalized and carefully monitored. The antidote for acute overdosage is **protamine sulfate** (Salmine) 1 mg/100 units heparin last given. When given alone, protamine sulfate has a strong anticoagulant effect, but when given in the presence of heparin (which is strongly acidic), it forms a stable salt, resulting in the loss of anticoagulant activity of both drugs. If the blood inactivates protamine sulfate before it is able to neutralize heparin, a "heparin rebound" occurs, necessitating larger doses of protamine. However, administration of an excessive amount of protamine (greater than that required to neutralize heparin) will have an anticoagulant effect, resulting in a tendency to hemorrhage.

The primary hemostatic defense in heparinized patients is the platelet aggregation reaction, which by itself is not sufficient to allow the patient to withstand subgingival débridement or oral surgical procedures.

Coumarins

Unlike heparin sodium, which acts directly as an antithromboplastin, the coumarins act indirectly to prevent coagulation by depressing the liver synthesis of vitamin-K-dependent clotting factors (II, VIII, IX, and X) and thus decreasing plasma concentrations. Prolonged prothrombin times are not observed during coumarin therapy until there is a significant depletion of these clotting factors from the plasma, which may require from 12 to 24 hours to occur. These agents are indicated for the prophylaxis and treatment of venous thrombosis, pulmonary embolism, and as an adjunct in the treatment of coronary occlusion.

The major advantage of using the coumarins instead of heparin sodium is that they are effective by mouth and are easier to take in maintenance doses. The effectiveness of a dose is monitored by measuring the prothrombin time, which should be maintained at between 1.5 and 3 times the control value. It is generally agreed that a dose that results in a PT of two times the control value provides adequate anticoagulation with less risk of uncontrolled hemorrhage than does a dose that yields a more prolonged PT value.

The major disadvantages of the coumarins are drug interactions (Chap. 11, Sec. 1) and uncontrollable hemorrhage. Potentially hemorrhagic conditions (e.g., pregnancy, ulcers, blood dyscrasias such as leukemia, and scorbutic gingivitis) contraindicate the use of these drugs, and conversely, patients taking these drugs should not undergo any elective surgery, dental extractions, or subgingival débridement and dental prophylaxis. Such patients should not even undergo a periodontal probing to record gingival pocket measurements unless prior clearance has been obtained from the patient's physician.

Although patients taking coumarin anticoagulants may show obvious dental neglect and advanced periodontal disease, they are taking the anticoagulant for an even more serious health problem, and their dental care must be deferred until their physicians indicate that it can be begun. Such patients will usually discontinue taking the drug for five days to restore clotting factors to normal levels and may be given between 1 and 10 mg **vitamin K$_1$** (phytonadione) orally or between 20 and 40 mg parenterally to accelerate the process. In emergency hospital situations the patient is given between 250 and 500 cc fresh normal plasma to immediately restore the clotting factors.

The coumarin drug of choice is **warfarin sodium** (Coumadin Sodium, Panwarfin) and the initial daily dose is between 40 and 60 mg, with average maintenance doses between 2 and 10 mg, given orally. This drug is available in injection form and as 2, 2.5, 5, 7.5, 10, and 25 mg tablets. Although **dicumarol** (bishydroxycoumarin) is the prototype agent for the group, it has erratic bioavailability due to its poor water solubility and is less commonly used. Alternate coumarin agents include **phenprocoumon** (Liquamar) and **adenocumarol** (Sintrom).

Indandiones

The **indandione** derivatives **phenindione** (Hedulin), **diphenadione** (Dipaxin), and **anisindione** (Miradon) are identical to the coumarins in mechanism of action; i.e., they selectively depress the hepatic synthesis of certain essential clotting factors by acting as vitamin K antimetabolites. They offer no clinical advantage over the coumarins and are associated with a wider spectrum of adverse effects, including hematopoietic, hepatic, renal, and cutaneous effects. For these reasons, they are seldom used.

The same precautions taken in approaching dental treatment of patients taking coumarin anticoagulants should also be exercised in treating those taking indandione derivatives (Chap. 5, Sec. 2).

SECTION 3: AGENTS THAT FACILITATE CLOTTING OR CLOT BREAKDOWN

Agents Used Locally to Control Bleeding

When blood vessels are injured, the subendothelial collagen becomes exposed, which attracts platelets and results in a temporary plug of aggregated platelets (the so-called "platelet plug"), and this is detected by measuring the bleeding time and is not prevented by any of the anticoagulant drugs. Several agents promote platelet disruption or form a matrix for fibrin deposition when the clotting mechanism is normal and bleeding is confined to capillary oozing.

Absorbable gelatin sponge (Gelfoam) is a sterile pliable surgical sponge that may be cut into small pieces, lightly crushed with the fingers, and inserted into fresh non-infected extraction sockets. It functions to provide a framework for fibrin deposition and a scaffolding into which granulation tissue may grow, thereby aiding healing. It is contraindicated with frank infection, in shallow wounds or sockets where it would protrude to the surface after suturing, and in extraction cases with suspected or confirmed antral perforation. It completely liquefies between two and five days after contact with a bleeding surface, and it is completely absorbed between four and six weeks following implantation in tissues. Dental packs are available in two sizes: size two (10 X 20 X 7 mm) and size four (20 X 20 X 7 mm). Both sizes are sold fifteen to a pack. Size two is preferable for most dental extraction cases.

The use of **oxidized cellulose** (Oxycel, Surgicel) in dentistry is limited to placement over a fresh extraction socket with application of pressure to the bleeding area. When it is placed within extraction sockets it may interfere with bone regeneration and delay healing, leading to cyst formation.

Topical thrombin is available in 1000, 5000, and 10,000 unit vials and may be prepared in sterile water or isotonic saline (0.9 per cent NaCl) to render solutions of various concentrations. Solutions containing 100 units/cc are used for oral surgery, but when profuse bleeding is expected solutions as high as 2000 units/cc may be used. Thrombin clots the fibrinogen of the blood directly. It may also be used orally to control hemorrhage of the upper gastrointestinal tract if stomach acids are neutralized prior to oral administration.

Negatol (Negatan) 45 per cent solution has a powerful coagulant effect on protein substances, including plasma clotting factors and other plasma and tissue proteins. In dilutions up to 1:100 it is also a strong germicide (Chap. 2, Sec. 1). Its principle use in dentistry is as a styptic (an astringent and hemostatic agent) during deep interproximal cavity preparation or during crown or bridge prosthesis preparations.

Aluminum chloride 25 per cent (Hemodent) may also be used as a styptic but has no germicidal action.

Tannic acid (found in tea) is a styptic commonly found in the home, and patients who experience excessive postoperative bleeding may be instructed to bite on a teabag for 30 minutes in lieu of treatment by a dentist.

Racemic epinephrine 8 per cent (Racord) is falling into disuse as a hemostatic and astringent in dentistry because of unwanted cardiovascular effects (Chap. 6, Sec. 2).

Proteolytic Enzymes

The inflammatory and edematous reaction associated with multiple dental extractions, or alveolectomy often results in deposition of fibrin and denatured protein macromolecules in the tissue spaces, and this can block the free flow of body fluids and the resorption of edema. Unsightly facial swelling or bruising may result. Healing action in these cases can be accelerated, and the macromolecular deposits can be decreased in size (depolymerized) by proteolytic digestion.

Tablets containing 50,000 units **trypsin** and 4000 units **chymotrypsin** (Orenzyme) may be given in a dose of one or two tablets q.i.d. Tablets containing twice as much trypsin and chymotrypsin (Orenzyme Bitabs) are given as a dose of one tablet q.i.d.

Trypsin and chymotrypsin are also available in a 6:1 ratio in forms containing 50,000 units of enzyme activity (Chymoral) or 100,000 units of enzyme activity (Chymoral-100). When only chymotrypsin is prescribed it is available in a dose of 50,000 units (Avazyme) or 100,000 units (Avazyme-100). The dosages for these products are the same as for Orenzyme (50,000 units 1 or 2 q.i.d. and 100,000 units q.i.d.).

Other agents less commonly used include bromelains (Ananase-50, Ananase-100) and carica papaya proteolytic enzymes (Papase).

All of the products just mentioned should be used sparingly owing to a lack of substantial evidence of effectiveness as adjunctive therapy for edema and inflammation secondary to surgical trauma; however, even though the mode of action of these agents has not been completely established, they should form part of every dentist's routine prescribing regimen.

Immune Globulin and Serum Hepatitis

It is well documented that blood-to-blood contact with as little as 10^{-4} cc (0.0001 cc) of infected blood can spread hepatitis B virus (serum hepatitis). Blood bank blood is rarely taken from a hepatitis carrier, but the dental profession more commonly contributes to the spread of the disease by failing to scrub and autoclave instruments properly or by failing to wear surgical gloves when necessary. When an adequate medical history is taken on all new patients and proper precautions are taken during all dental procedures involving hepatitis carriers, the incidence of serum hepatitis will decrease (Chap. 2, Sec. 1).

Hepatitis B immune globulin (H-BIG) is a sterile solution of between 10 and 18 per cent protein containing a high concentration of antibody against hepatitis B surface antigen, and when injected it will build the general resistance of the body to serum hepatitis. It is indicated following accidental "needle-stick" from a known hepatitis carrier and is given I.M., usually in the deltoid or gluteal region (Chap. 9, Sec. 2).

Previous estimates of the number of dentists who rely on only cold chemical disinfection of their penetrating instruments have been as high as 45 per cent, an alarming number considering that the mouth is the most highly contaminated area of the body. Any expanded-function dental hygienist is within his or her rights to require the dentist employer to furnish an adequate medical history on each new patient treated, to have surgical gloves available when needed, and to sterilize penetrating instruments between patients to insure minimum standards for patient and operator safety. Even though a dentist may have practiced without regard to these standards for years without having a problem arise, that is still no excuse, and would be considered negligence in a court of law. Many dentists have never been reprimanded for their laxity in this matter because the incubation period for serum hepatitis is extremely long (between 6 and 25 weeks), and septic transmission resulting from dental procedures is usually difficult to prove (Chap. 9, Sec. 2).

Postoperative Care Following Oral Surgery

Every patient should be given verbal and written instructions following subgingival curettage or periodontal or other oral surgery, regardless of whether or not an antibiotic or analgesic is prescribed, and these directions should include the following:

1. Bite on moistened gauze to apply pressure to the affected area for 30 minutes after treatment (gauze should be dispensed at the chair).

2. Avoid rinsing the mouth for 24 hours and report any unusual bleeding. Some oozing is normal.

3. The first day, apply an icebag to the affected area of the face, on 15 minutes and off 15 minutes. After the first day, warm saline (moist heat) should be held in the mouth over the area several times daily.

4. Take the medicine prescribed. If none is prescribed, aspirin may be taken every four hours.

5. Report any unusual reactions to medicine, persistent bleeding, a bad taste in the mouth, or persistent soreness after the third postoperative day.

Patients taking anticoagulants who have undergone oral surgery should have been pre-medicated with a sedative, analgesic, and vitamin C, they should bite on gauze for one hour after surgery, and they should avoid rinsing for 48 hours. Icebags are used for 48 hours, on 30 minutes and off 30 minutes. Postoperative discomfort is usually greater in these patients and extends over a longer period of time than is normal. Close cooperation with the patient's physician is needed owing to possible interactions of the anticoagulant with certain antibiotics or analgesics (Chap. 11, Sec. 1).

Management of Hemophiliacs

Classical hemophilia is a hereditary deficiency of antihemophilic globulin factor VIII (hemophilia A); when the hemophilia is due to plasma deficiency of thromboplastin component factor IX, the disorder is called hemophilia B. Together hemophilias A and B account for over 90 per cent of all hereditary coagulation disorders. Over 80 per cent of hemophiliac patients have hemophilia A.

The PTT is abnormal in all severe cases; when a normal PT is observed in the presence of an abnormal PTT, specific factor testing should be performed.

Because of the hazard of uncontrollable bleeding, oral surgery is approached with extreme caution in these patients. Patients are hospitalized and receive blood transfusions before and during the surgery. When extractions are performed, suturing is avoided and fine gauge needles are used, thrombin packs are employed, and protective acrylic splints are made. Every effort is made to minimize surgical trauma. In lieu of whole blood transfusions, antihemophilic factor (Factorate, Hemofil, Humafac, Koate, Profilate) and factor IX complex (Konyne, Proplex) may be given to maintain levels of these factors between 20 and 60 per cent above normal during surgery and for eight days afterwards.

Aminocaproic acid (Amicar) is available in injection form, as a syrup containing 250 mg/cc, and as 500 mg tablets. It acts to inhibit the activation of profibrinolysin (plasminogen), and it is usually prescribed to hemophiliacs prior to dental extractions. The plasma concentration necessary for the inhibition of profibrinolysin is 13 mg/per cent (0.13 mg/cc), a level which is often maintained with an I.V. infusion. Heparin sodium is often administered concurrently with aminocaproic acid in order to prevent disseminated thrombosis.

Hemophiliacs should begin regular and careful dental hygiene at an early age, and may require periodic recall for reinforcement of oral hygiene procedures by the hygienist.

SECTION 4: HISTAMINE AND ANTIHISTAMINES

Histamine

Histamine is a naturally occurring amine of which the precise physiological function and significance are not known. It is stored in mast cells and circulating basophils, where it is bound to heparin in an inactive form. There is a possibility that it may be a neurotransmitter in the central nervous system, where it is stored in synaptic vesicles. In humans its effects are (1) powerful vasodilation of arterioles, venules, and capillaries; (2) increased permeability of venules and capillaries; (3) stimulation of non-vascular smooth muscle, as occurs in bronchoconstriction; (4) stimulation of exocrine glands, such as salivary, pancreatic, bronchial, and lacrimal glands and gastric mucosa; and (5) stimulation of cutaneous nerve endings, resulting in axon reflexes (Chap. 5, Sec. 1).

Any drug that results in a release of histamine will also result in a release of heparin, which may affect clotting time; agents that will release histamine include morphine (Chap. 8, Sec. 1), succinylcholine chloride (Anectine) (Chap. 6, Sec. 2), epinephrine (Chap. 6, Sec. 2), and surprisingly enough, almost all antihistamines (Chap. 5, Sec. 4). Histamine is also liberated during antigen-antibody reactions (Chap. 1, Sec. 2; Chap. 12, Sec. 1) and during chemical, thermal, physical, or bacterial trauma (Chap. 2, Sec. 2; Chap. 9, Sec. 1).

The actions of histamine in humans appear to be mediated by two distinct histamine receptors, designated H_1 and H_2. When either an H_1 or H_2 receptor blocker is administered there is little effect on the histamine-induced vasodilation response, whereas combined administration of H_1 and H_2 receptor antagonists can reverse the hypotension. This suggests that both receptor types are involved in the cardiovascular response to histamine. The conventional antihistamines are H_1 receptor antagonists, whereas the recently developed H_2 receptor antagonists, such as cimetidine (Tagamet), have found use in inhibiting gastric acid secretion stimulated by histamine, food, caffeine, or insulin and may be used in short-term treatment of duodenal ulcer without resorting to anticholinergic agents. **Cimetidine** (Tagamet) is marketed as 300 mg tablets and in injection form containing 300 mg/2 cc; the usual oral dose for treatment of duodenal ulcer is 300 mg with meals and at bedtime.

Antihistamines

Antihistamines act by competitive antagonism of the H_1 histamine receptor on cell membranes, rather than by blocking the release of histamine. Like autonomic receptors (Chap. 6, Sec. 2), histamine receptors are postulated to exist solely to explain the action of antihistamines and have never been demonstrated histologically. Antihistamines have many important effects useful in dentistry and are often prescribed by dentists because of the side-effects, which include (1) sedation of varying effectiveness, (2) antiemetic action, (3) potentiation of many other drugs, and (4) anticholinergic action (drying). Although antihistamines do not antagonize all of the pharmacological effects of histamine, they have local anesthetic properties to varying degrees when injected into tissues. Because of these multiple actions they are often combined with analgesics or decongestants and used as pre-operative medication. They also find use in treatment of mild allergic reactions and toothache of sinus origin.

Ascorbate (vitamin C) is the naturally occurring antihistamine of mammalian cells, and it only detoxifies the end products of the histamine reaction (Chap. 3, Sec. 1). Megascorbic supplementation has been shown to induce improvement in mammals undergoing physiological histamine stress.

Both the **phenothiazine** and **diphenylmethane** tranquilizers have potent antihistaminic properties, which can make them the more valuable agents to dentists (Chap. 7, Sec. 2; Chap. 8, Sec. 2; Chap. 12, Sec. 1).

Chlorpheniramine maleate (Chlor-Trimeton) is used mainly as a pre-operative medication for children owing to its sedative and anticholinergic (drying) effects. It is available as 4 mg tablets, 8 and 12 mg sustained and time-release tablets, and as a syrup containing 2 mg/tsp. It is an ingredient in Pedo-Sol, which is available in tablet or elixir form (Chap. 8, Sec. 2).

An antihistamine-decongestant combination (Dimetapp Extentabs, Dimetapp Elixir) should be prescribed to dental patients complaining of unexplained pain emanating from maxillary posterior teeth when oral inspection shows no evidence of disease or occlusal traumatism, radiographic findings are negative, and there is a history of sinus trouble (Chap. 8, Sec. 2). If there has been no improvement after one week, a diabetic arteritis of the dental pulp should be suspected, and the patient should be referred to his physician. Extractions should be delayed until after physical examination. The author has personally relieved dental pain in this manner in a patient who previously had two bicuspids and a lateral incisor removed on the same quadrant in a desperate search for the offending tooth and who presented with a toothache referred to an edentulous space. The anatomical basis for such a toothache is that the fibers of the posterior superior alveolar nerve and the middle superior alveolar nerve (when present) innervating the maxillary bicuspids and molars travel along the wall of the maxillary sinus (antrum of Highmore) on their way to the brain; when this sinus cavity is inflamed or congested the pain sensation may be incorrectly interpreted by the brain as having arisen from peripheral tooth pulps whose afferent fibers have been stimulated midway along their axons, rather than at their terminal dendrites. **Brompheniramine maleate** (Dimetane) is marketed as 4 mg tablets, as 8 and 12 mg sustained-release tablets, and as an elixir containing 2 mg/tsp; it is also available in combination form with the decongestants **phenylephrine** and **phenylpropanolamine** (Dimetapp Extentabs, Dimetapp Elixir) (Chap. 8, Sec. 2). The average adult dose is between 4 and 12 mg t.i.d. or q.i.d. and 0.5 mg/kg/day in divided doses for children.

Dimenhydrinate (Dramamine) is a potent pre-operative sedative and antiemetic that is given for the prevention or treatment of nausea or vomiting secondary to drug therapy or anticipation of painful dental procedures. The usual adult dose is between 50 and 100 mg orally q.4h. and is available as 50 mg tablets and as a liquid containing 12.5 mg per 4 cc or per 5 cc; it is also marketed as 100 mg suppositories and in injection form in a concentration of 50 mg/cc. It is often combined with a phosphorated carbohydrate solution (Emetrol) and marketed as Dramitrol; its main advantage over the phenothiazines is that it has no effect on autonomic receptors.

The **catecholamines** (Chap. 6, Sec. 2) counteract some of the pharmacological properties of histamine and inhibit antigen-induced histamine release by stimulating cyclic AMP formation in white blood cells.

TEST QUESTIONS

1. Injury to skin and underlying vasculature results in a release of substances that arrest hemorrhage, including:
   (a) histamine or a histamine-like substance, or both
   (b) a vasoconstrictor, thought to be serotonin released from platelets
   (c) extrinsic thromboplastin
   √(d) all of the above

2. The possibility of thrombus formation within intact vessels may be reduced with:
   (a) anticoagulant therapy
   (b) long-term use of salicylates
   (c) vitamin E therapy
   (d) all of the above

3. An anticoagulant drug that inhibits the formation of fibrin clots by acting as an antithromboplastin and by inhibiting Stuart-Prower factor X and fibrin stabilizing factor XIII is:
   (a) heparin sodium
   (b) warfarin sodium
   (c) phenindione
   (d) both b and c

4. An anticoagulant drug that acts indirectly to prevent blood coagulation by depressing the liver synthesis of vitamin K-dependent clotting factors (II, VIII, IX, and X) is:
   (a) heparin sodium
   (b) warfarin sodium
   (c) phenindione
   (d) both b and c

5. A drug that notably does NOT cross the placenta is:
   (a) heparin sodium
   (b) warfarin sodium
   (c) phenindione
   (d) aminocaproic acid
   (e) protamine sulfate
   (f) cimetidine

6. Patients taking anticoagulants should discontinue therapy for _____ prior to dental procedures, and only with proper medical supervision.
   (a) two days
   (b) three days
   (c) four days
   (d) five days

7. Absorbable gelatin sponge is not suitable for placement into extraction sockets that:
   (a) are grossly infected
   (b) are so shallow that it would protrude to the surface after suturing
   (c) have a suspected antral perforation
   (d) all of the above

8. Unsightly facial bruising or swelling following traumatic oral surgery may be controlled with the use of:
   (a) topical thrombin and fibrin foam packs
   (b) trypsin and chymotrypsin orally
   (c) parenteral immune globulin
   (d) all of the above

9. A method of treatment for hepatitis B is to build the general resistance of the body to infections by parenteral administration of:
   (a) trypsin and chymotrypsin
   (b) aminocaproic acid
   (c) immune globulin
   (d) protamine sulfate

10. If no medicine was prescribed following oral surgery the patient should be instructed to take _____ every four hours.
    (a) vitamin C
    (b) aspirin
    (c) ice water
    (d) strong tea

11. A drug administered via I.V. infusion to hemophiliac patients prior to oral surgery and to which heparin sodium is often added is:
    (a) immune globulin
    (b) protamine sulfate
    (c) warfarin sodium
    (d) aminocaproic acid
    (e) phenindione
    (f) cimetidine

12. Any drug that results in the release of histamine from mast cells will also produce a release of:
    (a) insulin
    (b) heparin
    (c) extrinsic thromboplastin
    (d) parotin

13. A histamine H_2 receptor antagonist used to treat peptic and duodenal ulcer is:
    (a) aminocaproic acid
    (b) protamine sulfate
    (c) cimetidine
    (d) parotin
    (e) glucagon
    (f) warfarin sodium

14. An anticoagulant used as an antidote for overdosage of heparin sodium is:
    (a) aminocaproic acid
    (b) protamine sulfate
    (c) cimetidine
    (e) glucagon
    (f) warfarin sodium

15. All of the following are side-effects of antihistamine administration EXCEPT:
    (a) sedation of varying effectiveness
    (b) local anesthetic properties to varying degrees when the drug is given as an injection
    (c) antiemetic action
    (d) anticholinergic action (drying effects)
    (e) potentiation of many other drugs
    (f) prolongation of bleeding time

16. A patient reports pain in a maxillary molar, along with a head cold; clinical oral examination shows no dental restorations and occlusal traumatism is absent. Radiographic examination is also negative. Treatment would consist of:
    (a) oral tetracycline and recall in one week
    (b) an antihistamine-decongestant orally and recall in one week
    (c) extraction of the offending tooth under local anesthesia
    (d) endodontic therapy of the offending tooth, allowing drainage through the access opening

17. The naturally occurring antihistamine in nature is:
    (a) ascorbate
    (b) dicumarol
    (c) epinephrine
    (d) morphine

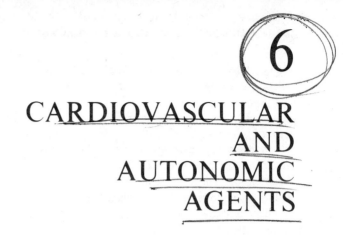

6

CARDIOVASCULAR
AND
AUTONOMIC
AGENTS

SECTION 1: CARDIOVASCULAR AGENTS

Categories of Shock

Any dental patient may suddenly go into shock in the dental chair at any time during treatment, and the cardiovascular agents help stabilize the patient in shock until he can be safely transported to a hospital. There are five types of shock: (1) neurogenic shock, or syncope (fainting); (2) cardiogenic shock, or cardiac arrest; (3) hypovolemic shock, or hemorrhage; (4) anaphylactic shock, or histamine shock; and (5) septic shock, or blood poisoning.

Neurogenic shock, or syncope (fainting), is the type of shock most frequently seen in a dental office. In some patients the fear of pain from dental procedures sets up an emotional disturbance that triggers excitation of the vasodilator nerves to skeletal muscle and to the splanchnic vessels, and excitation of the parasympathetic nerve to the heart (vagus nerve). This causes a reflex slowing of the heart rate and a decrease in arterial pressure resulting in cerebral anoxia and release of adrenalin (Chap. 6, Sec. 2). The adrenalin causes a peripheral vasoconstriction, a sudden rise in blood sugar and arterial pressure, and secretion by the sweat glands, causing the patient to appear pale, cold, and clammy and to report feeling ill or dizzy (Chap 12, Sec. 1).

In cardiogenic shock, or cardiac arrest, the heart stops beating and fails to circulate the blood, usually owing to an abnormal spread of excitation through the myocardial bundle of His or Purkinje's fibers. Arterial pressure falls to zero, and cerebral anoxia rapidly ensues. The patient's skin appears ashen grey, and the lips and nailbeds appear blue (cyanotic) (Chap. 12, Sec. 1).

During hypovolemic shock, or hemorrhage, the blood volume is decreased, with insufficient circulation to the brain and other vital organs. This type of shock usually results from violent accidents and left untreated will result in a powerful wave of sympathetic discharge (Chap. 6, Sec. 2), a last-resort effort to elevate arterial pressure (CNS ischemic response).

In anaphylactic shock, histamine or a histamine-like substance is liberated from cells damaged by the antigen-antibody reaction (Chap. 1, Sec. 2); the resulting arteriolar dilation decreases the peripheral resistance, and the resulting venous dilation increases the vascular capacity. This greatly reduces the arterial pressure and venous return (Chap. 12, Sec. 1). Left untreated anaphylactic shock can progress into cardiogenic shock.

In cases of septic shock, or blood poisoning, bacterial toxins cause a decrease in vascular resistance, which leads to a progressive deterioration of the circulation and to hypotension. Fever and chills are usually present, with a bounding pulse and rising and falling blood pressure (hyperdynamic syndrome).

Insulin "shock" (hypoglycemia), a complication of insulin treatment for diabetes mellitus (Chap. 12, Sec. 1), is not considered a form of actual shock because in shock states blood flow to peripheral tissues is always inadequate to sustain life because of maldistribution of blood flow or insufficient cardiac output (the product of the ventricular stroke volume and the heart rate).

Patients who experience neurogenic shock while in a dental chair often do not faint but merely feel ill suddenly or begin hyperventilating. These mild forms of syncope can be seen as often as once or twice a month in a general dental practice and are usually precipitated by anticipation of dental injections or extractions. In almost all cases the patient's blood sugar is abnormally low due to fasting or excessive consumption of sugar, caffeine, or refined carbohydrates two or three hours previously. For this reason, a can of lemon-lime soda or other sweetened drink should be stored in every dental office for use in such cases to rapidly elevate the blood sugar and sustain it long enough to complete the treatment for that day (Chap. 3, Sec. 1; Chap. 12, Sec. 1).

Epinephrine (Adrenalin Chloride) (Chap. 6, Sec. 2) has been traditionally used as an immediate treatment for all forms of shock except neurogenic (syncope); however, when it is rapidly administered it may produce arrhythmias, may further reduce venous return, and may constrict blood flow to the kidney, intensifying renal ischemia. For these reasons it cannot be considered the drug of choice for treatment of shock unless the patient has cardiac standstill, in which case drastic measures are needed in order to avoid permanent kidney and brain damage. Direct current countershock with a defibrillator cannot reverse cardiac arrest but can convert an arrhythmia induced with I.V. epinephrine to sinus rhythm. In cases of cardiac arrest it is much easier to manage an arrhythmia induced by a cardiotonic drug administered I.V. than to continue to cope with the effects of cardiac standstill.

Naturally released (endogenous) adrenalin is a mixture of 85 per cent epinephrine and 15 per cent norepinephrine by weight (Chap. 4, Sec. 1; Chap. 6, Sec. 2). Although most of the sweat glands have cholinergic receptors, some have adrenergic receptors and respond to norepinephrine, especially in the areas of the palm, soles, forehead, and axillae (Chap. 6, Sec. 2). When shock occurs and endogenous adrenalin is released, it is only the norepinephrine component of the adrenalin that triggers sweat gland secretion; epinephrine marketed as Adrenalin Chloride will not produce perspiration when administered. For these reasons the word "adrenalin" should be clearly defined in clinical discussions.

Coronary Vasodilators

Coronary vasodilators have a potent dilatory effect on the coronary arteries that feed the myocardium but have no effect on heart rate or heart muscle contractility; this serves to distinguish them from beta$_1$ stimulants, which also produce dilation of the coronary vessels (Chap. 6, Sec. 2). This group is composed of two types of antianginal agents: (1) rapid-acting nitrates used to relieve pain of acute angina pectoris and (2) long-acting nitrates used to prevent or decrease the severity of anginal attacks.

The rapid-acting nitrates are often stored in dental offices for use in emergencies (Chap. 12, Sec. 1). Amyl nitrite "pearls" (thin glass containers wrapped in gauze and containing 0.18 or 0.3 cc of amyl nitrite) may be broken underneath the nose and the patient may inhale vapor, which has a disagreeable odor but the most rapid action of the nitrates. Nitroglycerin sublingual tablets are available in doses of 0.15, 0.3, 0.4, and 0.6 mg and may be placed underneath the tongue or in the buccal pouch and allowed to dissolve. This appears to produce less nausea than inhalation of amyl nitrite but may produce a burning sensation, indicating potency (shelf-life not expired). **Isosorbide dinitrate** (Sorbitrate) sublingual tablets are available in doses of 2.5 and 5 mg and may also be dissolved underneath the tongue or in the buccal pouch; this drug is also available in 5 and 10 mg chewable tablets.

Long-acting nitrates are represented by (1) **isosorbide dinitrate** (Sorbitrate) oral, available in 5, 10, 20, 30, and 40 mg tablets and taken in doses of between 5 and 30 mg q.i.d.; (2) **nitroglycerin** sustained-release, available in 1.3, 2.5, and 6.5 mg tablets and taken in doses of one tablet b.i.d. or t.i.d.; (3) **erythrityl tetranitrate** (Cardilate), available in 5, 10, and 15 mg tablets and taken in doses of between 5 and 10 mg t.i.d.; (4) **pentaerythritol tetranitrate** (Peritrate), available in 10, 20, and 40 mg tablets and taken in doses of between 10 and 20 mg q.i.d.; and (5) **dipyridamole** (Persantine) 25 mg tablets, taken in a dose of 50 mg t.i.d. at least one hour before meals.

In patients in whom emotional excitement may contribute to the frequency of anginal attacks, coronary vasodilators are prescribed in multiple-entity combination products containing barbiturates (Chap. 7, Sec. 1), hydroxyzine hydrochloride (Chap. 7, Sec. 2), or meprobamate (Chap. 7, Sec. 2).

As a result of the vasodilation caused by the nitrates, any of them may produce headache, intracranial throbbing, or even syncope, especially nitroglycerin. Patients should be warned of this in advance and should receive their first dose in a sitting or reclining position.

Xanthines

The xanthines are central nervous system stimulants (analeptics) that have cardiovascular effects, sharing this dual function with the amphetamines (Chap. 7, Sec. 3). Xanthines increase cardiac output by increasing heart rate and contractility in a way similar to that of beta$_1$ stimulation (Chap. 6, Sec. 2) and produce diuresis by partially inhibiting renal reabsorption of sodium and chloride ions, promoting loss of these charged particles in the urine along with water molecules loosely attracted to them. Because of these actions the xanthines may find use in treatment of patients with any condition characterized by respiratory depression or with pulmonary edema secondary to congestive heart failure.

Caffeine is an ingredient in many commercial beverages (coffee, tea, colas, and cocoa) and is a weak diuretic. It is used primarily as an analeptic (Chap. 7, Sec. 3) due to the availability of better diuretics. Caffeine increases the release of endogenous epinephrine by increasing cyclic AMP levels, which readily mobilizes liver and muscle glycogen and upsets the blood sugar. Some dental patients are so habituated to the effects of caffeine on their blood sugar levels that they experience withdrawal symptoms when it is removed from their diet; because of these effects caffeine should probably be viewed for internal use with caution, as with alcohol, sugar, or any other refined carbohydrate (Chap. 3, Sec. 1; Chap. 6, Sec. 2).

Theophylline and its soluble salts and derivatives relax smooth muscle of the bronchi and pulmonary vessels in addition to inducing the typical effects of xanthine, producing a clinical response similar to the $beta_1$-$beta_2$ stimulant isoproterenol. It is specifically indicated for reversing bronchospasm associated with bronchial asthma, bronchitis, or emphysema. It is marketed in a wide variety of tablets, capsules, and pediatric elixirs. **Theophylline ethylenediamine** (aminophylline) is the most important of the derivatives and is available in various oral dosage forms and in injection form containing 250 mg (equivalent to 198 mg theophylline) or 500 mg (equivalent to 395 mg theophylline). I.M. injections of aminophylline are painful; it is usually given I.V. in a diluted form (25 mg/cc) and injected slowly to avoid hypotension related to sudden decreases in total peripheral resistance that can end in circulatory collapse. When it is injected at a rate greater than 25 mg/min the likelihood of hypotensive episodes drastically increases; should this occur, treatment would consist of administration of an alpha stimulant and a $beta_2$ blocker. The dosage of aminophylline for acute asthmatic attacks in adults is 500 mg stat., and for children 7.5 mg/kg stat., administered I.M. Maintenance doses are given orally in a range of 200 to 315 mg q.i.d. for adults and 3 to 6 mg/kg q.i.d. for children.

Cardiac Glycosides

All of the naturally occurring cardiac (digitalis) glycosides have qualitatively the same effects, differing only in their potency and rate of absorption and onset and duration of action. Their direct effects include (1) increasing the force of myocardial contraction (in a way similar to $beta_1$ stimulation but without an increase in heart rate); (2) increasing the total peripheral resistance (in a way similar to alpha stimulation); (3) increasing the refractory period of the **atrioventricular** (A-V) node, allowing more time for ventricular filling; and (4) depression of the firing frequency of the **sinoatrial** (S-A) node and prolongation of conduction in the A-V node by stimulating the vagus nerve. The cardiac glycosides are indicated for treatment of congestive heart failure, atrial flutter or fibrillation, paroxysmal atrial tachycardia, and pulmonary edema secondary to cardiogenic shock.

Cardiac glycosides may be divided into four groups like those of the barbiturates (Chap. 7, Sec. 1) based on the onset, peak, and duration of action: (1) the ultrashort-acting (onset within minutes, peaks in 2 hrs), such as **ouabain**; (2) rapid-acting (onset between 1 and 2 hrs, peak between 4 and 6 hrs), such as **digoxin** (Lanoxin) and **lanatoside C**; (3) intermediate-acting (onset between 2 and 4 hrs, peak between 8 and 12 hrs), such as **gitalin** and **acetyldigitoxin**; and (4) long-acting (onset between 2 and 4 hrs, peak between 12 and 24 hrs) such as **digitalis** and **digitoxin**. The agents most commonly used are **digoxin** (Lanoxin) and digitoxin.

The average digitalizing dose of digoxin (Lanoxin) in adults is between 1 and 1.5 mg with maintenance doses ranging from 0.125 to 0.5 mg (average 0.25 mg) q.i.d. or t.i.d. It is available as 0.125, 0.25, and 0.5 mg tablets, as a pediatric elixir containing 0.05 mg/cc (0.25 mg/tsp or as a 0.005 per cent solution), and in injection form containing 0.1 or 0.25 mg/cc.

Antihypertensive Agents

Some of the autonomic drugs and tranquilizers have potent blood-pressure-lowering effects, such as the ganglionic blocker **mecamylamine** (Inversine) (Chap. 6, Sec. 2); the alpha blockers, such as **phentolamine** (Regitine); or the beta blockers, such as **propanolol** (Inderal) and **metoprolol** (Lopressor) (Chap. 6, Sec. 2); Rauwolfia alkaloids, such as **reserpine** (Serpasil) (Chap. 7, Sec. 2); or monoamine oxidase inhibitors, such as **tranylcypromine** (Parnate) (Chap. 7, Sec. 2).

The thiazide diuretics have largely replaced the mercurial diuretics, the carbonic anhydrase inhibitors, and the xanthines for production of diuresis (Chap. 6, Sec. 1). All **thiazides** are approximately equal in diuretic potency at maximal therapeutic dosage, differing only in onset, peak, and duration of action. The antihypertensive effect of these agents is noted only after several days; they are indicated either as the sole therapeutic agent in cases of mild hypertension or to enhance the effect of other antihypertensive drugs in severe cases of hypertension. They also find use as adjunctive therapy for patients with pulmonary edema secondary to congestive heart failure. **Chlorothiazide** (Diuril) is available in 250 and 500 mg tablets, as an oral suspension containing 250 mg/tsp, and in injection form containing 500 mg/20 cc vial. The usual adult starting dose is between 500 and 1000 mg daily in single or divided dose and increased or decreased according to the response of the patient. **Hydrochlorothiazide** (Hydrodiuril) is available in 25, 50, and 100 mg tablets and may be given in an initial dose of 75 mg; the patient is then maintained on a dose between 25 and 100 mg daily based on his response. **Methyclothiazide** (Enduron) is available in 2.5 and 5 mg tablets and may be given in an initial dose between 2.5 and 10 mg; the patient is then maintained on a dose between 2.5 and 5 mg once daily based on response. Patients who complain of tooth hypersensitivity and who are taking a diuretic to remove excess sodium, chloride, and water from the body should not be given desensitizing dentifrices containing **sodium citrate** (Protect), which tend to add sodium to the body. In these cases it is best to prescribe a **strontium chloride** dentifrice (Sensodyne) or a **stannous fluoride** gel for home use (Gel-Kam) (Chap. 3, Sec. 2).

Hypertensive patients whose blood pressure cannot be adequately controlled with thiazides may be given **furosemide** (Lasix), a very potent diuretic. It is available in 20 and 40 mg tablets, as an oral solution containing 10 mg/cc, and in injection form containing 10 mg/cc. The usual adult dose is between 20 and 80 mg, followed by 40 mg b.i.d. Patients who do not respond favorably to thiazides will probably not respond to furosemide alone, and it is often given with other agents.

Triamterene (Dyrenium) is another diuretic useful in treating hypertension unresponsive to thiazides and is marketed in 50 and 100 mg capsules. The usual starting dose when the drug is used alone is 100 mg b.i.d. after meals; the patient is then maintained on an individualized dosage schedule not exceeding 300 mg daily. It is a component of the combination product Dyazide (Chap. 8, Sec. 2), which is taken in a dose between 1 and 2 capsules b.i.d.

Certain studies have suggested that hypertension may be related to increased sympathetic activity, with increased secretion of norepinephrine. In addition to the diuretics certain agents are in use that tend to reduce sympathetic activity in treating hypertension. **Guanethidine sulfate** (Ismelin) inhibits norepinephrine release and depletes norepinephrine stores at sympathetic nerve endings, thus lowering sympathetic tone. It is available in 10 and 25 mg tablets, and treatment is initiated with 10 mg daily and is increased according to patient response. It also is a component of the combination product Esimil

(Chap. 8, Sec. 2), which has the same dosage schedule and is gaining popularity owing to enhancement of the effectiveness of guanethidine sulfate by the thiazides. The major problem with guanethidine sulfate is orthostatic hypotension and dizziness, which the patient should be forewarned of prior to initiation of therapy. **Methyldopa** (Aldomet) has been shown to produce a net reduction of all the catecholamines in various tissues, and its antihypertensive effect is probably due to its metabolism to alpha-methyl-norepinephrine, which lowers arterial pressure by stimulation of central inhibitory alpha receptors and false neurotransmission. It is available as 125, 250, and 500 mg tablets and in injection form containing 250 mg methyldopate hydrochloride. The usual starting dosage is 250 mg b.i.d. or t.i.d. for 48 hrs.; this dosage is then increased or decreased depending on patient response.

In contrast with other hypertensive agents, which reduce renal blood flow, **hydralazine** (Apresoline) usually improves renal blood flow and lowers blood pressure by exerting a peripheral vasodilating effect similar to $beta_2$ stimulation (Chap. 6, Sec. 2). It has little effect on venous capacitance vessels but acts mainly on arteriolar smooth muscle, decreasing the total peripheral resistance. Because of reflex increases in cardiac function, hydralazine is often combined with drugs that inhibit sympathetic activity (beta blockers, guanethidine sulfate, or methyldopa). Therapy is begun with 10 mg q.i.d. for the first two to four days, and this is then increased to 25 mg q.i.d. for the rest of the week; during the second and subsequent weeks the dose is increased to 50 mg q.i.d. It is marketed as 10, 25, 50, and 100 mg tablets and in injection form containing 20 mg/cc.

Antiarrhythmic Agents

Certain autonomic drugs are currently in use for the treatment of disorders of cardiac rhythm; these include the $beta_1$-$beta_2$ stimulant isoproterenol (Chap. 6, Sec. 2) and the $beta_1$-$beta_2$ blocker propanolol (Chap. 6, Sec. 2).

Lidocaine (Xylocaine) is a local anesthetic that exerts an antiarrhythmic effect by increasing the electrical stimulation threshold of the ventricles during diastole; it produces no change in absolute refractory period, systolic pressure, or heart muscle contractility. It is specifically indicated in the acute management of life-threatening arrhythmias, such as those that occur secondary to myocardial infraction or during cardiac surgery (Chap. 9, Sec. 1; Chap. 12, Sec. 1). Constant EKG monitoring is essential for proper administration of lidocaine, and only without vasoconstrictors and clearly labeled for I.V. use should it be used for arrhythmias. The available solutions for I.V. use contain lidocaine in concentrations of 1, 2, 4, and 10 per cent. The usual dose is between 50 and 100 mg (1 mg/kg) I.V. with EKG monitoring. Isoproterenol is often given prior to lidocaine for correction of ventricular ectopic beats to accelerate the heart rate and to avoid production of more serious ventricular arrhythmias or the complete heart block that could occur in patients with sinus bradycardia or incomplete heart block. When normal sinus rhythm is established the patient is often maintained on an I.V. infusion of lidocaine in a concentration that results in a dose between 1 and 3 mg/min.

Procainamide (Pronestyl) is another local anesthetic that exerts an arrhythmic effect by depressing the excitability of heart muscle and slowing conduction in the atria, bundle of His, and ventricles. There is no increase in heart muscle contractility, but the heart rate may be accelerated, suggesting that the drug may have anticholinergic properties. It is indicated for treatment of atrial fibrillation, paroxysmal atrial tachycardia, ventricular tachycardia, and premature ventricular contractions (PCVs). Unlike lidocaine, procainamide hydrochloride is a peripheral vasodilator, and I.V. administration may produce a transient but severe hypotension; the effects of this drug are additive to those of lidocaine, and the two drugs should not be administered together, as ventricular tachycardia and severe hypotension could result, a fact many dentists must bear in mind (Chap. 11, Sec. 1; Chap. 13, Sec. 1). It is marketed as 250, 375, and 500 mg tablets and capsules and in injection form containing 100 and 500 mg/cc. Oral doses of 50 mg/kg/day in divided doses every three hrs is recommended; I.M. administration is the parenteral route of choice, whereas I.V. use should be reserved for extreme emergencies, and the 500 mg/cc solution should be diluted prior to use.

Quinidine has been found to decrease heart muscle contractility, excitability, and conduction velocity and to prolong the effective refractory period. It also exerts an anticholinergic effect, preventing the cardiac slowing of cholinergic drugs or vagal impulses. Like procainamide it is a peripheral vasodilator, and hypotension may result from parenteral use. It is indicated for a wide variety of cardiac disorders of rhythm, including atrial flutter, paroxysmal atrial tachycardia, paroxysmal atrial fibrillation, and premature atrial or ventricular contractions (PACs and PVCs). Adverse effects are common, and the usual oral dose between 200 and 600 mg may cause nausea and vomiting; large doses may produce "cinchonism" (tinnitus or "ringing in the ears," headache, impaired hearing, nausea, or disturbed vision) after a single dose. It is available as 100, 200, and 300 mg tablets, 200 mg capsules, 300 mg sustained-release tablets, and in injection form containing 200 mg/cc.

SECTION 2: AUTONOMIC AGENTS

Autonomic Physiology

The human nervous system is divided into two segments: (1) the central nervous system (CNS, neuroaxis) composed of brain and spinal cord and (2) the peripheral nervous system (PNS) composed of nerve fibers, ganglia, and end organs. The so-called visceral nervous system is that portion of the PNS that conveys impulses to and from the CNS and the viscera, and it is broken down into the visceral afferent and visceral efferent (autonomic) systems. The **visceral efferent** (autonomic) system contains a **thoracolumbar** (sympathetic) division and a **craniosacral** (parasympathetic) division; these antagonize each other physiologically and have morphological differences based on connections with the CNS and the location of ganglia.

Short preganglionic fibers of the sympathetic system leave the CNS and travel a short distance to nearby chain ganglia, where acetylcholine is released at the nerve terminal. At the ganglion the acetylcholine activates a nicotinic cholinergic receptor that produces an action potential in a long postganglionic fiber that leaves the ganglion and travels to the effector organ (Chap. 6, Sec. 2; Chap. 9, Sec. 1). Norepinephrine is released at the postganglionic nerve terminal (Chap. 6, Sec. 2), which then activates an adrenergic receptor at the effector organ cell (Fig. 6-1).

In a parasympathetic nerve the impulse transmission is identical to that in the sympathetic nerve except (1) preganglionic fibers are long instead of short and exit from craniosacral segments, (2) postganglionic fibers are short instead of long and release acetylcholine instead of norepinephrine at the nerve terminals, and (3) a muscarinic cholinergic receptor instead of an adrenergic receptor is activated at the effector organ cell.

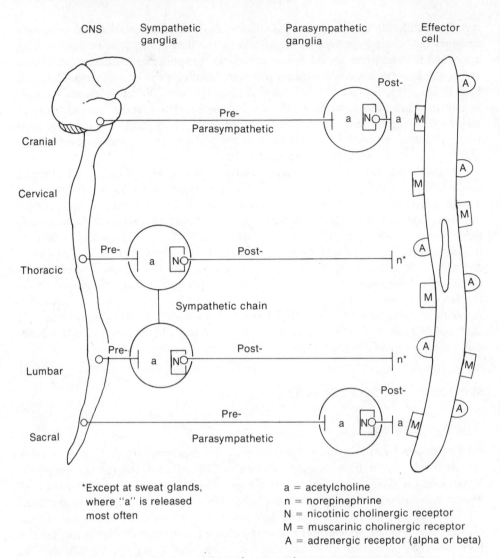

*Except at sweat glands,
where "a" is released
most often

a = acetylcholine
n = norepinephrine
N = nicotinic cholinergic receptor
M = muscarinic cholinergic receptor
A = adrenergic receptor (alpha or beta)

Figure 6–1. Diagram of visceral efferent (autonomic) system and postulated receptors.

Acetylcholine is the neurotransmitter substance at all preganglionic and parasympathetic postganglionic fibers and at most sympathetic postganglionic fibers that affect sweat glands. All other sympathetic postganglionics release norepinephrine (Chap. 6, Sec. 1).

The two types of cholinergic receptors are named nicotinic and muscarinic because they can be stimulated by nicotine and muscarine respectively. It has been postulated that there are also two different types of adrenergic receptors, alpha and beta, and these serve as a useful explanation for the effect of certain drugs on effector organs. They are also termed the smooth muscle excitatory (alpha) and smooth muscle inhibitory (beta) receptors; beta receptors are further subdivided into beta$_1$ (cardiac) and beta$_2$ (pulmonary) receptors.

Nicotinic cholinergic receptors are present not only at ganglia but also at neuromuscular junctions, which are also stimulated by acetylcholine; muscarinic cholinergic receptors are present only at the effector organs. Both alpha and beta receptors may be present in an effector organ, but usually one type of adrenergic receptor predominates. Alpha receptors are notably present in the dilator pupillae, uterus, ureter, intestine, and visceral and cutaneous blood vessels; they respond to both norepinephrine and epinephrine released from the adrenal medulla, resulting in the alpha response pattern (smooth muscle excitation and contraction, except in the intestine, which undergoes relaxation). $Beta_1$ receptors are located in the myocardium and coronary vessels; these receptors also respond to norepinephrine and epinephrine released from the adrenal medulla, resulting in the $beta_1$ response pattern (smooth muscle inhibition, and relaxation of coronary vessels and contraction of the myocardium). $Beta_2$ receptors are located in the bronchi, uterus, and skeletal muscle vessels; they respond only to epinephrine released from the adrenal medulla, resulting in the $beta_2$ response pattern (smooth muscle inhibition and relaxation).

It has been further postulated that activation of the cellular enzyme adenyl cyclase, which leads to increased cyclic AMP levels, is mediated by beta receptor stimulation, whereas inhibition of adenyl cyclase, which leads to decreased cyclic AMP levels, is mediated by alpha receptor stimulation. If this hypothesis proves to be true then the mode of action of all the autonomic drugs will be reduced to either increasing or decreasing the levels of intracellular cyclic AMP in the target tissues. At the present time the only agents that have been shown to produce some of their effects by way of an increase in the level of cyclic AMP and other effects by way of a decrease are the catecholamines (epinephrine, norepinephrine, dopamine, and isoproterenol) and the prostaglandins.

The fact that glucagon stimulates cardiac adenyl cyclase, increasing cyclic AMP levels in cardiac muscle, lends support to the idea that the cardiac effects of the catecholamines are mediated by cyclic AMP. Unlike glucagon, the catecholamines increase the levels of cyclic AMP and activate phosphorylase in all forms of muscle, as well as in the liver, resulting in increased blood sugar levels. In addition to their direct effects on muscle, they have also been shown to facilitate neuromuscular transmission, a function which may be either an alpha or a beta receptor effect mediated by cyclic AMP. Important hematological effects of the catecholamines are (1) improved platelet aggregation (decreased bleeding time) mediated by alpha stimulation, and increased plasma levels of antihemophilic globulin factor VIII mediated by beta stimulation (Chap. 6, Sec. 2; Chap. 5, Sec. 1).

The classification of the autonomic drugs is based on their action of either stimulating or blocking impulse transmission at the level of the ganglion or the effector cell, and there are thus four possible categories: (1) ganglionic stimulants, (2) ganglionic blockers, (3) effector cell stimulants, and (4) effector cell blockers. Receptor blocking agents take precedence over receptor stimulants when administered in combination; i.e., when an alpha stimulant is given with an alpha blocker, the result is alpha blockade, and so forth.

Neuromuscular stimulants and blockers are generally classed with the autonomic drugs because skeletal muscles are also internal organs receiving efferent impulses from the CNS. Neuromuscular blockers are also known as peripherally acting muscle relaxants, and may be either depolarizing or competitive in mechanism (Chap. 6, Sec. 2).

The theory of autonomic receptors fails to explain the cardiovascular and pulmonary effects of many drugs, such as the bronchodilatory effects of theophylline, atropine, and phenylephrine or the cardiotonic effects of digitalis glycosides. These inherent weaknesses are often overlooked in explanations about autonomic drugs and their actions, many of which cannot be explained without the autonomic receptor theory.

Neuromuscular and Ganglionic Stimulants

Skeletal muscle endplates and postganglionic neurons contain cholinergic receptors that can be stimulated by nicotine. Most cholinergic drugs are not purely nicotinic in action but also exercise a certain degree of muscarinic action upon the effector cell; conversely, muscarinic drugs often possess a certain degree of nicotinic action.

Acetylcholine (ACh) is the naturally occurring chemical mediator that stimulates nicotinic cholinergic receptors, and it is considered both nicotinic and muscarinic, since it can also stimulate muscarinic cholinergic receptors at the effector organ cell. It is the only neuromuscular and ganglionic stimulant of interest in dentistry. It is similar to epinephrine in that it stimulates both types of cholinergic receptors in the same fashion that epinephrine stimulates both types of adrenergic receptors. This property of stimulating two different receptors becomes useful when one of the two receptors is blocked with a second drug. For example, when muscarinic receptors are blocked with atropine, the effects of acetylcholine become purely nicotinic in character, producing an increase in blood pressure that would not occur without atropine. The major difference between acetylcholine and epinephrine, aside from the types of receptors they stimulate, is that acetylcholine is a local hormone, whereas epinephrine is a general hormone (Chap. 4, Sec. 1).

When it is deemed desirable for the effects of acetylcholine to persist, certain drugs are given to block the enzyme that terminates the action of acetylcholine, since administration of acetylcholine by injection results only in rapid plasma breakdown of the drug; the enzyme responsible for the breakdown is acetylcholinesterase, and the drugs that block the action of this enzyme are called cholinesterase inhibitors, or anticholinesterases (Chap. 7, Sec. 2). Blockade of acetylcholinesterase may be either reversible or irreversible.

Physostigmine salicylate administered in a dose between 1 and 3 mg I.V. will reverse the symptoms of dibenzazepine poisoning, and this drug is a naturally occurring reversible cholinesterase inhibitor. It is also the drug of choice for treatment of atropine toxicity and for this purpose can be given hourly in a dose between 1 and 4 mg. It is commonly used as a miotic in opthalmology as a 0.25 per cent solution given one or two drops into each eye as needed.

Neostigmine is another reversible cholinesterase inhibitor structurally similar to acetylcholine and therefore possessing a stimulatory effect of its own, in addition to its effect on acetylcholinesterase. It is used as an antidote for curare overdosage and as a drug to combat poisoning with anticholinergic drugs, and it is given in a dose of 0.5 mg q.2h. or q.3h. Its main use is in myasthenia gravis in doses between 15 and 375 mg daily in from four to eight divided doses.

Pyridostigmine can also be used as a reversible cholinesterase inhibitor to treat myasthenia gravis but has a slower onset and longer duration of action than neostigmine. The usual dose is between 360 and 1500 mg daily orally in from four to six divided doses.

Many organophosphorus insecticides, such as parathion, are irreversible cholinesterase inhibitors of no therapeutic use but of toxicological interest.

Neuromuscular Blockers

When dental patients are hospitalized and about to undergo general anesthesia it is necessary for their skeletal muscles to be completely relaxed so the endotracheal tube can be safely passed through the larynx and into the lumen of the trachea without producing laryngospasm. Neuromuscular blocking drugs have been developed to induce a temporary but profound paralysis of the laryngeal and other skeletal muscles to allow safe and efficient endotracheal intubation.

Succinylcholine chloride (Anectine) is an ultrashort-acting skeletal muscle relaxant that mimics acetylcholine by combining with the nicotinic receptors of the motor end-plate to produce depolarization followed by an initial muscle contraction visible as fasciculations. The patient's entire body begins to twitch and jump as the drug takes effect, and this ends in paralysis of all muscles, including the diaphragm, and breathing ceases. Prior to administration of the drug the patient's lungs are well ventilated and he is given an intravenous general anesthetic, sufficient time is allowed to elapse before injecting succinylcholine chloride and robbing him of his ability to breathe, and when the fasciculations end and he is further ventilated he is then intubated and placed on a respirator. Succinylcholine chloride is usually given I.V. in a dose between 25 and 75 mg but may be given I.M. when a suitable vein is not available. When the drug is given I.V. paralysis lasts from two to four minutes, and the effect of a single paralyzing dose disappears within eight to ten minutes as the drug is hydrolyzed at the receptor sites, resulting in repolarization of the skeletal muscles.

Curare preparations, such as tubocurarine chloride, also block neuromuscular junctions, resulting in flaccid paralysis of skeletal muscles, but these drugs are less commonly used prior to general anesthesia because the duration of paralysis is longer (between 25 and 90 minutes) and because of interactions with inhalation anesthetics (Chap. 11, Sec. 1). These agents raise the threshold of the receptor at the neuromuscular junction and prevent its activation by the acetylcholine normally released at the somatic motor nerve terminals, producing a non-depolarizing blockade. There is no antidote for excessive dosage of curare except administration of a cholinesterase inhibitor, such as neostigmine (Chap. 6, Sec. 2).

Ganglionic Blockers

Ganglionic blocking agents are potent hypotensive agents and will lower blood pressure in both normotensive and hypertensive individuals. Much of this effect is due to a decrease in cardiac output secondary to a decrease in venous return. Since these agents act on nicotinic cholinergic receptors of ganglia, both sympathetic and parasympathetic ganglia are affected. They are only infrequently used as antihypertensive agents because of the many side-effects that occur during their administration.

Mecamylamine hydrochloride (Inversine) is indicated in moderately severe to severe essential hypertension and in uncomplicated cases of malignant hypertension. The average daily dose is 25 mg in three divided doses, but as little as 2.5 mg daily may be sufficient to control hypertension in some cases. It is available as 2.5 and 10 mg tablets. If this agent is suddenly discontinued, hypertensive levels may return, and this may occur abruptly and produce a cerebrovascular accident (stroke) or congestive heart failure. The dose of this agent must be critically adjusted, and the patient must be educated and closely supervised during administration. This drug may be combined with other agents, and the dosage may be reduced to avoid excessive hypotension.

Although nicotine stimulates ganglionic transmission in low doses, it also has the interesting property of blocking ganglionic transmission in high doses, and it therefore has a dual function. The exact mechanism for this is currently unknown.

Effector Cell Stimulants

Drugs that stimulate both muscarinic and adrenergic receptors are generally lethal because such stimulation leads to a confusion of signals at the effector cell, with cancellation of one response pattern by its opposite, resulting in zero organ activity. There are eight possible types of useful effector cell stimulants remaining: (1) muscarinic receptor stimulants, (2) alpha stimulants, (3) $beta_1$ stimulants, (4) $beta_2$ stimulants, (5) alpha-$beta_1$ stimulants, (6) alpha-$beta_2$ stimulants, (7) $beta_1$-$beta_2$ stimulants, and (8) alpha-$beta_1$-$beta_2$ stimulants (Table 6–1).

Although acetylcholine is considered both a nicotinic and muscarinic stimulant, muscarine was the first muscarinic stimulant to be used (Chap. 6, Sec. 2). The muscarinic stimulants encourage outward dentinal fluid movement and have been shown to produce a caries reduction of between 95 and 100 per cent, even when the parotid glands are excised and the diet contains high amounts of sugar (Chap. 4, Sec. 2); this would suggest that the dental pulp may contain muscarinic receptors that respond to parasympathetic stimulants, as well as to parotin. The most commonly used muscarinic stimulant is **pilocarpine hydrochloride**, which (1) lowers intraocular pressure by increasing the outflow of aqueous humor, (2) produced moisis (constricted pupil) by contracting the ciliary muscle, and (3) stimulates accommodation by contracting the ciliary body. This drug finds its greatest use in treating glaucoma; acetylcholine is not used for this purpose owing to its short duration of action. The most widely used pilocarpine hydrochloride ophthalmic solutions are the 1 and 2 per cent, but solutions are available in a range of concentrations from 0.5 to 6 per cent. The dose is one or two drops into each affected eye, repeated up to six times daily as needed.

The alpha stimulant **methoxamine hydrochloride** (Vasoxyl) is used as a vasopressor, and its main advantage, as with all alpha stimulants, is that it does not directly stimulate the heart. Its vasopressive action results from increasing venous tone and total peripheral resistance, and it is indicated for hypotensive states, notably vasovagal syncope (Chap. 12, Sec. 1). Dosage is adjusted based on patient response, with an initial dose in the range of 2 to 10 mg I.M. or 5 mg I.V. **Phenylephrine** (Neo-Synephrine) is another alpha stimulant and is somewhat superior to methoxamine hydrochloride because it relaxes bronchioles. It is present alone or in combination in many over-the-counter and prescription nasal sprays, but when it is used as a vasopressor the usual adult dose is between 1 and 10 mg I.M. or Sub-Q, or between 0.1 and 0.5 mg I.V.

Dopamine hydrochloride (Intropin) is a catecholamine and a potent $beta_1$ stimulant indicated for correction of hemodynamic imbalances in various forms of shock secondary to trauma, septicemia, renal failure, or myocardial infarction (Chap. 6, Sec. 1). It is administered in a dilute form at a rate between 5 and 50 μg/kg/min.

Metaproterenol sulfate (Metaprel) and **terbutaline sulfate** (Brethine) are $beta_2$ stimulants used in the management of asthma and reversible bronchospasm associated with bronchitis and emphysema. Metaproterenol sulfate is marketed as 10 and 20 mg tablets and as a syrup containing 10 mg/tsp; the usual adult dose is between 10 and 20 mg q.i.d.

Terbutaline sulfate is available as 2.5 and 5 mg tablets and in injection form containing 1 mg/cc; the usual adult dose is between 2.5 and 5 mg P.O. t.i.d. or between 0.25 and 0.5 mg Sub-Q q.4h.

Norepinephrine, or levarterenol bitartrate (Levophed), is a powerful naturally occurring alpha-beta$_1$ stimulant related to epinephrine, dopamine, and isoproterenol (catecholamines). When any blood volume deficits are corrected, norepinephrine raises blood pressure to optimal levels through both peripheral vasoconstriction and myocardial stimulation; it also helps to limit myocardial ischemia by dilating the coronary arteries. This drug is found with epinephrine in significant concentrations in the adrenal medulla and has a therapeutic index four times that of epinephrine (Chap. 1, Sec. 1). It can be used as an adjunct in the treatment of cardiogenic shock (Chap. 6, Sec. 1), but when used as a vasoconstrictor in local anesthetic solutions, it is associated with a higher incidence of ischemic necrosis and sloughing of tissue than epinephrine (Chap. 9, Sec. 3). As **levarterenol bitartrate** (Levophed), norepinephrine is marketed in 4 cc ampuls in a concentration of 0.1 per cent which is added to 1000 cc of 5 per cent dextrose solution for proper dilution (4 µg/cc) and to help prevent loss of potency due to oxidation; the initial dose of this dilution is between 2 and 3 cc (between 8 and 12 µg) and the flow rate is adjusted to maintain a low normal blood pressure (between 80 and 100 mm mercury systolic pressure) and to maintain circulation to vital organs. **Metaraminol bitartrate** (Aramine) is another alpha-beta$_1$ stimulant that acts to deplete norepinephrine at sympathetic nerve endings. Its advantage over norepinephrine is that it may be given I.M. or Sub-Q in addition to I.V., but its major disadvantage, compared to norepinephrine, is that the maximal effect is not immediately apparent, and therefore at least ten minutes should elapse before increasing the dose. The average adult dose is between 2 and 10 mg I.M. or Sub-Q, or between 0.5 and 5 mg I.V. followed by I.V. infusion of between 15 and 100 mg in infusion fluid. **Mephentermine sulfate** (Wyamine) is another alpha-beta$_1$ stimulant that produces a release of endogenous norepinephrine and that can be administered I.M. or I.V. without fear of local irritation at the injection site. It is available in 1.5 and 3 per cent solutions, and the usual adult dose for hypotension is between 15 and 60 mg I.V.

Blood pressure maintenance is a function of five variables, four of which are under autonomic control: (1) blood volume, (2) venous tone (alpha), (3) total peripheral resistance (alpha), (4) heart rate (beta$_1$), and (5) myocardial contractility (beta$_1$). Therefore, any agent that stimulates both alpha and beta$_1$ receptors would be a more potent vasopressor than either an alpha stimulant alone or a beta$_1$ stimulant alone. The pressor response to norepinephrine, metaraminol bitartrate, mephentermine sulfate, epinephrine, ephedrine sulfate, amphetamine sulfate, or levonordefrin would be expected to be more dramatic than the pressor response to methoxamine hydrochloride, phenylephrine, dopamine, or isoproterenol.

Isoproterenol hydrochloride (Isuprel) is a synthetic catecholamine and a powerful beta$_1$-beta$_2$ stimulant that increases cardiac output and lowers total peripheral resistance; these actions are reflected in increased systolic and mean arterial pressures and in decreased diastolic pressures (Chap. 12, Sec. 1). This drug is indicated as an adjunct in the management of cardiogenic shock, carotid sinus hypersensitivity, ventricular tachycardia or arrhythmias, and Stokes-Adams attacks (syncope secondary to infranodal A-V heart block). It is available as 10 and 15 mg glossets for sublingual or rectal use, as 15 and 30 mg sustained-release tablets, and as a 1:5000 solution for injection. When given as an I.V. infusion, the solution should be diluted by adding 1 mg isoproterenol (5 cc) to 500 cc 5 per cent dextrose solution to produce a 1:500,000 solution. Concentrations up to ten times greater may be used. The initial dose for cardiac arrest or arrhythmia is 0.2 mg I.M. or Sub-Q, 0.02 mg for intracardiac injection, between 0.02 and 0.06 mg I.V., or 5 μg/min by I.V. infusion. The phenothiazine tranquilizers are also known to be weak $beta_1$-$beta_2$ stimulants (Chap. 7, Sec. 2).

Epinephrine (Adrenalin Chloride) is a powerful naturally occurring alpha-$beta_1$-$beta_2$ stimulant related to norepinephrine and dopamine (catecholamines). When injected slowly I.V., it produces a moderate rise in systolic pressure and a decrease in diastolic pressure that are very similar to those observed with isoproterenol administration; there is usually no great elevation in mean blood pressure because the predominate effects of the drug are on beta receptors. When injected rapidly I.V., it produces a rapid rise in blood pressure, mainly systolic. This drug is indicated for relief of bronchospasm and allergic reactions, and is used to prolong the absorption and duration of local anesthetics, decreasing their toxicity (Chap. 9, Sec. 1). It has also found use in decreasing the secretion of aqueous humor and improving the clinical course of glaucoma, in resuscitation in cardiogenic shock, and as a hemostatic agent (Chap. 5, Sec. 3; Chap. 12, Sec. 1; Chap. 12, Sec. 2). Epinephrine should not be used as a vasoconstrictor in local anesthetic solutions if the patient is taking certain drugs, owing to the possibility of potentially fatal reactions (Chap. 6, Sec. 2; Chap. 7, Sec. 2; Chap. 11, Sec. 1). It is not the drug of choice for the treatment of shock because it may produce ventricular fibrillation in the ischemic and irritable myocardium, may further reduce venous return, and may intensify renal ischemia (Chap. 6, Sec. 1). It is available as a 1:1000 or 1:10,000 solution, and it is administered in a small initial dose (between 0.2 and 1.0 cc of a 1:1000 solution) and can be increased as needed. **Ephedrine sulfate** is another powerful alpha-$beta_1$-$beta_2$ stimulant that also acts to release tissue stores of norepinephrine. It causes a rise in blood pressure and increased heart rate but a decrease in total peripheral resistance because $beta_2$ stimulation more than compensates for alpha stimulation. Ephedrine is also a potent CNS stimulant and is indicated in hypotensive states and Stokes-Adams attacks. It is available in injection form as 25 or 50 mg/cc. **Amphetamine sulfate** is another alpha-$beta_1$-$beta_2$ and CNS stimulant that elevates systolic and diastolic pressures. Its beta effects are weak, and it is indicated as a short-term adjunct to treat obesity when other dietary measures have failed (Chap. 7, Sec. 3). Amphetamine sulfate (Benzedrine) is available in 5 and 10 mg tablets and in 15 mg sustained-release tablets. **Levonordefrin** (Neocobefrin) is another alpha-$beta_1$-$beta_2$ stimulant similar in action to epinephrine but much less potent; it finds its most common use as a vasoconstrictor in local anesthetic solutions (Chap. 9, Sec. 1).

Effector Cell Blockers

Drugs that block both muscarinic and adrenergic receptors are also generally lethal because such a blockade robs the body of both parasympathetic and sympathetic control of its visceral functions. There are also eight possible types of useful effector cell blockers remaining: (1) muscarinic receptor blockers, (2) alpha blockers, (3) $beta_1$ blockers, (4) $beta_2$ blockers, (5) alpha-$beta_1$ blockers, (6) alpha-$beta_2$ blockers, (7) $beta_1$-$beta_2$ blockers, and (8) alpha-$beta_1$-$beta_2$ blockers (Table 6–1).

The best known muscarinic receptor blockers, or anticholinergic agents, are the **belladonna alkaloids**. They are indicated for treatment of certain stomach and intestinal disorders and as pre-operative medication to reduce secretions, relax bronchioles, and

Table 6–1. EFFECTOR CELL STIMULANTS AND BLOCKERS

RECEPTORS	STIMULANTS	BLOCKERS
Muscarinic	muscarine pilocarpine hydrochloride acetylcholine	atropine sulfate scopolamine hydrobromide mathantheline bromide
Alpha	phenylephrine methoxamine hydrochloride	phentolamine
Beta$_1$	dopamine hydrochloride	metoprolol tartrate
Beta$_2$	metaproterenol sulfate terbutaline sulfate	–
Alpha-beta$_1$	nonrepinephrine metaraminol bitartrate mephentermine sulfate	–
Alpha-beta$_2$	–	–
Beta$_1$-beta$_2$	isoproterenol hydrochloride	metoprolol tartrate propanolol
Alpha-beta$_1$-beta$_2$	epinephrine ephedrine sulfate amphetamine sulfate levonordefrin	–

inhibit parasympathetic slowing of the heart mediated through the vagus nerve, thereby regulating the pulse. **Atropine sulfate** is often administered with meperidine (Demerol) and hydroxyzine (Vistaril) prior to general anesthesia for dental procedures (Chap. 8, Sec. 1; Chap. 7, Sec. 2; Chap. 10, Sec. 1), and the usual adult dose is between 0.4 and 0.6 mg I.M. and for children between 0.1 and 0.6 mg I.M., depending on body weight. The greater use of **scopolamine hydrobromide** as pre-operative medication for pediatric use is related to a degree of amnesia induced by this agent, in addition to the effects just mentioned. Scopolamine is often combined with a barbiturate and an antihistamine for this purpose (Pedo-Sol), and the usual dose is between 0.4 and 0.8 mg P.O. (Chap. 8, Sec. 2). In patients who produce unusually copious amounts of saliva that cannot be adequately managed with conventional methods (cotton rolls, saliva ejector, or rubber dam) **methantheline bromide** (Banthine) may be drawn into the anesthetic syringe and injected into the area previously chosen for infiltration anesthesia to reduce salivary flow (Chap. 9, Sec. 2). Methantheline bromide is available as 50 mg tablets and as a 5 per cent solution (50 mg/cc); the usual adult dose is 50 mg, and the dose for children is between 12.5 and 50.0 mg. All of these agents are contraindicated for treatment of patients with a history of glaucoma, asthma, or ulcerative colitis. The tricyclic anti-depressants also block muscarinic receptors (Chap. 7, Sec. 2), as do the phenothiazines (Chap. 7, Sec. 2).

Phentolamine (Regitine) is an alpha blocker indicated for the treatment of dermal necrosis secondary to I.V. administration of norepinephrine and for prevention and control of hypertensive episodes during surgical excision of adrenal medullary tumors (pheochromocytomas). Conversely, norepinephrine is the antidote for accidental overdosage of phentolamine (Regitine); administration of epinephrine should be avoided in such overdosage to prevent a paradoxical fall in blood pressure (epinephrine reversal)

(Chap. 11, Sec. 1). It is available as 50 mg tablets and in injection form as phentolamine mesylate 5 mg with lactose 5 mg/cc. Dosage is variable depending on the condition being treated. The phenothiazine tranquilizers are also weak alpha blockers, and can also initiate epinephrine reversal. Droperidol (Inapsine) is also associated with weak alpha blocking activity.

There are many agents used in other countries to block beta receptors; in the United States the only beta blockers available at this time are **metoprolol tartrate** (Lopressor) and **propanolol** (Inderal). Metoprolol tartrate (Lopressor) is primarily a beta$_1$ blocker, but in high doses behaves as a beta$_1$-beta$_2$ blocker. It is used to treat hypertension and is often combined with other antihypertensive agents, especially thiazide diuretics (Chap. 6, Sec. 1). Its effects can be reversed by administration of beta receptor agonists, such as isoproterenol. It is available as 50 and 100 mg tablets, and dosage varies with the individual; the usual initial dose is 50 mg b.i.d. and is increased after one week to between 100 and 450 mg b.i.d. Beta$_1$ selectivity diminishes as the dose is increased. Propanolol (Inderal) is a beta$_1$-beta$_2$ blocker at any dose and is indicated to treat hypertension, cardiac arrhythmias, and angina pectoris due to coronary atherosclerosis. Its effects can also be reversed by isoproterenol. It is available as 10, 40, and 80 mg tablets and in injection form in a concentration of 1 mg/cc. Dosage of this agent is also individualized depending on the condition being treated; for hypertension the initial dose is 80 mg daily in divided doses ranging up to 640 mg daily, for angina pectoris the dose is initially between 10 and 20 mg q.i.d. and is increased to 160 mg daily in divided doses, and for arrhythmias the dose is between 10 and 30 mg q.i.d. before meals and at bedtime. There is some evidence that propanolol (Inderal) in a dose of 120 mg daily is an effective treatment of anxiety and essential tremor. At the present time there is no advantage to using beta$_2$ blockers, alpha-beta$_1$ blockers, alpha-beta$_2$ blockers, or alpha-beta$_1$-beta$_2$ blockers instead of the available agents, and for this reason they have not been developed.

TEST QUESTIONS

1. All of the following are states in which blood flow is inadequate to sustain life because of maldistribution of flow or inadequate cardiac output EXCEPT:
   (a) neurogenic shock
   (b) cardiogenic shock
   (c) hypovolemic shock
   (d) anaphylactic shock
   (e) septic shock
   (f) insulin shock
2. The form of shock most frequently seen during dental procedures is _(1)_ , in which a reflex _(2)_ causes a reduction in arterial pressure.
   (a) (1) cardiogenic and (2) vasoconstriction
   (b) (1) cardiogenic and (2) vasodilation
   (c) (1) neurogenic and (2) vasoconstriction
   (d) (1) neurogenic and (2) vasodilation
   (e) (1) anaphylactic and (2) vasoconstriction
   (f) (1) anaphylactic and (2) vasodilation
3. The word "adrenalin" should be clearly defined in clinical discussions because it can mean any of the following EXCEPT:
   (a) the endogenous secretion from the adrenal cortex
   (b) epinephrine (Adrenalin Chloride) U.S.P.
   (c) 85 per cent epinephrine and 15 per cent norepinephrine
   (d) all of the above

4. Epinephrine (Adrenalin Chloride) is the drug of choice for treatment of cardiogenic shock and of any other condition that progresses rapidly into cardiogenic shock, but its undesirable effects include:
   (a) further reducing venous return
   (b) producing arrhythmias
   (c) intensifying renal ischemia
   (d) all of the above

5. The most rapid-acting coronary vasodilator is:
   (a) isosorbide dinitrate
   (b) glyceryl trinitrate (nitro-glycerin)
   (c) amyl nitrate
   (d) pentaerythritol tetranitrate
   (e) dipyridamole
   (f) erythrityl tetranitrate

6. A xanthine that is specifically indicated to reverse bronchospasm associated with bronchial asthma, bronchitis, and emphysema is:
   (a) caffeine
   (b) digoxin (Lanoxin)
   (c) theophylline ethylenediamine
   (d) hydrochlorothiazide

7. A xanthine that increases the release of endogenous epinephrine, and that upsets the blood sugar is:
   (a) caffeine
   (b) digoxin (Lanoxin)
   (c) theophylline ethylenediamine
   (d) hydrochlorothiazide

8. The direct effects of the cardiac glycosides include:
   (a) increasing myocardial contractility
   (b) increasing total peripheral resistance
   (c) stimulation of the vagus nerve
   (d) all of the above

9. Antihypertensive agents useful as the sole therapeutic agents in cases of mild hypertension are the:
   (a) xanthines
   (b) thiazide diuretics
   (c) cardiac glycosides
   (d) coronary vasodilators

10. All of the following are antihypertensive agents EXCEPT:
    (a) mecamylamine
    (b) phentolamine
    (c) propanolol
    (d) reserpine
    (e) tranylcypromine
    (f) hydrochlorothiazide
    (g) furosemide
    (h) triamterene
    (i) guanethidine sulfate
    (j) methyldopa
    (k) procainamide
    (l) hydralazine

11. All of the following are antiarrhythmic agents EXCEPT:
    (a) lidocaine
    (b) procainamide
    (c) quinidine
    (d) isoproterenol
    (e) propanolol
    (f) mephentermine sulfate

12. A disadvantage to using lidocaine intravenously would be that:
    (a) myocardial contractility is increased
    (b) systolic pressure is increased
    (c) constant EKG monitoring is needed
    (d) all of the above

13. When it is deemed desirable for the effects of acetylcholine to persist, an anticholinesterase is given because administration of acetylcholine by injection results in:
    (a) laryngospasm
    (b) neostigmine
    (c) rapid breakdown of the drug
    (d) toxic reaction to the drug

14. The anticholinesterase drug of choice for atropine toxicity is:
    (a) physostigmine salicylate   (c) pyridostigmine
    (b) neostigmine   (d) none of the above
15. The anticholinesterase drug of choice for curare toxicity is:
    (a) physostigmine salicylate   (c) pyridostigmine
    (b) neostigmine   (d) none of the above
16. Laryngospasm during general anesthesia is best prevented or treated with the use of:
    (a) acetylcholine   (c) succinylcholine chloride
    (b) epinephrine   (d) tubocurarine chloride
17. A ganglionic blocking agent that will lower blood pressure in both normotensive and hypertensive individuals is:
    (a) succinylcholine chloride   (c) mecamylamine
    (b) reserpine   (d) methyldopa
18. Acetylcholine, muscarine, and pilocarpine hydrochloride are all examples of:
    (a) muscarinic stimulants   (c) alpha stimulants
    (b) muscarinic blockers   (d) alpha blockers
19. Phenylephrine and methoxamine hydrochloride are examples of:
    (a) muscarinic stimulants   (c) alpha stimulants
    (b) muscarinic blockers   (d) alpha blockers
20. Phentolamine is an example of a(n):
    (a) muscarinic stimulant   (c) alpha stimulant
    (b) muscarinic blocker   (d) alpha blocker
21. Atropine sulfate, scopolamine hydrobromide, and methantheline bromide are all examples of:
    (a) muscarinic stimulants   (c) alpha stimulants
    (b) muscarinic blockers   (d) alpha blockers
22. All of the following are alpha-beta$_1$, beta$_2$ stimulants EXCEPT:
    (a) epinephrine   (d) amphetamine sulfate
    (b) norepinephrine   (e) levonordefrin
    (c) ephedrine sulfate   (f) all of the above are stimulants
23. All of the following are alpha-beta$_1$ stimulants EXCEPT:
    (a) epinephrine   (c) metaraminol bitartrate
    (b) norepinephrine   (d) mephentermine sulfate
24. Metoprolol tartrate and propanolol are examples of:
    (a) alpha stimulants   (c) beta$_1$-beta$_2$ stimulants
    (b) alpha blockers   (d) beta$_1$-beta$_2$ blockers
25. The advantage of using phenylephrine and methoxamine hydrochloride as vasopressors is that:
    (a) they do not increase venous tone and total peripheral resistance
    (b) they do not directly stimulate the heart
    (c) they do not directly stimulate the CNS
    (d) all of the above
26. Blood pressure maintenance is a function of all of the following variables EXCEPT:
    (a) blood volume   (d) heart rate
    (b) venous tone   (e) myocardial contractility
    (c) total peripheral resistance   (f) cardiac output

27. Epinephrine reversal may occur whenever epinephrine is administered to a patient who is taking a drug that:
    (a) stimulates alpha receptors
    (c) stimulates beta$_1$ receptors
    (b) blocks alpha receptors
    (d) blocks beta$_1$ receptors

28. Epinephrine is preferred to norepinephrine as a vasoconstrictor in local anesthetic solutions because:
    (a) it does not dilate the coronary arteries
    (b) the incidence of ischemic necrosis and tissue sloughing is less
    (c) the therapeutic index for epinephrine is much less
    (d) all of the above

7

SEDATIVE-HYPNOTICS, TRANQUILZERS, AND CNS STIMULANTS AND DEPRESSANTS

SECTION 1: SEDATIVE-HYPNOTICS

Barbiturates

Barbiturates are derivatives of barbituric acid and are the most important sedative-hypnotics used in dentistry. Working on a relaxed dental patient can be a pleasant experience for both the patient and the operator, but with some patients proper dosage and prescription of sedatives may be a matter of life or death. Some drugs can produce **sedation** (reduced activity with drowsiness) and in higher doses produce **hypnosis** (sleep); the two classes of sedative-hypnotics are (1) barbiturates and (2) non-barbiturates.

Barbiturates are divided into four groups based on onset and duration of action: (1) ultrashort-acting (onset between 30 and 40 sec after I.V. injection), represented by thiopental sodium (Pentothal) and methohexital sodium (Brevital); (2) short-acting (onset after 30 min, duration up to three hrs), represented by pentobarbital (Nembutal) and secobarbital (Seconal); (3) intermediate-acting (onset between 40 and 60 min, duration between 3 and 6 hrs), represented by amobarbital (Amytal) and butabarbital (Butisol); and (4) long-lacting (onset after two to three hrs, duration of over six hrs), represented by phenobarbital (Luminal). Although any of the barbiturates can induce a general anesthetic state in a dose that is high enough, the ultrashort-acting members are most often used for this purpose; the short and intermediate-acting members are often used in sedative doses as pre-operative medication to allay anxiety, and the long-acting members are often used as both sedatives and anticonvulsants, particularly in infants prone to febrile seizures or in epileptic patients.

Sedative and hypnotic doses of the barbiturates act at the level of the thalamus and the reticular activating system to depress transmission of impulses to the cerebral cortex. Since depression of the cerebral cortex impairs mental and physical skills to some degree, patients under sedation should be advised not to drive back and forth to the dental office but to have someone else drive for them. In elderly patients in whom the cerebral cortex has already undergone physiological atrophy, a sedative dose of a barbiturate may cause a paradoxical excitement, or even delirium. Patients in pain may also become agitated or delirious if barbiturates are administered without analgesics; for this reason, barbiturates are not prescribed to patients in pain without also prescribing analgesics.

Anesthetic doses of barbiturates are very close to the dose that results in lethal blood levels. As little as eight to ten times the usual hypnotic dose is all that is needed to result in lethal poisoning due to respiratory depression; it is therefore unwise to prescribe more than six hypnotic doses or ten sedative doses to a patient at any one time.

The ultrashort-acting barbiturates are also known as intravenous general anesthetics (Chap. 10, Sec. 1). Although they can be used in the office for short procedures, they find their greatest use in providing smooth induction (unconsciousness) prior to inhalation anesthesia in hospitalized dental patients.

Pentobarbital sodium (Nembutal) is available as 30, 50, and 100 mg capsules, 90 and 100 mg time-release tablets, and as an elixir containing 20 mg/tsp. The usual adult sedative dose given prior to dental procedures is 100 mg taken 90 min. before the appointment, and the dose is individualized for children. **Secobarbital sodium** (Seconal) is available as 30, 50, 60, and 100 mg capsules, as 100 mg time-release capsules, and as an elixir containing 22 mg/tsp. Sedative dosage is the same as with pentobarbital sodium.

The dosage of **amobarbital sodium** (Amytal) and **butabarbital sodium** (Butisol) for sedation prior to dental procedures is identical to that of pentobarbital sodium. Amobarbital sodium is more commonly given as a pre-anesthetic sedation in a 200 mg dose, whereas butabarbital sodium is often administered to children as an elixir containing 30 mg/tsp. It is a component of Pedo-Sol (Chap. 8, Sec. 2), in which it is combined with an antihistamine and a belladonna alkaloid.

Phenobarbital is most commonly prescribed in an elixir form containing 20 mg/tsp to children prone to febrile or epileptic seizures, because of its long-acting properties. It is seldom used for pre-operative sedation due to its slow onset (two to three hrs after administration). Children who have a history of taking phenobarbital for prolonged periods will have developed a tolerance to barbiturates and when pre-operative sedation is needed, a non-barbiturate should be chosen.

Barbiturate Intoxication

Individual patients differ in their susceptibility to the depressant action of barbiturates, and this is most noticeable in the elderly or debilitated, the dehydrated, the hypertensive, or the pediatric patient. Too rapid an I.V. injection in these patients can result in coughing, hiccoughing, laryngospasm, or a peripheral vasodilation and fall in blood pressure that is termed barbiturate intoxication. Brochospasm may occur in patients with a history of bronchial asthma or allergic reactions. Respiration and reflexes are depressed; the body temperature may decrease with a return of fever later. The patient eventually develops pulmonary edema and lapses into a coma.

Treatment of this condition consists of maintaining respiration and body temperature, performing gastric lavage, and supporting circulation with vasopressors (alpha stimulants, such as phenylephrine, mephentermine, and methoxamine) and I.V. fluids. The condition can be prevented by injecting the barbiturate slowly or by using alternate agents when the patient's history reveals hypertension, dehydration, debilitation, or extreme age or youth and when the surgical procedures that follow will result in appreciable trauma or blood loss.

Picrotoxin is a non-nitrogenous central nervous system stimulant that exerts inhibitory action on certain cells in the medullary area of the brain and that is occasionally used as an antidote for barbiturate intoxication (Chap. 7, Sec. 3).

Non-Barbiturates

Non-barbiturate sedative-hypnotics are generally weaker than the barbiturates and are less often used for sedation in dentistry.

Ethyl alcohol (ethanol) is an effective agent equal to pentobarbital or diazepam when administered in a dose that results in a blood alcohol level not exceeding 50 mg/dl. Eighty proof distilled neutral spirits can be given orally to patients in a suitable vehicle (fruit or vegetable juice) in a ratio of one part alcohol to two parts vehicle. Side-effects are seldom observed, metabolism is rapid, and the effects wear off in about 80 minutes. No other agents should be administered with ethyl alcohol in combination, and the suggested trial dose is 30 cc (for up to 140 lbs body weight) or 60 cc (for up to 220 lbs).

Although any of the **tranquilizers** (ataractics) produce reduced activity with drowsiness and may be used as sedative-hypnotics, they are primarily indicated for treatment of anxiety, tension, and psychiatric disorders. They are gaining popularity as preoperative sedatives in dentistry because of the difficulty patients may have in separating fear of pain from the dental experience and because of the burden this tension adds to tensions already generated by the complexities of living in today's world. These agents are sometimes combined with barbiturates or analgesics, as in the useful combination of Nembutal 100 mg with Mepergan Fortis (Chap. 8, Sec. 2); commonly used tranquilizing pediatric elixirs are Phenergan Syrup and Phenergan Fortis Syrup (Chap. 8, Sec. 2). Benadryl elixir is also gaining popularity for this purpose (Chap. 8, Sec. 2). Other agents often used include diazepam, chlordiazepoxide, hydroxyzine, and meprobamate (Chap. 7, Sec. 2).

Chloral hydrate (Noctec) has an advantage over barbiturates and other sedatives in that "hangover" and depressant after-effects are only rarely encountered, and blood pressure and respiration are depressed only slightly more than in regular sleep; the patient can therefore be promptly and completely aroused. The average adult sedative dose is 500 mg given 90 min before dental appointments, and for children the dose is 25 mg/kg. It is available as 250 and 500 mg capsules and as a syrup containing 250, 267, and 500 mg/tsp.

Other non-barbiturate sedative-hypnotics are rarely used in dentistry because they are usually given in hypnotic doses to treat insomnia, but the benzodiazepine compound flurazepam (Dalmane) has found some use as a hypnotic to be taken the night before the dental patient is scheduled to receive a general anesthetic (Chap. 7, Sec. 2).

SECTION 2: TRANQUILIZERS

Phenothiazines and Antiemetics

The **phenothiazine tranquilizers** are all derivatives of phenothiazine, and they possess sedative, antiemetic, antihistaminic, autonomic, and potentiating properties to varying degrees. Their multiple actions make them very useful agents for the physician and dentist alike. The available evidence suggests that the phenothiazines act on the cerebral cortex, limbic system, basal ganglia, hypothalamus, brain stem, and medulla by blocking postsynaptic dopamine receptors. They are believed to depress parts of the reticular activating system controlling basal metabolism, body temperature, wakefulness, emesis, hormone balance, and vasomotor tone. Their peripheral autonomic effects include anticholinergic action, weak alpha-blocking and weak beta-stimulating actions (Chap. 6, Sec. 2). Because of their alpha-blocking action, they can initiate epinephrine reversal (Chap. 11, Sec. 1). They are used principally as antipsychotic agents and have as their most predominate side-effects, sedation, orthostatic hypotension, anticholinergic effects, and extrapyramidal symptoms (trismus, dysphagia, restlessness, rolling back of the eyes, spasm of neck muscles). Administration of manganese chelate can be a preventive measure to reduce the possibility of extrapyramidal symptoms associated with phenothiazines; the drug of choice for treating these symptoms is diphenhydramine (Benadryl) (Chap. 7, Sec. 2).

Promethazine (Phenergan) is without question the most important single-entity multiple-action drug used in dental practice, in both the pre-operative and the postoperative phases of treatment. Its use can be considered whenever a sedative, antihistamine, antiemetic, antisialogogue, or narcotic synergist is indicated and is to be administered by the oral route. It is available as 12.5, 25, and 50 mg tablets, 50 mg capsules, and in injection form containing 25 and 50 mg/cc. It is also marketed in elixir forms containing 6.25 mg/tsp (Phenergan Syrup) and 25 mg/tsp (Phenergan Fortis Syrup), which can be given pre-operatively to children requiring restorative dentistry when a dry field cannot be obtained by conventional means (cotton rolls, saliva ejector, rubber dam). As an ingredient in Mepergan Fortis (Chap. 8, Sec. 2), it not only counteracts nausea and vomiting often experienced with meperidine but also allows the effective dose of meperidine to be lower, reducing the addicting potential. The usual dose for adults is between 25 and 50 mg and for children between 6.25 and 25 mg, depending on body weight and degree of sedation desired. Care must be taken to prescribe antiemetic drugs for no longer than 48 hours at a time, because nausea and vomiting can be indicative of serious illnesses, e.g., appendicitis.

Prochlorperazine (Compazine) is particularly useful in management of drug-induced nausea and vomiting associated with intravenous sedation (Chap. 10, Sec. 2) or with postoperative analgesic administration. It is available in several forms but the most useful are the 10, 15, 30, and 75 mg sustained-release capsules ("spansules") and the syrup containing 5 mg/tsp. More than one day's therapy is usually unnecessary, and control is usually obtained with one dose; the usual dose for adults is 10 mg q.12h. and for children between 2.5 and 5 mg once or twice daily. The injection form is usually available in dental offices for parenteral emergency use, and it contains 5 mg/cc.

Chlorpromazine (Thorazine) is often used in the management of psychiatric disorders for relief of tension, anxiety, and agitation. Patients are initially given between 10 and 25 mg t.i.d. for between 24 and 48 hours, and the dosage is then increased by

25 to 50 mg semiweekly until the patient becomes calm and cooperative; dosage is continued at optimal levels for two weeks and is then gradually reduced to a maintenance level between 200 and 400 mg daily. It is marketed as 10, 25, 50, 100, and 200 mg tablets; as 30, 75, 150, 200, and 300 mg timed-release capsules; as a syrup containing 10 mg/tsp.; and in injection form containing 25 mg/cc.

Trifluoperazine (Stelazine) is also used in the management of psychotic disorders but is given in a dose between 1 and 2 mg b.i.d. to outpatients; for those who are hospitalized or under close supervision the usual starting dose is between 2 and 5 mg, which can be increased up to 40 mg daily in divided doses.

Thioridazine (Mellaril) is indicated for short-term treatment of depressive neurosis. The usual starting dose is between 50 and 100 mg t.i.d., this is gradually increased to a maximum of 800 mg daily divided into two or four doses, which is subsequently reduced to a minimal maintenance level. It has found some use in the treatment of senility, intractable pain, and alcohol withdrawal syndrome.

Methotrimeprazine (Levoprome) not only produces sedation and tranquilization but also antihistaminic, anticholinergic, and antiadrenalin effects. It also produces a degree of amnesia similar to that resulting from scopolamine and diazepam administration, and it raises the pain threshold in a fashion comparable to that of morphine and meperidine (Chap. 8, Sec. 2). An important advantage to using this agent is that respiratory depression occurs infrequently with it, but the greatest disadvantage is that orthostatic hypotension, dizziness, and fainting can occur. It is indicated for sedation and analgesia in non-ambulatory patients when respiratory depression is to be avoided. The usual dose is between 10 and 20 mg I.M. into a large muscle mass q.4h. p.r.n. pain and is available in a form for injection containing 20 mg/cc.

The phenothiazines together with the Rauwolfia alkaloids and butyrophenones are used in the management of psychoses and are therefore classified as major tranquilizers. The propanediols, benzodiazepines, and diphenylmethanes are used in the management of neuroses and therefore classified as minor tranquilizers. The monoamine oxidase inhibitors and dibenzazepines (tricyclic antidepressants) are collectively termed antidepressants and are also used in the management of neuroses.

The **antiemetics** include peripherally acting agents, such as Coca-Cola syrup and phosphorated carbohydrate solution (Emetrol), and certain centrally acting agents, including the phenothiazine tranquilizers, antihistamines (dimenhydrinate, diphenhydramine, hydroxyzine pamoate), and the miscellaneous drug trimethobenzamide hydrochloride.

Just as syrup of ipecac is a common household product used to induce vomiting (emesis), **Coca-Cola syrup** is commonly kept in the home to calm an upset stomach and both products are available without a prescription in any pharmacy. Coca-Cola syrup should be kept in every dental office and given in a dose of 3 teaspoons orally to any patient who has recently vomited; a **phosphorated carbohydrate solution** (Emetrol) that may be substituted requires no refrigeration and is given orally to adults in doses between 3 and 6 teaspoons or to children in doses between 1 and 2 teaspoons. These may be repeated every 15 minutes as needed.

The **phenothiazines** appear to act directly on the vomiting center, the chemoreceptor trigger zone (CTZ), the cerebral cortex, or, during motion sickness, on the vestibular apparatus, rather than on peripheral areas, such as the gastric mucosa. These agents are chemically similar to the dibenzazepines (tricyclic antidepressants), but although these two groups are known as "tricyclic" compounds, the latter have no entiemetic activity.

Antihistamines with potent antiemetic action include dimenhydrinate (Dramamine) (Chap. 5, Sec. 4) and the diphenylmethane tranquilizers diphenhydramine hydrochloride (Benadryl) and hydroxyzine pamoate (Vistaril) (Chap. 7, Sec. 2).

Trimethobenzamide hydrochloride (Tigan) is a miscellaneous drug chemically un-related to any other drugs and possessing the unique property of being a pure antiemetic (without multiple actions). It acts solely by inhibiting the chemoreceptor trigger zone (CTZ) of the medulla oblongata. It is marketed as 100 and 250 mg capsules, 200 mg suppositories, 100 mg pediatric suppositories, and in injection form containing 100 mg/cc; the usual adult dose is 200 mg I.M. q.i.d. or 250 mg P.O. q.i.d. Its particular advantage is that its limited action renders it virtually devoid of hazardous drug inter-actions (Chap. 11, Sec. 1).

Rauwolfia Alkaloids

The rauwolfia derivatives are believed to exert their antihypertensive effects by inhibiting storage of norepinephrine in sympathetic postganglionic nerve endings, and their tranquilizing effects are thought to be due to depletion of amines in the CNS. Since several days of therapy with these drugs are required to deplete norepinephrine stores, the onset of antihypertensive action is delayed and may require as long as one week or more to appear. When therapy is discontinued, antihypertensive effects may persist for several weeks. Although these agents are indicated for relief of mild essential hypertension, they have also been used as antipsychotic agents, particularly in patients who cannot tolerate phenothiazines or who require antihypertensive medication. Caution must be used in prescribing these agents to patients with a history of mental depression because drug-induced depression may persist several months after drug with-drawal and may be of sufficient intensity to result in suicide.

Reserpine (Serpasil) is available as 0.1, 0.25, 0.5, and 1 mg tablets, as 0.5 mg capsules, as an elixir containing 0.25 mg/tsp, and in injection form containing 2.5 mg/cc. Although it is the most important Rauwolfia alkaloid, reserpine is falling into disuse owing to its slow onset, unpredictable latent period upon discontinuance, tendency to induce suicide, and the availability of better drugs. Dosage is individualized and ranges from 0.1 to 5 mg daily depending on the condition being treated.

Butyrophenones

Droperidol (Inapsine) is a potent sedative and tranquilizer with antiemetic effects that render it a useful agent for pre-medication prior to general anesthesia and as an adjunct to certain surgical and diagnostic procedures. Being a weak alpha blocker, it is capable of initiating epinephrine reversal (Chap. 11, Sec. 1). It may reduce the incidence of epinephrine-induced arrhythmias by decreasing peripheral resistance in a way similar to that of beta$_2$ stimulation, thereby lowering the pressor effect of epinephrine; it does not prevent other arrhythmias. Droperidol is often combined with a potent narcotic, such as **fentanyl** (Sublimaze), in a 1:50 ratio (1 part fentanyl:50 parts droperidol), to form an agent that is called Innovar. Because of its intense activity, droperidol is termed a neuroleptic agent; when administered to a patient in combination with fentanyl as Innovar, it produces a state of neuroleptanalgesia characterized by profound analgesia and tranquilization. When nitrous oxide oxygen sedation is combined with Innovar, a general anesthetic state is produced. In patients who are poor risks for general anesthesia,

Innovar is a most advantageous adjunct to local anesthesia, but it is not recommended for ambulatory patients. Patients pre-medicated with Innovar must be carefully monitored for signs of hypoxia, and agents for managing respiratory depression and hypotension should be readily available (positive pressure oxygen, narcotic antagonists, and vasopressors other than epinephrine). Droperidol is available in injection form containing 2.5 mg/cc and the usual dose for pre-medication prior to surgery is between 2.5 and 10 mg injected I.M. between 30 and 60 minutes pre-operatively; for children, between 1 and 1.5 mg/20 to 25 lbs is recommended.

Propanediols and Centrally Acting Muscle Relaxants

Meprobamate (Equanil, Miltown) is a carbamate derivative of propyl alcohol that exerts effects at several sites in the CNS, including the thalamus and limbic system, and is indicated to promote sleep in nervous patients and to relieve anxiety and tension. Although it is an excellent alternative for use as a sedative-hypnotic when barbiturates are contraindicated, it may produce oral lesions (Chap. 1, Sec. 2), precipitate seizures in epileptics (Chap. 7, Sec. 3), and when combined with analgesics (Equagesic), may result in the perception of greater postoperative pain than would be present without any analgesic (Chap. 8, Sec. 2). It is available as 200, 400, and 600 mg tablets and as 200 and 400 mg sustained-release capsules. The usual dose is between 1200 and 1600 mg daily in divided doses for adults, and for children between ages 6 and 12, 100 and 200 mg 2 or 3 times daily. It is not recommended for children under age six. Since meprobamate is a centrally acting muscle relaxant, it may also be used as an adjunct in the treatment of tetanus. Meprobamate for I.M. injection (Intramuscular Miltown) is marketed as 400 mg/5 cc ampul, and it is administered by deep I.M. injection in the gluteal region. It is never given I.V. because the vehicle may cause hemolysis or thrombosis.

The benzodiazepine tranquilizer **diazepam** (Valium) appears to act on portions of the thalamus, hypothalamus, and limbic system to induce calming effects and muscle relaxation (Chap. 7, Sec. 2). It is indicated for relief of muscle spasm associated with tetanus or mandibular subluxation (Chap. 12, Sec. 1).

Benzodiazepines

The benzodiazepine compounds have anticonvulsant and muscle-relaxing properties to varying degrees and produce a calming action on certain subcortical levels of the CNS, particularly the limbic system. Although these drugs are associated with a wide margin of safety between therapeutic and toxic doses, mild paradoxical reactions (hyperexcited states) have been observed in some psychiatric patients. Recent estimates claim that 60 million Americans are currently under treatment with these agents, making them the most widely prescribed group of drugs in the United States at the present time.

Chlordiazepoxide hydrochloride (Librium) can be used for pre-operative sedation prior to dental procedures, and the usual dose for relief of anxiety and tension is between 5 and 25 mg t.i.d. or q.i.d. It is marketed as 5, 10, and 25 mg capsules and as a powder that can be reconstituted with bacteriostatic water or sterile saline to produce an injection containing 20 mg/cc.

Diazepam (Valium) has enjoyed the widest use by dentists for pre-operative sedation and is the drug of choice for certain recurrent or prolonged epileptic seizures (Chap. 7, Sec. 3; Chap. 12, Sec. 1) or for subluxation (Chap. 12, Sec. 1) when manual efforts have failed to reposition a dislocated temporamandibular joint. Specific receptors for diazepam have not been found in skeletal muscle but have been found in the CNS, suggesting that the drug's effects are accomplished there rather than at the muscular level. Diazepam has been found to have certain advantages over chlordiazepoxide in that it has a shorter duration of action and therefore a wider margin of safety during dental procedures, it is a more potent muscle relaxant, and when administered I.V. it produces a degree of amnesia similar to that produced by scopolamine; however, phlebitis is commonly associated with I.V. administration, and it has been found to have undesirable side-effects interfering with muscle tissue formation (myoblast fusion and expression of muscle-specific protein synthesis). The usual adult dose is between 2 and 10 mg b.i.d., t.i.d., or q.i.d. depending on the severity of the condition treated, and it is available as 2, 5, and 10 mg tablets and in injection form containing 5 mg/cc.

Chlorazepate dipotassium (Tranxene) is indicated for anxiety and tension and symptomatic relief of acute alcohol withdrawal. The usual daily dose is 30 mg, adjusted gradually in the range of 15 to 60 mg daily based on patient response. In the elderly or debilitated patient, treatment is begun with between 7.5 and 15 mg. It is marketed as 3.75, 7.5, and 15 mg capsules and as 11.25 and 22.5 mg tablets.

Flurazepam hydrochloride (Dalmane) increases the arousal threshold to stimulation of the amygdala and hypothalamus and is used effectively in patients with recurrent insomnia, poor sleeping habits, or in medical situations requiring restful sleep, such as the night before general anesthesia. It is available as 15 and 30 mg capsules, and the usual adult dose taken before retiring is between 15 and 30 mg. In the elderly or debilitated, therapy is begun with a 15 mg dose, which is continued until individual responses are determined to preclude the development of oversedation, dizziness, staggering, and an increasing number of falling incidents.

Diphenylmethanes

Hydroxyzine pamoate (Vistaril) is not a cortical depressant, as are the barbiturates, but its ataractic properties may be due to a suppression of activity in certain key regions of the subcortical areas of the CNS. It not only induces a calming effect in tense patients without impairing mental alertness but also has been shown to possess antihistaminic, antispasmodic, antiemetic, and analgesic effects (Chap. 8, Sec. 2). Primary skeletal muscle relaxation has been observed, in addition to secondary relaxation induced by ataraxia. It is often administered pre-operatively with meperidine (Demerol) and atropine prior to general anesthesia. The usual dose is between 25 and 100 mg for adults and 0.5 mg/lb for children, which can be given three or four times daily as needed. It is marketed as 25, 50, and 100 mg capsules, as an oral suspension containing 25 mg/tsp, and in injection form containing 25 or 50 mg/cc.

Diphenhydramine hydrochloride (Benadryl) is a weak tranquilizer with potent antihistaminic properties that render it ideally suited for treatment of mild allergic reactions (Chap. 12, Sec. 1) or of extrapyramidal symptoms associated with phenothiazines in elderly patients who are unable to tolerate more potent agents (Chap. 7, Sec. 2). When injected into tissues it has been shown to possess weak local anesthetic properties (Chap. 9, Sec. 1). The usual dose is between 25 and 50 mg t.i.d. or q.i.d. for adults and for children, between 12.5 and 25 mg t.i.d. or q.i.d. or 5 mg/kg/24 hrs in divided doses. It is available as 25 and 50 mg capsules, 50 mg tablets, as an elixir containing 10 mg/tsp, and as a syrup containing either 12.5 or 13.3 mg/tsp. This agent has antitussive effects similar to those of codeine (Chap. 8, Sec. 1) and can be used as a non-narcotic cough suppressant. The syrup formulations are specifically indicated for this purpose and also contain ammonium chloride and sodium citrate, inactive ingredients that have been traditionally used as expectorants; for this reason diphenhydramine syrup is not prescribed in maintenance doses to any patients who must restrict intake of sodium, such as those patients being treated for hypertension with a diuretic (Chap. 6, Sec. 1).

Monoamine Oxidase Inhibitors

Certain proteins in the body (enzymes) act as chemical catalysts to allow accelerated breakdown and metabolism of various substances in order to preserve a steady state (homeostasis). The enzyme acetylcholine esterase metabolizes acetylcholine within cholinergic neurons; if a cholinesterase inhibitor (physostigmine, neostigmine, or pyridostigmine) is administered (Chap. 6, Sec. 2), acetylcholine accumulates at neuromuscular junctions and at preganglionic, parasympathetic postganglionic, and sympathetic postganglionic fibers affecting some of the sweat glands. The counterpart to acetylcholine esterase, monoamine oxidase, metabolizes catecholamines and other biogenic amines within adrenergic neurons; biogenic amines can accumulate at all sympathetic postganglionic fibers, except some of the sweat glands, if a monoamine oxidase inhibitor (tranylcypromine, isocarboxazid, or phenelzine sulfate) is administered.

Therapy with monoamine oxidase inhibitors results in buildup of epinephrine, norepinephrine, dopamine (catecholamines), as well as serotonin, tyramine, and tryptamine, in various tissues; the resulting euphoric stimulation has caused these agents to be labeled as mood elevators. They should be reserved as a last resort for use with patients who do not respond to psychotherapy because they inhibit not only monoamine oxidase but also many other enzyme systems and can modify the action of virtually every drug known; serious and often lethal drug interactions have resulted with other agents are used with them in combination (Chap. 11, Sec. 1).

Tranylcypromine (Parnate) is the most potent of the monoamine oxidase inhibitors and is marketed as 10 mg tablets to be administered in a dose of 10 b.i.d.

Isocarboxazid (Marplan) is also available as 10 mg tablets, and the usual dose is 30 mg daily, which is reduced to a maintenance level of 10 mg daily or less when clinical improvement is seen.

Phenelzine sulfate (Nardil) is supplied as 15 mg tablets, and the dose is 15 mg t.i.d. and initially is adjusted according to clinical observations, decreasing to 15 mg every other day.

Although monoamine oxidase inhibitors are associated with antihypertensive effects, the use of these drugs to treat hypertension is questionable due to the availability of better agents (Chap. 6, Sec. 1).

Dibenzazepines

The **tricyclic antidepressants** are structurally related to the phenothiazines and have similar side-effects of sedation and anticholinergic action. These tricyclic compounds are characterized by their amine-uptake blocking activity, which is specific for norepinephrine and serotonin at the pre-synaptic neuron in the CNS, in contrast with the phenothiazines, which act on dopamine receptors (Chap. 7, Sec. 2). In addition to inhibiting the uptake of norepinephrine and serotonin, they have been shown to inhibit the activity of acetylcholine and histamine, to increase the pressor effect of norepinephrine, and to produce mild peripheral vasodilation similar to that resulting from beta$_2$ stimulation (Chap. 6, Sec. 2). Even though adverse cardiovascular effects (orthostatic hypotension or arrhythmias) can occur with these agents, they are generally preferred over monoamine oxidase inhibitors for the treatment of depression because their spectrum of adverse effects is smaller.

It has been suggested that depression may be divided into two subtypes characterized by a deficiency of either norepinephrine or serotonin. Patients with a norepinephrine deficiency are more likely to respond to nortriptyline (Aventyl), desipramine (Norpramin), or protriptyline (Vivactil), whereas those with a serotonin deficiency are more likely to respond to amitriptyline (Elavil). Imipramine (Tofranil) is effective for both subtypes.

Patients taking a tricyclic antidepressant should not be given local anesthesia with epinephrine because the tricyclic compounds potentiate all of the catecholamines (epinephrine, norepinephrine, and dopamine) (Chap. 6, Sec. 2; Chap. 11, Sec. 1).

Nortriptyline hydrochloride (Aventyl) is marketed as 10 mg capsules and as a solution containing 10 mg/tsp; it is given in a dose of 25 mg t.i.d. or q.i.d.

Desipramine hydrochloride (Norpramin) is available as 25, 50, 75, 100, and 150 mg tablets and as 25 and 50 mg capsules; the usual dose is between 75 and 200 mg daily in a single dose or divided doses.

Protriptyline hydrochloride (Vivactil) is available as 5 and 10 mg tablets, and the daily dose is between 15 and 40 mg divided into three or four doses.

Amitriptyline hydrochloride (Elavil) is marketed as 10, 25, 50, 75, 100, and 150 mg tablets and in injection form containing 10 mg/cc; the usual dose is between 75 and 150 mg daily in divided doses.

Imipramine hydrochloride (Tofranil) is available as 10, 25, and 50 mg tablets and in injection form containing 25 mg/2 cc with ascorbate, anhydrous sodium sulfite, and sodium bisulfite. As imipramine pamoate, it is also marketed as 75, 100, 125, and 150 mg capsules. Dosage is the same as for amitriptyline hydrochloride (Elavil) (between 75 and 150 mg daily in divided doses).

Since these drugs block muscarinic receptors, as do the belladonna alkaloids (Chap. 6, Sec. 2), treatment of overdosage consists of administration of a cholinesterase inhibitor, such as physostigmine salicylate (Chap. 6, Sec. 2).

SECTION 3: CNS STIMULANTS AND DEPRESSANTS

Miscellaneous Neurotropic Agents

The CNS stimulants (analeptics) are a heterogeneous group of compounds that by stimulating the medullary area, produce an improvement in the rate and depth of breathing and possibly a return of consciousness or of reflexes that have been depressed. Since the effect of this drug on the medulla is non-specific and widespread, respiratory stimulation is often accompanied by nausea, vomiting, increased motor activity, and changes in blood pressure and heart rate. The use of these agents in cases of drug-induced respiratory depression is questionable because the difference between a respiratory-stimulant dose and a convulsant dose is usually very small, and should such use result in muscle tremors or convulsions during administration, the resulting postconvulsive depression could add to the respiratory depression already present. For this reason, specific antagonists are indicated in these cases rather than non-specific physiological antagonists (analeptics).

Doxapram hydrochloride (Dopram) is indicated to hasten arousal and return of laryngopharyngeal reflexes and stimulate respiration in patients who have apnea or respiratory depression in the postanesthesia period, other than that induced by muscle relaxant drugs. It is associated with a pressor effect secondary to the improved cardiac output that results from increased release of catecholamines (epinephrine, norepinephrine, and dopamine). It is generally used as an adjunct to supportive measures and resuscitative techniques, rather than as the primary treatment for drug-induced depression, and I.V. short-acting barbiturates (Chap. 7, Sec. 1; Chap. 10, Sec. 1), positive-pressure oxygen, and resuscitative equipment should be available to manage doxapram overdosage, which is characterized by excessive pressor effect, tachycardia, and skeletal muscle hyperactivity. This drug is marketed only in injection form containing 20 mg/cc and is given either as a single I.V. injection of between 0.5 and 1 mg/kg or as an infusion of between 1 and 5 mg/min, diluted as 250 mg doxapram in 250 cc dextrose 5 per cent or saline solution (0.9 per cent NaC1). Respiratory stimulation appears to be mediated through the peripheral carotid chemoreceptors and to progress gradually to the CNS as the dose is increased.

Nikethamide (Coramine) acts directly on the CNS and secondarily on peripheral carotid chemoreceptors and is indicated to overcome respiratory depression secondary to drugs, shock, coronary occlusion, newborn asphyxia, or carbon monoxide poisoning. It is available in 25 per cent parenteral and oral solutions, and the usual initial dose is between 2 and 10 cc, repeated as needed.

Picrotoxin (Cocculin) has traditionally been used as an antidote for barbiturate intoxication (Chap. 7, Sec. 1), but its use for this purpose is controversial. A 0.3 per cent solution in saline is used, and 3 mg of this dilution is given at five minute intervals until muscle twitches or increased respiration is observed.

Strychnine is a CNS convulsive agent of toxicological interest but not of therapeutic usefulness; the minimum lethal dose is between 100 and 120 mg orally and between 30 and 40 mg parenterally. In some patients lower doses have been lethal.

Some of the CNS stimulants have been associated with subjective reasons described as psychotomimetic and have been misused for this reason (Chap. 11, Sec. 1). Agents in this category include cocaine, cannabinols, lysergic acid diethylamide (LSD), and mescaline (peyote). Other therapeutic agents known to be used for non-therapeutic purposes by abusers include alcohol, sedative-hypnotics, narcotic analgesics and antagonists, anticholinergics, and nitrous oxide (Chap. 11, Sec. 2). There is a small but growing number of physicians and dentists, medical and dental students, and other individuals in health professions who are guilty of misuse of such drugs, particularly cocaine, amphetamines, and nitrous oxide.

Cocaine is legally classified as a narcotic to help prevent its misuse, but technically it is a CNS stimulant and local anesthetic (Chap. 9, Sec. 1). It produces intense vasoconstriction, which has made it somewhat advantageous for use during the pre-anesthesia period; a 1 or 2 per cent solution of cocaine can be sprayed into a patient's nose and larynx prior to intubation, and this will block sensory nerve endings and constrict local blood vessels in preparation for passage of the nasotracheal tube. The spray tends to inhibit laryngeal reflexes and to reduce hemorrhage from the nasal mucosa, both desirable effects. Concentrations as high as 20 per cent have been used to anesthetize the nose and throat. The dose-related effects cocaine produces can be described as euphoria, aphrodisia, indifference to pain, antifatigue action that often provokes the user to exceed his physical limitations, or even an amphetamine-type psychosis marked by paranoia, delusions of persecution, visual or auditory disturbances, or violent temperament.

Amphetamines

The amphetamines can be classified either as autonomic drugs with central stimulating activity (Chap. 6, Sec. 2) or as CNS stimulants with autonomic effects. The peripheral actions of the amphetamines include weak respiratory stimulation, weak bronchodilation, and elevation of systolic and diastolic pressures. Because of the high potential for abuse, the clinical use of the amphetamines is limited to producing anorexia for short-term weight reduction, managing narcolepsy, and managing minimal brain dysfunction (MBD). These drugs may be combined with amobarbital or prochlorperazine to limit the stimulation that could occur in some patients taking amphetamines alone (Chap. 7, Sec. 1; Chap. 7, Sec. 2).

The average dose for any of the amphetamines is for narcolepsy, between 5 and 60 mg daily in divided doses; for MBD, between 2.5 and 5 mg once or twice daily; and for obesity, between 5 and 30 mg daily in divided doses 60 minutes before meals. Treatment of amphetamine intoxication is symptomatic but includes gastric lavage and sedation with a barbiturate.

Amphetamine sulfate (Benzedrine) is marketed as 5 and 10 mg tablets and as 15 mg sustained-release capsules.

Dextroamphetamine sulfate (Dexedrine) is available as 5 and 10 mg tablets, as 15 mg capsules, as 5, 10, and 15 mg sustained-release capsules, and as an elixir containing 5 mg/tsp.

Methamphetamine hydrochloride (Desoxyn) is available as 2.5, 5, and 10 mg tablets and as 5, 10, and 15 mg gradumets (long-acting tablets).

Amphetamines cause a release of endogenous catecholamines (epinephrine, norepinephrine, and dopamine), which accounts in part for their sympathomimetic activity; when catecholamines are depleted, the amphetamines are still active centrally but are not peripherally. A syndrome resembling paranoid schizophrenia may appear in patients taking amphetamines, and this is characterized by visual and auditory disturbances, delusions of persecution, and anxiety similar to that induced by cocaine (Chap. 7, Sec. 3).

Xanthines

The xanthines share a dual function with the amphetamines in that both drug groups are CNS stimulants with cardiovascular effects (Chap. 6, Sec. 1).

Caffeine is used primarily as a CNS stimulant because its cardiovascular and bronchodilator effects are not potent enough to be useful clinically without its stimulating effects; in this respect it differs from theophylline ethylenediamine (aminophylline). The average amount of caffeine contained in a cup of coffee made by percolation, drip, or vacuum methods is between 100 and 150 mg/cup; made with instant coffee, between 52 and 67 mg/cup; made with decaffeinated coffee, between 13 and 35 mg/cup. A cup of tea may contain between 43 and 110 mg, depending on strength. Caffeine has been used as an aid in staying awake and as a respiratory stimulant in cases of morphine- and alcohol-induced depression. It has also found some use in restoring respiration following electric shock or in relieving headache secondary to spinal puncture. It is not an effective analeptic in most cases of severe drug-induced depressions because it can further depress an already depressed patient, and better drugs are available.

Caffeine is marketed as 100, 200, and 250 mg tablets, and 100 and 250 mg time-release capsules; citrated caffeine is available in 65 mg tablets; caffeine with sodium benzoate is available only in injection form containing 250 mg/cc. The usual oral dose between 65 and 250 mg, whereas the parenteral dose is 500 mg I.M. or I.V. Single doses of caffeine and sodium benzoate should not exceed 1000 mg; short-acting barbiturates are used to counteract adverse reactions (Chap. 7, Sec. 1).

Anticonvulsants and Epilepsy

Epilepsy is a recurrent disorder of cerebral function that is characterized by sudden brief attacks of altered consciousness, motor activity, or sensory phenomena. There are many recurrent epileptic patterns, but the most common form is the convulsive seizure, which begins with a loss of motor control and consciousness and progresses into muscular jerking of the extremities. Such seizures can be precipitated in susceptible patients by convulsant drugs, such as picrotoxin or strychnine (Chap. 7, Sec. 2); or by drug allergy, or any increase in sensory input, such as a mild toothache or anxiety over having one's teeth cleaned. If such a seizure begins in a dental office, a dental auxiliary often notices it first and can begin supportive treatment.

The convulsive seizure is believed to be initiated by an ectopic focus of neuron depolarization beginning as an orderly arrangement of firing instead of the random pattern of firing seen in the normal brain. This orderly pattern of excitation spreads throughout the brain, resulting in excessive impulse to the skeletal muscles. The convulsion usually lasts between two and five minutes; if the convulsion continues and is left untreated (status epilepticus), it may persist for hours or days and is often fatal.

Prior to some types of seizures there is a specific sensory, motor, or psychic aberration called the "aura," which reflects the location in the brain where the seizure begins. Sometimes a seizure occurs so rapidly that there is not time for an aura to begin.

Grand mal seizures usually begin with an aura (a sinking or rising sensation in the epigastrium), followed by an outcry and a sudden loss of consciousness. If the patient is standing he will fall to the floor, muscle spasms will occur, and he may be seen biting his tongue. He either will not remember the convulsion when he awakens or will lapse into a deep sleep. When he does awaken he often complains of headache or muscle soreness.

Petit mal seizures are not preceded by an aura and consist of a brief loss of consciousness, between 10 and 30 seconds long, with a number of minor eye and muscle movements. The patient suddenly stops whatever he is doing and resumes his activity after the attack. Petit mal seizures never begin after age 20 and occur predominately in young children. The attacks often occur several times daily and often begin when the patient sits quietly, such as when in a dental chair. In about half the cases of petit mal epilepsy, grand mal epilepsy develops later in life.

Psychomotor seizures are preceded by an aura and consist of a stereotyped pattern of movement and loss of contact with the surroundings that last between one and two minutes. The patient may stare and stagger, utter meaningless sounds, perform purposeless movements, and fail to understand what is said. He may also resist aid. Mental confusion continues for between one and two minutes after the seizure.

Jacksonian seizure, or "marching" epilepsy, either begins in a hand or foot and "marches" up the extremity or begins at the corner of the mouth and progresses to involve the entire body. Like petit mal or psychomotor seizures, it is preceded by an aura and usually progresses into grand mal seizure.

Epilepsy affects 2 per cent of the population, and about 90 per cent of these experience grand mal seizures, either alone or in combination with other types of seizures; petit mal attacks are experienced by 25 per cent of such patients, and psychomotor attacks, by 18 per cent, either alone or in combination. Management of convulsions is limited to preventing injury.

No single drug controls all types of seizures, and patients may require several drugs; medication is usually continued for at least five seizure-free years. When seizures are infrequent, long-acting barbiturates, such as phenobarbital, can be given to adults orally in a dose of 100 mg once daily (Chap. 7, Sec. 1). The short- and intermediate-acting barbiturates have also been used for this purpose.

When seizures are frequent, the hydantoins are used either alone or in combination with the barbiturates, and this combination is the most effective against grand mal seizures. The hydantoins inhibit the spread of seizure activity in the motor cortex and are associated with a number of adverse reactions involving mainly the CNS. **Phenytoin sodium** (Dilantin) is marketed as a powder, as 30 and 100 mg capsules, and as 250 mg time-release capsules; the usual adult dose is 100 mg t.i.d. or 5 mg/kg/day in two or three divided doses. Phenytoin sodium for parenteral administration is available only as a 50 mg/cc ready-mixed solution, and I.V. administration should not exceed 50 mg/min; between 150 and 250 mg can be administered for status epilepticus and can be followed by between 100 and 150 mg 30 minutes later if needed. A dosage consisting of phenytoin, between 300 and 400 mg daily, plus phenobarbital, between 100 and 200 mg daily, is often more effective in prevention of grand mal seizures than increased doses of either drug alone. Gingival hyperplasia (Dilantin fibromatosis) occurs frequently in patients taking phenytoin and has been observed in even mouths free of local irritants. Treatment of this condition includes frequent brushing, recall examinations with sub-gingival débridement and dental prophylaxis every four months, removal of occlusal disharmonies, restoration of unfilled cavities, correction of overhanging and underhanging restorations, and in severe cases, gingivectomy. Dietary sodium ascorbate (Chap. 3, Sec. 1) has been used as an adjunct to phenytoin in the treatment of seizures; animals deprived of ascorbate while on phenytoin have recurrent seizures that disappear when ascorbate is put into the diet again.

Diazepam (Valium) is indicated as adjunctive therapy for recurrent or prolonged seizures (Chap. 7, Sec. 2) but has not proven useful as the sole therapy because of its short life following I.V. administration; once seizures are brought under control with diazepam, longer acting agents should be considered for maintenance.

TEST QUESTIONS

1. Barbiturate pre-medication is contraindicated for dental procedures that will result in appreciable trauma or blood loss for patients who are:
   (a) elderly or debilitated
   (b) hypertensive
   (c) dehydrated
   (d) all of the above

2. Patients in pain may become agitated or delirious if barbiturate pre-medication is given without concomitant administration of:
   - (a) antihistamines
   - (b) analgesics
   - (c) antibiotics
   - (d) antihypertensive agents

3. All of the following are non-barbiturate sedative-hypnotics which are used for dental pre-operative sedation EXCEPT:
   - (a) ethyl alcohol
   - (b) promethazine
   - (c) diazepam
   - (d) chlordiazepoxide
   - (e) dimenhydrinate
   - (f) hydroxyzine pamoate
   - (g) meprobamate
   - (h) pentobarbital
   - (i) chloral hydrate

4. Barbiturates used for oral sedation are classified as:
   - (a) long-acting
   - (b) intermediate- and short-acting
   - (c) ultrashort-acting

5. Promethazine is only used in dentistry as a(n):
   - (a) antihistamine
   - (b) antiemetic
   - (c) antisialogogue
   - (d) sedative
   - (e) narcotic synergist
   - (f) all of the above

6. All of the following are antiemetics EXCEPT:
   - (a) promethazine
   - (b) prochlorperazine
   - (c) phosphorated carbohydrate solution (Emetrol)
   - (d) dimenhydrinate
   - (e) syrup of Coca-Cola
   - (f) diphenhydramine
   - (g) syrup of ipecac
   - (h) trimethobenzamide hydrochloride
   - (i) hydroxyzine pamoate

7. A patient presenting for routine subgingival débridement and dental prophylaxis has a history of taking reserpine for hypertension. Of the following, the best choice for a pre-operative sedative for this patient would be:
   - (a) pentobarbital
   - (b) phenobarbital
   - (c) meprobamate
   - (d) diphenhydramine

8. Innovar contains fentanyl citrate and droperidol in a ratio of:
   - (a) 5 parts fentanyl:1 part droperidol
   - (b) 50 parts fentanyl:1 part droperidol
   - (c) 500 parts fentanyl:1 part droperidol
   - (d) 1 part fentanyl:5 parts droperidol
   - (e) 1 part fentanyl:50 parts droperidol
   - (f) 1 part fentanyl:500 parts droperidol

9. Disadvantages of using meprobamate as a sedative when barbiturates are contra-indicated include:
   - (a) precipitation of oral lesions
   - (b) precipitation of seizures in epileptics
   - (c) possible perception by the patient of greater postoperative pain when the drug is given with analgesics than would be present without an analgesic
   - (d) no I.V. administration
   - (e) all of the above

10. All of the following are benzodiazepines EXCEPT:
    - (a) chlordiazepoxide
    - (b) diazepam
    - (c) chlorazepate dipotassium
    - (d) flurazepam
    - (e) amitriptyline

11. The most potent of the MAO inhibitors is:
    (a) tranylcypromine
    (b) isocarboxazid
    (c) phenelzine sulfate

12. All of the following are dibenzazepines (tricyclic antidepressants) EXCEPT:
    (a) nortriptyline
    (b) desipramine
    (c) protriptyline
    (d) amitriptyline
    (e) atropine
    (f) imipramine

13. Cocaine is classified as a narcotic to help prevent its misuse, but technically it is a:
    (a) CNS stimulant
    (b) local anesthetic
    (c) vasoconstrictor
    (d) all of the above

14. Amphetamines cause a release of endogenous:
    (a) catecholamines
    (b) triiodothyronine
    (c) cocaine
    (d) all of the above

15. The xanthines include:
    (a) caffeine
    (b) theophylline ethylenediamine
    (c) phenytoin sodium
    (d) all of the above
    (e) both a and b

16. Epileptic seizures preceded by an "aura" include:
    (a) grand mal
    (b) petit mal
    (c) psychomotor
    (d) Jacksonian
    (e) a, b, and c
    (f) a, c, and d

17. Gingival hyperplasia frequently occurs with administration of:
    (a) diazepam
    (b) pentobarbital
    (c) phenytoin sodium
    (d) phenobarbital

8

ANALGESICS

SECTION 1: NARCOTICS

Naturally Occurring Opiates and Morphine Index

The narcotics play an important role in dental practice by raising the pain threshold and relieving pain of untreated oral disease or recent surgical wounds. All narcotics have undesirable side-effects, notably, respiratory depression; nausea or vomiting secondary to stimulation of the chemoreceptor trigger zone (CTZ) of the medulla oblongata, which radiates impulses into the vomiting center; dimness of vision; decreased mental alertness and lethargy; pupils become somewhat constricted with usual therapeutic doses and are fixed and non-reactive in overdosage. Patients who have vomited during narcotic administration and claim to be allergic to narcotics have often experienced only an undesirable side-effect; certain of the antiemetics are sometimes prescribed concurrent with narcotics (Chap. 7, Sec. 2). Narcotics are divided into three classes: (1) naturally occurring opiates, (2) synthetic opiates, and (3) opioids.

Since there is some variation among patients in the perception of painful stimuli of a fixed intensity, pain intensity is almost impossible to quantify; therefore, the analgesic potency of any analgesic drug can be assessed only by comparison with a similar drug chosen as a standard. This ratio should not be learned as a fixed number but rather as a general indicator of analgesic strength. The *morphine index* is the ratio of the analgesic potency of morphine (mg in numerator) compared to an equal quantity of another analgesic drug (mg in denominator) (Fig. 8–1).

The opium alkaloids obtained from the seeds of the poppy plant number over 25, constitute 25 per cent of the opium by weight, and are divided into the phenanthrene and benzylisoquinoline groups; morphine and codeine belong to the former group and constitute its most clinically used agents.

The analgesic activity of powdered opium extract (pantopon) is due primarily to its **morphine** content. Although morphine produces analgesia, sedation, and muscle relaxation, the systemic availability from oral administration is limited, and it should be given parenterally. It is hardly ever needed in dental practice because other less addicting agents

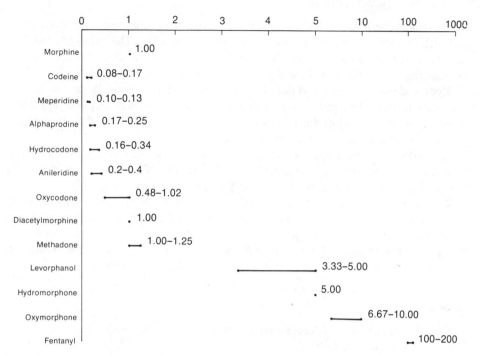

Figure 8-1. Morphine index of various narcotic analgesics. (Data based on efficacy at standard adult doses.)

are available. Morphine sulfate is marketed as 10, 15, and 30 mg tablets and in injection form containing 8, 10, and 15 mg/cc. The usual adult dose for pain is between 5 and 15 mg orally q.4h. or between 5 and 20 mg I.M. or Sub-Q as needed.

Codeine resembles morphine chemically and its effects are similar, but its action is weaker and causes less severe adverse reactions. It is the most widely prescribed narcotic in dental practice and is usually prescribed as codeine sulfate or codeine phosphate, which are both available as 15, 30, and 60 mg tablets. When given alone to an adult for treatment of dental pain codeine should be taken in a dose of 60 mg q.4h. p.r.n.; when it is used in combination with certain non-narcotics, a dose of 30 mg should be sufficient (Chap. 8, Sec. 2). It also has antitussive effects useful in the treatment of cough.

Synthetic Opiates

The group of synthetic opiates contains drugs that are all derivatives of either morphine or codeine and that have very similar chemical structures, analgesic properties, and adverse effects.

Diacetylmorphine (heroin) is as potent as morphine as an analgesic, but its usefulness is almost non-existent because it is a Schedule I drug that is highly addicting and illegal to prescribe, manufacture, or import into the United States.

Hydromorphone (Dilaudid) is more potent than morphine, with a correspondingly higher potential for adverse effects. Its principle use is for acutely severe pain of short duration, and it is often prescribed to terminally ill cancer patients. In dentistry it finds use following oral surgery when there has been considerable trauma to soft tissue or bone. The usual adult dose is 2 mg P.O. q.4h.

Oxymorphone (Numorphan) is also more potent than morphine, and it has a high potential for adverse effects, notably, respiratory depression. The usual adult dose is between 1 and 1.5 mg I.M. or Sub-Q q.4h. It is generally not used in dentistry because less addicting agents are available with fewer side-effects (Chap. 8; Sec. 1).

Hydrocodone (Dicodid) is about as effective as codeine as an analgesic, but it has a greater antitussive effect and is as addicting as morphine. Although its principle use is as an antitussive given in adult doses between 5 and 10 mg P.O. q.i.d., it finds its way into some combination products for use as an analgesic.

Oxycodone is more potent an analgesic and is more addicting than codeine but is available only as an analgesic in the multiple-entity product Percodan (Chap. 8, Sec. 2). It is useful in dentistry for relief of moderately severe pain.

Levorphanol (Levo-Dromoran) is chemically related to morphine, is a more potent analgesic, and has a similar spectrum of adverse effects. Its particular advantages are that it is compatible with a wide range of anesthetics, that it reduces thiopental requirements during induction (Chap. 10, Sec. 1), and that recovery time is shorter than with other drugs. The average adult dose is between 2 and 3 mg P.O., I.V., or Sub-Q.

Opioids

Opioids are narcotic analgesics that are pharmacologically similar to morphine and codeine but chemically unrelated.

Meperidine (Demerol) is the most used narcotic analgesic in dentistry, except for codeine, and is about equal to codeine in potency. It is available in injection form and as 50 and 100 mg tablets, and the average adult dose is between 50 and 150 mg I.V., I.M., Sub-Q, or P.O. q.4h. Its value in dentistry is not only as a good alternate drug in cases of codeine allergy but also as pre-operative medication when both analgesia and sedation are desirable. Meperedine is often combined with other agents that potentiate analgesic effects, resulting in pain relief at a substandard dosage or in antipyresis.

Alphaprodine (Nisentil) is chemically similar to meperidine but is only administered parenterally and has a shorter duration of action. This property makes it useful in dentistry for I.V. sedation, and the average adult dose for dental procedures is between 20 and 30 mg I.V., combined with a narcotic antagonist (Chap. 8, Sec. 4).

Anileridine (Leritine) is pharmacologically similar to meperidine and is available in injection form and as 25 mg tablets. It is a good alternate drug when meperidine is contraindicated. The usual adult dose is between 25 and 50 mg P.O., I.M., or Sub-Q q.4h.

Methadone (Dolophine) is equal to morphine in analgesic potency and finds its major use in alleviating the opiate withdrawal syndrome. The addict is given methadone in high doses to make withdrawal from morphine or heroin tolerable; if he becomes addicted to methadone in the process, he can stop taking methadone more easily than an opiate. Methadone is available in injection form and as 5 and 10 mg tablets. The usual adult dose for relief of pain is between 2.5 and 10 mg P.O., I.M., or Sub-Q q4h.

Fentanyl (Sublimaze) is the most potent narcotic and finds use prior to or during general anesthesia when analgesic action of short duration is beneficial. It also produces a degree of sedation, and the usual adult dose for hospitalized patients is between 0.05 and 0.1 mg I.M. or I.V. When given as pre-anesthetic medication, it is often combined with droperidol as fentanyl citrate in the combination product **Innovar** (Chap. 7, Sec. 2; Chap. 10, Sec. 1). Recent studies suggest that fentanyl may be preferable to meperidine for ambulatory dental patients who expect to work shortly after treatment, since recovery from fentanyl is faster. Studies comparing equivalent doses of fentanyl and meperidine given postoperatively by I.M. injections to general surgery patients have shown that (1) blood pressure dropped with meperidine but not with fentanyl; (2) meperidine produced tachycardia in 80 per cent of the cases, whereas fentanyl produced bradycardia in about 75 per cent of the cases treated; and (3) meperidine significantly depressed respiration, whereas fentanyl did not. Severe fentanyl-induced bradycardia may be treated with atropine (Chap. 6, Sec. 2).

Narcotic Antagonists and Nalorphine Index

Narcotic antagonists are drugs that reverse the respiratory depression of concurrent narcotic administration but that have no pharmacological activity in the absence of a narcotic agonist. Most narcotic antagonists also possess morphine-like properties and are correctly termed narcotic agonist-antagonists. Narcotic agonist-antagonists behave as narcotics in many respects, but in the presence of a strong narcotic effect, they behave as narcotic antagonists.

Narcotic antagonist potency is measured by the *nalorphine index*, or the ratio of the antagonist potency of nalorphine (mg in numerator) with an equal quantity of another narcotic antagonist (mg in denominator) (Fig. 8–2).

Naloxone (Narcan) has no agonist, or morphine-like, properties and is a pure narcotic antagonist. It is given in a dose of 0.4 mg I.V. to adults to rapidly reverse narcotic depression induced by narcotics, propoxyphene (Darvon), or pentazocine (Talwin) overdose (Chap. 8, Sec. 1; Chap. 8, Sec. 2). Longer lasting effects can be obtained with supplemental I.M. or Sub-Q injections. Naloxone has enjoyed the greatest use of the narcotic antagonists because it has the highest potency and no agonist properties to complicate the clinical picture.

Narcotic Agonist-Antagonists

Nalorphine (Nalline) has a morphine index of about 0.1 but has never achieved any popularity as an analgesic alone because of the frequency and severity of adverse reactions. It can be injected I.V. in a dose between 5 and 10 mg to reverse respiratory depression in known or suspected cases of narcotic-induced depression; this may be repeated in 10 to 15 min as needed, not exceeding three doses.

Pentazocine (Talwin) is a potent narcotic and a weak antagonist that was first developed in a search for a potent analgesic for use in cases of codeine and meperidine

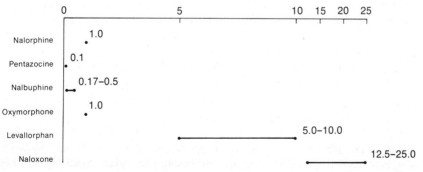

Figure 8–2. Nalorphine index of various narcotic antagonists. (Data based on efficacy at standard adult doses.)

allergy. The morphine index of pentazocine is between 0.25 and 0.5, and the usual adult dose is between 50 and 100 mg P.O. q.4h. or 30 mg I.M. or Sub-Q. Dental patients taking this drug for the first time should be forewarned of the possibility of severe adverse reactions of the psychogenic type.

Nalbuphine (Nubain) is a new drug with a morphine index between 0.75 and 1.5 and with a higher therapeutic index and fewer side-effects than pentazocine. It should prove to be a valuable drug in relieving severe pain and particularly useful in patients who are at a high risk of addiction to opiates. It is chemically related to naloxone and oxymorphone.

Oxymorphone (Numorphan, butorphanol), previously discussed as a synthetic opiate, is a potent antagonist approximately equal in strength to nalorphine. Since adverse reactions are common during its administration and more suitable drugs are available, it is used rarely as an analgesic and even less as an antagonist.

Levallorphan (Lorfan) has a morphine index of about 0.1 and is a very potent antagonist. It is given in a dose of 1 mg I.V., followed by one or two additional 0.5 doses at 10 to 15 minute intervals, if needed, to reverse respiratory depression induced by narcotics. The total dose should not exceed 3 mg. It is gaining popularity for use during I.V. sedation by dentists (Chap. 10, Sec. 2).

SECTION 2: NON-NARCOTICS

Antipyretics and Aspirin Index

Although not as potent as the narcotics, the non-narcotic analgesics play an equally important role in relieving pain of dental origin, and they may be divided into (1) the antipyretics and (2) the non-antipyretics.

Non-antipyretics produce only analgesia, whereas antipyretics also have fever-reducing potential. The *aspirin index* is the ratio of the analgesic potency of aspirin (mg in numerator) to an equal quantity of another analgesic drug (mg in denominator). Antipyretics may be further subdivided into (1) salicylates and (2) non-salicylates (Fig. 8–3).

The salicylates other than aspirin are salicylic acid, sodium salicylate, methyl salicylate, and salicylamide, and they find their way into certain combination products (Chap. 8, Sec. 2). **Acetylsalicylic acid** (aspirin) is the most widely recommended drug in dental practice, but it owes its analgesic effect to rapid plasma hydrolysis to form salicylic acid, which provides analgesia.

Aspirin has classically been associated with (1) antipyresis, (2) analgesia, and (3) antiinflammatory effects, but it also provides a decreased blood glucose level (antidiabetic effect), increased circulating thyroid hormone level (thyroid stimulating effect), decreased platelet adhesiveness and prolonged bleeding time (antithrombotic effect), and increased uric acid secretion with decreased plasma urate concentration (uricosuric effect). The usual dose is between 325 and 650 mg q.4h. for adults and 65 mg/kg/24 hrs in divided doses q.6h. for children. Aspirin is available only in tablet or capsule form or as rectal suppositories for enteral administration.

The principle adverse reaction to aspirin is painless gastric erosion and bleeding, which contraindicates the use of aspirin in patients who have a history of ulcers, gastritis, or hiatal hernia. With large doses or prolonged therapy, salicylate intoxication (salicylism) may ensue, characterized by headache, dizziness, tinnitus, fever, sweating, hyperventilation, or tachycardia.

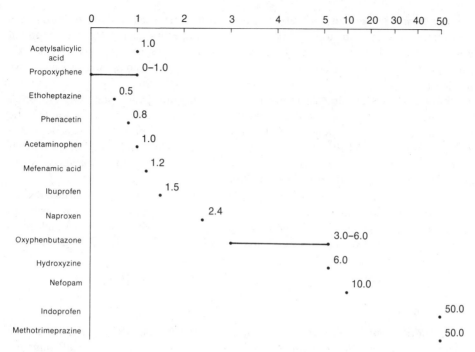

Figure 8–3. Aspirin index of various non-narcotic analgesics. (Data based on efficacy at standard adult doses.)

As an ingredient is combination products, aspirin is combined with antacids, other analgesics, sedatives, antihistamines, anticholinergic agents, or caffeine (Chap. 8, Sec. 2).

Acetaminophen (Tylenol, Tempra, Phenaphen, Datril, Nebs) has become the accepted alternative to aspirin in cases of aspirin allergy or when aspirin is contraindicated. It has no anti-inflammatory effects, and adult and child doses are the same as with aspirin. There is some evidence to suggest that doses of 1000 mg q.4h. are superior to regular 650 mg doses.

Unlike aspirin, acetaminophen has therapeutic effects of only analgesia and anti-pyresis. Persistently high fevers are often treated by administering aspirin and acetaminophen alternating every two hours and thereby obtaining peak blood levels of one while the blood levels of the other are lowering.

Phenacetin or acetophenetidin, is identical in effects to acetaminophen but has no particular advantage over the latter and is more prone to induce renal impairment and methemoglobinemia, a condition characterized by conversion of the ferrous iron in hemo-globin to the oxidized state (ferric), resulting in decreased ability to transport oxygen. Phenacetin is generally found in combination with other drugs (as the P in APC—aspirin, phenacetin, and caffeine). There is little justification for including it in multiple-entity products because it contributes additively rather than synergistically and has a narrower margin of safety than aspirin.

Mefenamic acid (Ponstel) possesses antipyretic, analgesic, and anti-inflammatory properties like aspirin and is available as 250 mg capsules. The usual adult dose is 500 mg, then 250 mg q.i.d. This agent has not become popular owing to troublesome and some-times serious adverse reactions often involving the gastrointestinal tract.

Oxyphenbutazone (Tandearil) also possesses antipyretic, analgesic, and anti-inflammatory effects like those of aspirin, mild uricosuric properties, and it has been reported useful following oral surgery. The usual adult dose is 100 mg q.i.d. and the drug is available as 100 mg tablets. Adverse reactions are commonly seen, among which are ulcerative stomatitis and parotitis.

Ibuprofen (Motrin) also has analgesic, anti-inflammatory, and antipyretic properties and causes less occult bleeding than does aspirin. It is marketed primarily for arthritic conditions but is gaining popularity for treatment of dental pain. It is available as 300 and 400 mg tablets and the usual adult dose is 300 or 400 mg t.i.d. or q.i.d. Although it is not devoid of adverse reactions, ibuprofen produces less gastric upset than does aspirin and shows promise as a future aspirin substitute.

Naproxen (Naprosyn) is identical to ibuprofen (Motrin) in its pharmacological effects but is slightly more potent as an analgesic. The usual adult dose is 250 mg b.i.d., and it is available as 250 mg tablets. Like aspirin, naproxen decreases platelet adhesiveness and prolongs bleeding time, but it has a higher incidence of adverse reactions than does ibuprofen.

Non-Antipyretics

In contrast with aspirin and its classic properties, the non-antipyretics (1) do not reduce body temperature in febrile states, (2) may or may not possess anti-inflammatory properties, and (3) provide analgesia in most cases but not all.

Propoxyphene hydrochloride (Darvon, Dolene) is sometimes included as a narcotic because it has a chemical structure similar to the narcotic methadone (Dolophine). Its only therapeutic effect is analgesia, and studies show considerable variation in its effectiveness. It is certainly no more, and probably less, effective than the usual doses of aspirin or APC. Some studies have shown that used by itself, propoxyphene is no more effective against pain than a placebo, and even inferior to a placebo. **Propoxyphene napsylate** (Darvon-N) is unlike the hydrochloride salt just discussed in that it is only slightly soluble in water, allowing more stable preparations to be made. Since the molecular weights of the two agents are different, 100 mg of propoxyphene napsylate is required to supply propoxyphene equivalent to 65 mg of propoxyphene hydrochloride, and these quantities are also the standard adult doses taken q.4h.

Although there are many combination products containing propoxyphene in its two forms, it is falling into disuse owing to its limited usefulness and the increasing potential for drug interactions and abuse (Chap. 11, Sec. 1). The following are the more commonly used preparations:

1. propoxyphene hydrochloride 32 mg (Darvon 32 mg)

2. propoxyphene hydrochloride 65 mg (Darvon 65 mg, Dolene)

3. propoxyphene hydrochloride 32 mg, APC (Darvon Compound)

4. propoxyphene hydrochloride 65 mg, APC (Darvon Compound 65)

5. propoxyphene hydrochloride 65 mg, 325 mg aspirin (Darvon with ASA)

6. propoxyphene hydrochloride 65 mg, 650 mg acetaminophen (Dolacet)

7. propoxyphene napsylate 100 mg (Darvon-N)

8. propoxyphene napsylate 100 mg, 325 mg aspirin (Darvon-N with ASA)

9. propoxyphene napsylate 50 mg, 325 mg acetaminophen (Darvocet-N 50)

10. propoxyphene napsylate 100 mg, 650 mg acetaminophen (Darvocet-N 100)

Ethoheptazine citrate (Zactane) is a weak analgesic like propoxyphene, but it has a chemical structure similar to the narcotic meperidine (Demerol). It is available as 75 mg tablets, which is the average adult dose, but it is usually combined with aspirin to increase its usefulness. Like propoxyphene, it offers no advantage over aspirin for relief of dental pain. It is administered q.4h. and is available as in the following forms:

1. ethoheptazine citrate 75 mg (Zactane)

2. ethoheptazine citrate 75 mg, 325 mg aspirin (Zactirin)

3. ethoheptazine citrate 100 mg, APC (Zactirin Compound-100)

4. ethoheptazine citrate 75 mg, 250 mg aspirin, 150 mg meprobamate (Equagesic)

In addition, the use of Equagesic, or any other analgesic combination product containing significant amounts of meprobamate, is questionable, since recent studies have shown that meprobamate in a 200 mg dose in combination with analgesics often causes the perception of greater postoperative pain than would be present without an analgesic. The effectiveness of meprobamate is statistically worse than that of a placebo in this regard.

Hydroxyzine (Vistaril, Atarax), previously discussed as a sedative, antihistamine, antispasmodic, and antiemetic in the diphenylmethane group of tranquilizers, also has potent analgesic properties of its own (Chap. 7, Sec. 2) and has been shown to be non-addicting and to potentiate potent analgesics. When given as a single dose of 100 mg I.M., hydroxyzine has effects equivalent to those produced by 8 mg morphine, and its analgesic activity appears to be additive to that of morphine when the two drugs are given together. Further studies of this agent as a potent analgesic certainly are indicated.

Nefopam hydrochloride is a new analgesic with a unique chemical structure unrelated to that of any known analgesic agent. It has no abuse potential and is not a respiratory depressant, but it is extremely potent in relieving pain. In addition, it has a faster onset than aspirin, and it causes no gastric bleeding. Adverse reactions appear to be fewer than with morphine, and like ibuprofen, it may prove to be a future aspirin substitute. The usual adult dose is 60 mg t.i.d.

The two most potent non-narcotic analgesics are indoprofen and methotrimeprazine (Levoprome). **Indoprofen** is a new phenylpropionic acid derivative with analgesic and anti-inflammatory properties, and it has been shown to be effective against cancer pain when given in an oral dose between 100 and 200 mg. **Methotrimeprazine** (Levoprome) is a phenothiazine tranquilizer with potent analgesic effects and no abuse or addiction potential (Chap. 7, Sec. 2). When it is used as an analgesic, 15 mg is equivalent to 10 mg of morphine. Both of these agents show promise in reducing the need for narcotics in the future.

Combination Products

It is often desirable to combine two or more agents in the same pharmaceutical product to provide enhancement of effect (Chap. 1, Sec. 1), and there are thousands of such combination products on the market. Most of those of interest to the dental profession contain narcotic and non-narcotic analgesics, but some contain antibiotics, vitamins, antihistamines, proteolytic enzymes, diuretics, antihypertensive agents, sedative-hypnotics, or tranquilizers. Further particulars regarding the actions of the ingredients in commonly used products will be found elsewhere in the text. The following is a list of such products:

ANTIBIOTICS:

Triple Sulfa, per tablet or teaspoon, contains

167 mg sulfadiazine
167 mg sulfamerazine
167 mg sulfamethazine

VITAMINS:

Vicon-C, per capsule, contains

20 mg thiamine
10 mg riboflavin
100 mg niacin
20 mg pantothenate
5 mg pyriodoxine
300 mg ascorbate
50 mg magnesium sulfate
50 mg zinc sulfate

ANTIHISTAMINES:

Dramitrol, per teaspoon, contains

12.5 mg dimenhydrinate
invert sugar (levulose and dextrose)
orthophosphoric acid

Dimetapp extentabs, per tablet, contains

12 mg brompheniramine maleate
15 mg phenylpropanolamine hydrochloride
15 mg phenylephrine hydrochloride

Dimetapp elixir, contains one third the above dose per teaspoon.

PROTEOLYTIC ENZYMES:

Orenzyme, per tablet, contains

50,000 units trypsin
4000 units chymotrypsin

ANTIHYPERTENSIVE AGENTS:

Dyazide, per capsule, contains

50 mg triamterene
25 mg hydrochlorothiazide

Esimil, per tablet, contains

10 mg guanethidine sulfate
25 mg hydrochlorothiazide

ANALGESICS, SEDATIVE-HYPNOTICS, TRANQUILIZERS

Empirin Compound (APC), per tablet or capsule, contains

227 mg aspirin
162 mg phenacetin
32 mg caffeine

Empirin Compound No. 1, 2, 3, or 4, per tablet, contains APC in the above dose and the following doses of codeine phosphate:

No. 1: 7.5 mg (1/8 gr)
No. 2: 15 mg (1/4 gr)
No. 3: 30 mg (1/2 gr)
No. 4: 60 mg (1 gr)

Tylenol No. 1, 2, 3, or 4, or Phenaphen No. 1, 2, 3, or 4, per tablet (Tylenol) or capsule (Phenaphen), contains 300 mg acetaminophen and the same doses of codeine phosphate as does Empirin Compound (above).

Darvon Compound 65, per capsule, contains 65 mg propoxyphene hydrochloride and Empirin Compound.

Fiorinal, per capsule, contains

200 mg aspirin
130 mg phenacetin
40 mg caffeine
50 mg butabarbital

Fiorinal with codeine No. 1, 2, 3, per capsule, contains Fiorinal in the above dose and the following doses of codeine phosphate:

No. 1: 7.5 mg (1/8 gr)
No. 2: 15 mg (1/4 gr)
No. 3: 30 mg (1/2 gr)

Synalgos, per capsule, contains

194 mg aspirin
162 mg phenacetin
30 mg caffeine
6.25 mg promethazine hydrochloride

Synalgos-DC, per capsule, contains Synalgos in the above dose and 16 mg dihydrocodeine bitartrate.

Percodan, per tablet, contains

224 mg aspirin
160 mg phenacetin

32 mg caffeine
4.5 mg oxycodone hydrochloride
0.38 mg oxycodone terephthalate

Vicodin, per tablet, contains

500 mg acetaminophen
5 mg hydrocodone bitartrate

Mepergan Fortis, per capsule, contains

50 mg meperidine hydrochloride
25 mg promethazine hydrochloride

Equagesic, per tablet, contains

250 mg aspirin
75 mg ethoheptazine citrate
150 mg meprobamate

Pedo-Sol, per tablet or teaspoon, contains

30 mg butabarbital
1.5 mg chlorpheniramine maleate
0.1 mg scopolamine

(This product was discontinued in January, 1979.)

The student should note that most of the analgesic combination products in this list contain aspirin (except Tylenol with Codeine, Phenaphen with Codeine, Vicodin, and Mepergan Fortis) and would be contraindicated in patients allergic to aspirin or having a history of ulcers, gastritis, or hiatal hernia.

Controlling Postoperative Discomfort

Patients who enter a dental office for the first time in pain usually have nothing to blame for their discomfort except a disease process; if they continue to suffer pain other than surgical soreness following their first contact with the dentist or hygienist, they will be very likely to direct that blame to something more tangible than a disease process, such as the dental operator, to convince themselves that they are not really sick anymore and thereby preserve their self-esteem. For this reason, it is especially important to effectively treat this particular type of patient at the first sitting, if possible, and to maintain him in a state of reasonable comfort immediately thereafter.

The human desire on the part of dentists to find an easy answer to the problems of patient infection, pain, and sedation and the fear of having to manage complications resulting from prescribing have contributed to widespread reliance on only a limited number of drugs to solve these problems and have led some dentists away from prescribing those drugs altogether. This pattern helps to explain the present tendency toward overuse of penicillins, propoxyphene, and nitrous oxide by the average general dentist. The dangers inherent in such laxity or in reliance on making clinical problems fit a limited drug vocabulary are (1) that the proper drug may be administered only after a delay or when the healing process is nearing completion, which can result in unnecessary suffering, and (2) visceral repercussions secondary to emotional distress resulting from prolonged unabating pain.

Analgesics may be considered in a general dental practice to decrease postoperative discomfort following (1) subgingival débridement; (2) subgingival curettage or soft tissue oral surgery; (3) dental extractions, bone surgery, or a combination of the two; (4) periapical irritations secondary to endodontic therapy; (5) gingival irritations secondary to crown and bridge retraction; or (6) pressure sores secondary to insertion of new dentures. Assuming minimal trauma, rigidly enforced aseptic conditions, and an uncompromised patient health status, non-narcotic single-entity drugs may be all that are required to provide reasonable postoperative comfort for any of these conditions. However, dental extractions, with or without bone surgery and periapical irritations secondary to endodontic therapy, often require the employment of a narcotic or multiple-entity combination product to supply sufficient analgesia, and nothing more potent that a Schedule III product, such as acetaminophen with codeine (Tylenol No. 3), Synalgos-DC, or Vicodin, should be employed first. Percodan, Mepergan Fortis, Dilaudid, and other Schedule II preparations should be reserved for limited use in cases unresponsive to agents in Schedule III.

TEST QUESTIONS

1. Undesirable effects of narcotics include all of the following EXCEPT:
   (a) respiratory depression
   (b) nausea and vomiting
   (c) dimness of vision
   (d) decreased mental alertness
   (e) lethargy
   (f) prolonged bleeding time
2. The most commonly used naturally occurring opiates are:
   (a) meperidine and methadone
   (b) morphine and codeine
   (c) fentanyl and alphaprodine
   (d) oxymorphone and oxycodone
3. All of the following are synthetic opiates EXCEPT:
   (a) hydromorphone
   (b) hydrocodone
   (c) oxymorphone
   (d) oxycodone
   (e) levorphanol
   (f) meperidine
4. All of the following are opioids EXCEPT:
   (a) meperidine
   (b) alphaprodine
   (c) codeine
   (d) anileridine
   (e) methadone
   (f) fentanyl
5. All of the following are narcotic agonist-antagonists EXCEPT:
   (a) naloxone
   (b) nalorphine
   (c) pentazocine
   (d) nalbuphine
   (e) oxymorphone
   (f) levallorphan
6. The most widely recommended drug in dental practice is:
   (a) codeine sulfate
   (b) penicillin V potassium
   (c) aspirin
   (d) propoxyphene hydrochloride
7. The most potent narcotic analgesic is:
   (a) hydromorphone
   (b) fentanyl
   (c) oxymorphone
   (d) levorphanol
   (e) methadone
   (f) methotrimeprazine

8. All of the following are antipyretic analgesics EXCEPT:
   - (a) aspirin
   - (b) acetaminophen
   - (c) phenacetin
   - (d) mefenamic acid
   - (e) oxyphenbutazone
   - (f) ibuprofen
   - (g) naproxen
   - (h) propoxyphene hydrochloride

9. Non-antipyretic analgesics include all of the following EXCEPT:
   - (a) propoxyphene hydrochloride
   - (b) ethoheptazine citrate
   - (c) acetaminophen
   - (d) hydroxyzine
   - (e) nefopam hydrochloride
   - (f) methotrimeprazine
   - (g) indoprofen
   - (h) propoxyphene napsylate

10. An undesirable effect of APC (aspirin, phenacetin, caffeine) is:
    - (a) gastric erosion and bleeding
    - (b) prolonged bleeding time
    - (c) renal impairment with chronic use
    - (d) unnecessary CNS stimulation
    - (e) alterations in blood surgar levels
    - (f) all of the above

11. Dental patients with a history of ulcers, gastritis, or hiatal hernia should NOT be given:
    - (a) aspirin
    - (b) Empirin Compound
    - (c) Darvon Compound 65
    - (d) Fiorinal
    - (e) Synalgos
    - (f) Percodan
    - (g) Equagesic
    - (h) a, b, and c
    - (i) a, d, and e
    - (j) a, d, e, f, and g
    - (k) any of the above

12. The most potent non-narcotic analgesics are:
    - (a) indoprofen and methotrimeprazine
    - (b) hydroxyzine and nefopam hydro-chloride
    - (c) naproxen and oxyphenbutazone
    - (d) morphine and codeine
    - (e) meperidine and methadone
    - (f) fentanyl and droperidol

13. Narcotic combination products that notably do NOT contain aspirin are:
    - (a) Tylenol with codeine
    - (b) Phenaphen with codeine
    - (c) Vicodin
    - (d) Mepergan Fortis
    - (e) Synalgos-DC
    - (f) Fiorinal with codeine
    - (g) Empirin Compound with codeine
    - (h) a, b, and c
    - (i) a, b, c, and d
    - (j) a, d, e, f, and g
    - (k) any of the above

14. Schedule II narcotics should not be prescribed for routine postoperative care following oral surgery until the patient's response is verified with a Schedule III narcotic, such as:
    - (a) Tylenol No. 3
    - (b) Phenaphen No. 3
    - (c) Vicodin
    - (d) Synalgos-DC
    - (e) Empirin Compound No. 3
    - (f) any of the above

15. The most widely prescribed narcotic in dental practice is:
    - (a) meperidine hydrochloride
    - (b) codeine
    - (c) propoxyphene hydrochloride
    - (d) pentazocine

16. The second most widely prescribed narcotic in dental practice is:
    - (a) meperidine hydrochloride
    - (b) codeine
    - (c) propoxyphene hydrochloride
    - (d) pentazocine

9

LOCAL ANESTHESIA

SECTION 1: MECHANISM AND AGENTS

Resting Membrane Potential

The membranes of all cells of the body create a minute electrical potential due to an uneven distribution of ionic charges on both sides of the membrane. When the total molar concentrations of ions on either side of a semipermeable membrane are known, the membrane potential at body temperature ($37°$ C) can be determined from the following equation:

$$EMF = 61 \log \frac{C_i}{C_o} = 61 \, (\log C_i - \log C_o)$$

EMF = electromotive force or membrane potential (millivolts)
C_i = ion concentration on the inside (moles)
C_o = ion concentration on the outside (moles)

It can be seen from this equation that when the total ion concentration on the inside of a cell is ten times that on the outside, the potential difference across the membrane is 61 mv (the log of ten is one and the log of one is zero). Conversely, when the total ion concentration on the outside of a cell is ten times that on the inside, the potential difference across the membrane is –61 mv.

Specialized excitable cells, such as nerve, muscle, and odontoblasts, allow passive diffusion and active transport of sodium ions (Na^+) and potassium ions (K^+) and carry the highest membrane potentials of any cells. It has been shown that in excitable cells sodium ions are metabolically extruded out of the cell and potassium ions metabolically intruded into the cell by active transport mechanisms that are as yet unidentified. This process requires energy and occurs against a concentration gradient (Chap. 1, Sec. 1). This active transport mechanism (called the sodium pump) produces a surplus of positive

135

charges on the outside of the membrane relative to the charges on the inside; micro-electrodes have been inserted into nerve axons and other tissue preparations and have shown that the resting membrane potential for nerve and muscle cells is about −85 mv and for odontoblasts about −40 mv, indicating a surplus of ions (mainly sodium) on the outside of the membrane.

Passive diffusion of sodium and potassium ions also occurs through membrane pores about 8 angstroms (Å) in diameter in most membranes. This process occurs along a concentration gradient and does not require energy (Chap. 1, Sec. 1). Membranes are more permeable to diffusion of potassium ions than of sodium ions because the diameter of a hydrated potassium ion (3.96 Å) is less than the diameter of a hydrated sodium ion (5.12 Å). Membrane pores are lined with positive charges that tend to repel small positively charged ions and to allow passage of larger negatively charged particles. Because of the influence of these positive charges along the inside of membrane pores, sodium ions leak through membranes only with great difficulty, whereas potassium ions pass through much more readily.

External stimuli or disturbances of the membrane produce a change in the membrane permeability to sodium, allowing sodium to enter the cell more readily. If the stimulus disturbs an excitable membrane of a neuron, there is a decrease in the potential difference of the membrane, termed a "local excitatory state." If the local excitatory state is of sufficient intensity to reach a certain threshold value, a rapid influx of sodium ions will occur, and this is propagated from the stimulus along the nerve fiber in both directions; this is followed by rapid extracellular diffusion of potassium ions to balance the charge outside the cell. This sequence of events is termed an "action potential," or nerve impulse.

Action potentials normally occur in a matter of a few milliseconds and proceed down the nerve fiber at velocities in the range of 0.5 to 130 m/sec. The velocity is proportional to the diameter of the fiber. The number of ions exchanging places along the membrane with each action potential is extremely minute but has been measured as 4×10^{-12} moles/cm^2.

A nerve impulse passes down a nerve fiber only if the strength of the local excitatory state is greater than the threshold potential. The safety factor is defined as the ratio of the action potential amplitude to the threshold potential, a ratio which in the normal nerve membrane is always a number greater than one. If a drug that reduces membrane permeability to sodium ions (local anesthetic) is deposited in solution in the vicinity of the nerve membrane, the resting membrane potential would remain unaltered, but the action potential amplitude would be decreased, and the threshold potential would be increased; this would reduce the safety factor to a number less than one, and the impulse would fail to pass across the affected area of the fiber.

Local anesthetics are used to prevent afferent impulses from reaching the CNS by virtue of their ability to produce a reversible blockade of peripheral nerves. They can also affect the functioning of any tissue or organ dependent on impulse conduction (heart, brain, ganglia, or neuromuscular junctions), and some can be used as cardiac anti-arrhythmic agents (Chap. 6, Sec. 1). Drugs that are associated with local anesthetic activity include benzoic acid esters, certain non-ester anilide drugs, cocaine, and certain antihistamines, such as diphenhydramine (Benadryl). Although there are other agents that have been shown to possess weak local anesthetic activity when injected into tissues, they are of no clinical importance.

Membrane-Stabilizing Drugs

The local anesthetics are classified according to the route of administration and are either topical or injectable. The injectable anesthetics include (1) esters of benzoic acid, meta-aminobenzoic acid, and para-aminobenzoic acid and (2) non-ester (anilide) derivatives of xylidine, toluidine, and other agents. Clinically, the most important drugs in this group are the para-aminobenzoic acid esters procaine, chloroprocaine, propoxycaine, and tetracaine, and the anilide drugs lidocaine, mepivacaine, and prilocaine.

Procaine hydrochloride (Novocain) 2 per cent is used in dentistry for peripheral nerve block but has vasodilating properties that result in rapid absorption and short duration of action. Its use is often supplemented with use of other anesthetics (e.g., propoxycaine) when anesthesia will be difficult to obtain or longer duration is needed. It is relatively ineffective when used topically, and the maximum dosage should not exceed 400 mg. Like all local anesthetics, it is capable of stimulating or depressing the CNS, and large doses cause a decrease in peripheral resistance, blockade of autonomic ganglia, myocardial depression, and profound hypotension (Chap. 6, Sec. 1; Chap. 12, Sec. 1).

Chloroprocaine hydrochloride (Nesacaine) is twice as potent as procaine and is also used in a 2 per cent solution for nerve block in dentistry. It has a short duration similar to that of procaine, and its use is often supplemented with that of a vasoconstrictor (Chap. 9, Sec. 1). The maximal dose should not exceed 800 mg.

Propoxycaine hydrochloride (Ravocaine) also has vasodilating properties but has a more rapid onset and produces a greater depth of anesthesia than procaine. It is more potent that chloroprocaine and therefore more toxic, and for this reason it is not used alone, but instead a small amount is mixed with procaine 2 per cent and a vasoconstrictor. When used in this fashion as a 0.4 per cent solution, the maximal dose should not exceed 30 mg.

Tetracaine hydrochloride (Pontocaine) is about ten times as potent and toxic as procaine but seems more like cocaine in pharmacological action. It is even more potent than propoxycaine and is generally mixed with procaine 2 per cent and a vasoconstrictor when given by injection. It may also be administered topically, as cocaine is. A 1 per cent solution is used for spinal anesthesia, and this is diluted to 0.15 per cent for nerve blocking. The maximal dose should not exceed 30 mg.

Procaine, chloroprocaine, propoxycaine, and tetracaine are all para-aminobenzoic acid (PABA) derivatives and should not be administered to patients taking sulfonamides (Chap. 2, Sec. 2; Chap. 11, Sec. 1).

Lidocaine hydrochloride (Xylocaine, Octocaine) is a non-ester (anilide) derivative of xylidine and is the most commonly used local anesthetic in dentistry. It is about twice as potent as procaine but more toxic, and it has a duration of between 1 and 1.5 hours when used as a 2 per cent solution with a vasoconstrictor. Like procaine, it can be used as an antiarrhythmic agent (Chap. 6, Sec. 1), and the maximal dose should not exceed 300 mg.

Mepivacaine hydrochloride (Carbocaine, Isocaine) is another non-ester (anilide) derivative of xylidine and is very similar to lidocaine in pharmacological action. It is used as a 2 per cent solution with a vasoconstrictor and as a 3 per cent solution without a vasoconstrictor. The duration of the 3 per cent solution without a vasoconstrictor is between 2 and 2.5 hours, and the maximal dose should not exceed 300 mg.

Prilocaine hydrochloride (Citanest) is another non-ester (anilide) derivative of toluidine and has a duration of anesthesia similar to mepivacaine (between 2 and 2.5 hours).

It is only about 60 per cent as toxic as lidocaine and is more effective with less vaso-constrictor than is lidocaine. Prilocaine hydrochloride is used as a 4 per cent solution for nerve blocking, and the maximal dose should not exceed 400 mg. In some patients methemoglobinemia will develop after administration of more than 400 mg prilocaine, a condition characterized by conversion of the ferrous iron (Fe^{++}) in hemoglobin to the ferric state (Fe^{+++}), resulting in decreased oxygen binding capacity and cyanosis of the lips and nailbeds.

The injectable local anesthetics that are most commonly used and that are available in a 1.8 cc dental cartridge are procaine-propoxycaine (Ravocaine-RNL), lidocaine (Xylocaine, Octocaine), mepivacaine (Carbocaine, Isocaine), and prilocaine (Citanest). Patients who are allergic to conventional local anesthetics and in whom general anes-thetics are contraindicated may, for nerve blocking, be given injectable antihistamines, such as diphenhydramine (Chap. 9, Sec. 2; Chap. 5, Sec. 4) supplemented with (1) oral, I.M., or I.V. sedation using narcotic analgesics, such as meperidine (Chap. 8, Sec. 1; Chap. 10, Sec. 2); (2) inhalation sedation using nitrous oxide oxygen (Chap. 10, Sec. 3); (3) hypnosis (Chap. 10, Sec. 3); or (4) hyperstimulation analgesia (Chap. 10, Sec. 3) to raise the pain threshold.

Vasoconstrictors

Vasoconstrictors are autonomic drugs that are added to local anesthetic solutions to stimulate alpha receptors in the vicinity of the injection, resulting in vasoconstriction (Chap. 6, Sec. 2). This vasoconstriction is desirable (1) to slow the systemic absorption of the anesthetic, thus decreasing its toxicity; (2) to prolong the duration of anesthesia; (3) to increase visibility at the surgical site by reducing hemorrhage; and (4) to permit smaller volumes of solution to be used. The disadvantages of using vasoconstrictors in local anesthetic solutions are that (1) local postoperative ischemia can develop; (2) there may be unwanted hyperglycemic effects, particularly with diabetic patients; (3) there may be mild CNS stimulation producing tachycardia; and (4) there are unwanted cardio-vascular effects made evident by inadvertent I.V. injection, and these include hyper-tensive action, tachycardia, and arrhythmias. Careful aspiration before injecting will virtually eliminate unwanted cardiovascular effects.

Vasoconstrictors are indicated for use in local anesthetic solutions when adding them will contribute to adequate anesthesia in patients who have cardiac disease. According to the American Heart Association, the adrenalin released in response to painful stimuli occurring when dental operations are performed under inadequate local anesthesia presents a greater hazard to the cardiac patient than does the minimal amount of vaso-constrictor contained in the usual local anesthetic solution, especially when proper caution is taken to prevent inadvertent I.V. injection (Chap. 13, Sec. 1). Although vaso-constrictors do not have any effect on the profoundness of anesthesia, their use in cardiac patients insures that the duration of anesthesia is satisfactory without resorting to re-peated injections.

Because of potentially fatal interactions, vasoconstrictors should not be given to patients who are diabetic or hyperthyroid or who are taking drugs causing blood pressure alterations (phenothiazines, MAO inhibitors, or tricyclic antidepressants) or who have recently been given or will soon receive a gaseous anesthetic or oxytocic drug (Chap. 11, Sec. 1; Chap. 13, Sec. 1).

The vasoconstrictors most commonly used in dental local anesthetic solutions are epinephrine (Adrenalin Chloride), norepinephrine (Levophed), and levonordefrin (Neo-Cobefrin). Under ordinary circumstances there is no need to administer a quantity of epinephrine in a concentration greater than 1:100,000 for dental local anesthesia, although the 1:50,000 concentration is occasionally used. Norepinephrine and levonordefrin when used are added in concentrations of 1:30,000 and 1:20,000 respectively (Chap. 6, Sec. 2).

The following are the usual local anesthetic solutions that can be stocked in a dental office:

1. Procaine-propoxycaine (Ravocaine-RNL, with Levophed 1:30,000)

2. Lidocaine 2 per cent plain

3. Lidocaine 2 per cent, with epinephrine 1:50,000

4. Lidocaine 2 per cent, with epinephrine 1:100,000

5. Mepivacaine 3 per cent plain

6. Mepivacaine 2 per cent, with Neo-Cobefrin 1:20,000

7. Prilocaine 4 per cent plain (Citanest)

8. Prilocaine 4 per cent, with epinephrine 1:200,000 (Citanest Forte)

The solutions in this list become outdated when their shelf-lives expire, which is usually three or four years after the solutions are manufactured. Injections of outdated anesthetic may result in local anesthesia lasting for several days.

Topical Anesthetics

Since there are so many over-the-counter mouthwashes, sprays, ointments, troches, and lozenges containing local anesthetics in varying concentrations, this text will focus only on those products of particular clinical interest when used in the oral cavity (Chap. 9, Sec. 1).

Although topical anesthetics have been used to inhibit the gag reflex prior to making maxillary impressions or periapical radiographs of maxillary teeth, their most common use is for providing surface anesthesia of the oral mucosa just prior to needle insertion. A pressurized spray is no more effective for this purpose than is a liquid applied with a cotton applicator. Topical anesthetics are not effective treatment against the cause of many disease states associated with pain in an area of the mouth, and they can actually complicate diagnosis by interfering with pain perception. Patients who request an "anesthetic mouthwash" or other similar product for routine home use should have an oral examination to uncover the cause of the discomfort. The treatment of some oral lesions, such as recurrent **aphthous stomatitis** (canker sores), with a steroid in an emollient base (triamcinolone acetonide 0.1 per cent in Orabase) is more effective than administration of a topical anesthetic ad libitum, which only treats a symptom of the underlying condition.

The use of any topical anesthetic in the mouth results in saliva carrying a small amount of it into the pharynx, which can temporarily anesthesize portions of the pharyngeal wall. This may interfere with normal sensory perception of the location of the food bolus during swallowing, especially in children. Patients who have had a topical anesthetic placed in their mouths should not have anything to eat for 60 minutes following its application. Since the average dental appointment lasts between 30 and 60 minutes, topical anesthetics are usually placed at the beginning of the procedure, and since the ambulatory dental patient usually has no access to food for at least 60 minutes after the scheduled time of his appointment, no verbal instructions need be given under these conditions. Advice about not eating after application of a topical anesthetic should be reserved for those who have had an extremely short procedure requiring topical anesthesia before the noon hour or at the end of the day in order to avoid generating unnecessary concern in the majority of patients about trapping food in the trachea.

The actions and use of cocaine as a topical local anesthetic have been described previously (Chap. 7, Sec. 2). As an anesthetic, it is generally considered too toxic to be given by injection.

Ethyl aminobenzoate, or Benzocaine, is a PABA ester similar to tetracaine but is less potent and less toxic than either tetracaine or lidocaine. It is marketed as a liquid or gel (Hurricaine, Gingicaine), as an ointment (Benzodent), as a spray, ointment, or liquid combined with tetracaine (Cetacaine), and as a liquid combined with phenol, iodine, and ethyl alcohol (Anbesol). The disadvantages of using it are that it is sensitizing and can produce methemoglobinemia (Chap. 9, Sec. 1), as can prilocaine.

Lidocaine is available both as a liquid and as an ointment (Xylocaine) for topical application. A special preparation in carboxymethylcellulose (Xylocaine Viscous) can be used as adjunctive therapy for severe pharyngitis associated with infectious mononucleosis or strep throat as well as non-specific tonsillar infections. It is also available as a dental spray (Chap. 6, Sec. 1; Chap. 9, Sec. 1).

SECTION 2: INTRAORAL INJECTIONS

Dental Needles

Local anesthesia and conscious pain control in dentistry are primarily accomplished through peripheral nerve block using local anesthetic drugs administered by means of needle injections. Such dental injections may be either intraoral or extraoral in their approach; most so-called "infiltrations" are intraoral in approach and are the type most commonly performed by the hygienist for mucosal anesthesia during deep scaling or root planing. Many states are now permitting the expanded-function dental hygienist to perform infiltration injections, and the time may come when block injections will also be allowed.

Dental injections are most tolerable to a patient when (1) topical anesthetics are used prior to needle puncture, (2) the needle is sharp, (3) the needle is the proper gauge, (4) direct thrusts of the needle in penetrating tissue are avoided, (5) vigorous aspiration is avoided, and (6) the solution is injected slowly into tissue (Chap. 9, Sec. 2).

The gauge of any needle is measured by means of gauge numbers indicating the lumen diameter of the shank; the larger gauge numbers indicate the smaller diameter needles. The length of a needle is measured from the hub to the point of the bevel. Dental needles range from 20 to 27 gauge and from $\frac{1}{2}$ to 4 inches in length; the most commonly used needles are 25 gauge (0.45 mm in diameter) $1\frac{1}{4}$ inch needles for infiltration injections and 23 gauge (0.57 mm diameter) $1\frac{5}{8}$ inch needles for nerve block injections. A heavier and longer needle is desirable for block injections when the insertion will be deep into tissue, because the needle will be rigid enough to be guided to the target area without bending, breakage is less likely to occur, aspiration is easier through the larger lumen, and the needle is less likely to penetrate smaller blood vessels.

In this day and age of high quality control and mass production there is no reason to resterilize a dental needle after an injection is made; it should be discarded altogether to rule out completely the problem of cross-contamination of patients with septic needles.

Septic Transmission of Serum Hepatitis

The problem of transmission of serum hepatitis by means of septic dental procedures has been described previously (Chap. 5, Sec. 3). As just stated, no dental needles should be resterilized after use; they should be discarded. It should be remembered that no matter how well the external surface of a needle is scrubbed and rinsed free of soap, blood, or mucus, the interior of the needle cannot be cleaned free of coagulated blood. This fact alone should be sufficient to persuade practitioners to discard needles after use; fortunately, it is economically feasible to do so today because of technological advances made in mass production and quality control. The slight additional cost of using a new needle with each patient is vastly outweighed by the operator's peace of mind in knowing that the needle is sharp, guaranteed sterile, and guaranteed rust-free on the inside.

Types of Injections

The approach of dental injections may be either extraoral or intraoral. Extraoral injections of local anesthetics in dentistry may be used to anesthetize (1) the temporo-mandibular joint, (2) the upper jaw, (3) the lower jaw, (4) the infraorbital nerve, (5) the mental nerve, (6) the entire maxillary nerve and its branches, and (7) the entire mandibular nerve and its branches. Intraoral injections of local anesthetics in dentistry are more commonly used and are divided into the (1) supraperiosteal (infiltration) injections, which rely mainly on diffusion; (2) block injections, which rely very little on diffusion; and (3) miscellaneous injections, which rely on diffusion to a certain extent but not as much as do infiltrations.

Supraperiosteal (infiltration) injections may be used to anesthetize the anterior, middle, or posterior superior alveolar nerves, as well as any individual teeth except the mandibular molars. The block injections include (1) the zygomatic block, (2) the infraorbital block, (3) the mental block, and (4) the mandibular block. The miscellaneous injections include (1) the long buccal, (2) the lingual, (3) the nasopalatine, (4) the posterior palatine, (5) the partial palatine, (6) the intraseptal, and (7) the intrapulpal injections.

Infiltration injections to anesthetize the mandibular molars are usually unsuccessful because the buccal cortical plate of bone in this area is extremely dense and inhibits diffusion of the local anesthetic solution. Infections also inhibit diffusion; injecting into infected tissue is contraindicated because anesthesia will usually be incomplete and because the needle may succeed in penetrating deeper into uninfected tissue and contribute to the spread of infection.

When profound local anesthesia cannot be obtained with supraperiosteal injections supplemented by block anesthesia or other injections, there are a number of alternatives other than performing painful dentistry: (1) a small amount of hyaluronidase may be added to the local anesthetic solution and the injections repeated (Chap. 9, Sec. 2), (2) parenteral sedation or relative analgesia can be considered for future appointments, (3) a general anesthetic may be administered, or (4) extraoral injections to block the upper or lower jaw may be given. There have been reports that a solution of 0.3 cc dexamethasone (Decadron) 4 per cent, 0.3 cc procaine hydrochloride (Novocain) 2 per cent, and 0.3 cc Vitamin B_{12} 0.1 per cent (0.9 cc in all) injected Sub-Q 0.5 cm anterior to the tragus of the ear will produce immediate anesthesia of the upper jaw on the affected side, whereas injection of this solution at the juncture of the ear lobe with the face will produce anesthesia of the lower jaw on the affected side. This procedure has been shown to bring relief to the pain of pulpalgia, periapical or periodontal abscess, local trauma, and other conditions that manifest themselves as toothaches (such as sinusitis or ear infection) in about 99 per cent of cases, but it is not known to what extent it is effective in the absence of pain. It has been postulated that the relief of pain by this solution is secondary to reduction of inflammation triggered by dexamethasone, which is helped in this capacity by the local anesthetic properties of procaine and the neurotropic effects of Vitamin B_{12}. In the studies published in the preliminary reports on this combination, the solution was administered with a 26 gauge needle and a tuberculin syringe, and repeated injections for relief of pain were not needed in the majority of patients so treated.

The intraoral approach to nerve block anesthesia of the entire maxillary nerve and its branches is accomplished by entering the greater palatine foramen, traversing the pterygopalatine canal with the needle, and then depositing the solution into the superior portion of the pterygopalatine fossa, where the main trunk of the maxillary division of the trigeminal nerve is located. This approach is particularly useful for sinus operations or in cases of facial trauma.

Procedure for Infiltration Anesthesia

There are many recommended methods for the proper administration of local anesthetics by injection; the author has used the following general guidelines to administer thousands of intraoral injections in a manner comfortable to the patient.

The preferred method of beginning an injection is to dry the puncture site with a gauze square and apply a disinfecting agent. This will minimize the number of bacteria pushed into muscle but will not totally eliminate the possibility of a postoperative reaction in the area of the needle puncture. Clinically, the incidence of postoperative infectious complications secondary to needle insertions performed without such disinfection is almost non-existent.

The point of needle placement for all supraperiosteal (infiltration) injections, for all block injections except the mandibular block, and for the long buccal injection is in the deepest point of the mucobuccal fold. A cotton applicator lightly saturated with topical anesthetic should be placed in this area for between one and two minutes prior to needle insertion. During this time, the subject of needles and injections should be avoided in conversation, and the operator should create conversation designed to keep the patient's attention distracted by dwelling on such topics as the weather, food, and movies. During this time the cotton applicator is withdrawn from the mouth, the lip or cheek is lightly retracted with the fingers, and the aspirating syringe is grasped as the dental assistant removes the needle sheath behind the patient's head. The needle point is positioned at the deepest point of the mucobuccal fold and held there while the lip is gently moved over the needle to puncture the mucosa; a "stab" with a direct thrust of the needle is more unpleasant to the patient than if the tissues are brought to the needle and the lip is moved up and down about once a second as the needle is advanced. This maneuver may succeed in tricking the patient into thinking that only movement of his lip is occurring and that the operator wants only to loosen up the lip for some reason.

After the needle initially punctures the mucosa a small amount of anesthetic solution (about 0.1 cc) is injected very slowly while the lip continues to be wiggled; the operator should next wait between 10 and 15 seconds for diffusion to begin and then deposit the remainder of the solution slowly. The tissues should not be ballooned out rapidly on the assumption that it is best to "get in and get out"; while this short cut may save a small amount of time, the injection site will be very sore when the anesthesia wears off, and the injection itself is most uncomfortable.

Recent studies claim that in between 2 and 3 per cent of all intraoral injections, blood will be drawn into the syringe during aspiration (pulling back on the plunger), and the injection will result in I.V. administration unless the needle is withdrawn and redirected into the tissues. In the author's experience the incidence of vascular penetration is somewhat less than two or three per cent, but it occurs with enough frequency to justify aspiration before any solution is deposited into tissue. Aspiration should be done gently, so that no more than $\frac{1}{2}$ ounce of negative pressure is created inside the needle lumen; additional aspiration is not required to determine the presence or absence of blood in the dental cartridge and can result in additional postoperative discomfort. Hemorrhage from the puncture point secondary to vessel rupture can be controlled by rolling a gauze square and placing it in the mucobuccal fold for a few minutes.

The most common errors made by dental hygiene students during administration of local anesthetics are (1) approaching the face of the patient with a trembling syringe, (2) injecting solution into the mouth before needle penetration, and (3) making too many needle insertions. These errors can be minimized by understanding fully the anatomy involved, checking to be sure the needle is indeed into tissue before injecting, and practicing injections on manikins, cadavers, or fellow students when such opportunities are available. The patient will not appreciate being injected by anyone who has to be "talked through" the procedure by an instructor, and the patient will be less likely to develop syncope when the beginner makes the injection unassisted.

Profound gingival anesthesia sufficient for deep scaling, root planing, or soft tissue curettage can be expected about five minutes after administration of a supraperiosteal injection.

Complications

Local complications have been known to occur with administration of injectable local anesthetics and most commonly involve (1) broken needles, (2) trismus, (3) tissue desquamation, (4) bacterial contamination, and (5) soft tissue trauma during the postoperative period.

The following precautions are suggested: (1) do not attempt to force a needle against a resistance when it is embedded in tissue, (2) do not use a needle with too fine a gauge or a needle that has been used before on another patient, (3) do not attempt to change the direction of the needle while it is embedded in tissue, (4) do not bury a needle in tissue all the way to the hub—always have at least one third of the needle shank visible, (5) do not attempt injections when uncertain about the anatomy of the area, (6) do not hurry during the injection sequence, (7) avoid anesthetizing both sides of the mouth at the same time, (8) advise the patient to eat carefully on the unaffected side of his mouth until the anesthetic wears off, and (9) maintain aseptic technique.

Hyaluronidase, Antisialagogues, and Antihistamines

Hyaluronic acid is a substance present in all tissues that tends to block diffusion of foreign substances and that can be responsible for failure to obtain profound local anesthesia by means of supraperiosteal injections in a certain percentage of cases. Some bacteria owe their invasiveness to their ability to manufacture an enzyme (hyaluronidase) that hydrolyzes hyaluronic acid, promoting diffusion of the bacterial toxic products. Whenever supplemental local injections fail to produce satisfactory local anesthesia, a small amount of **hyaluronidase** (Wydase, Alidase) may be drawn into the syringe with a small quantity of anesthetic solution and injected into the previously anesthetized area to promote diffusion of the local anesthetic. Hyaluronidase is marketed as 150 units of powder to which must be added 1 cc of sterile saline (0.9 per cent NaC1) for proper reconstitution for injection. The approximate effective dose of hyaluronidase solution needed to enhance local anesthesia in the oral cavity is 75 units (0.5 cc). Its effectiveness is increased when between 0.5 and 1 cc of anesthetic solution is injected simultaneously, since the rate and extent of diffusion is proportional to the volume of solution used. Hyaluronidase is most effective when combined with anesthetic solutions containing no vasoconstrictor, which if present would reduce diffusion of the mixture and increase the loss of enzyme activity. The rationale for using the mixture with a vasoconstrictor is questionable, because hyaluronidase increases absorption of the anesthetic, which is an effect opposite to that of the vasoconstrictor. By shortening the duration of anesthesia, hyaluronidase also increases the toxicity of the anesthetic (Chap. 12, Sec. 1). It may be given over a previous injection containing a vasoconstrictor, but such polypharmacy would be difficult to justify in a court of law. For this reason it is best to give patients needing this drug a second appointment and to use no vasoconstrictor at the next sitting. Hyaluronidase is seldom associated with allergic reactions and is often effective in the presence of a vasoconstrictor.

An anticholinergic drug used primarily to reduce salivary flow is termed an antisialagogue; the most commonly used agent in this category is methantheline bromide (Banthine), and its use for this purpose has been described previously (Chap. 6, Sec. 2). This drug also is supplied in a vial that contains 50 mg of powder to which must be added 1 cc of bacteriostatic water to reconstitute the drug for injection. About five minutes are required for the effects of the drug to become apparent. Unlike hyaluronidase, the effectiveness of this agent is not increased by injecting a small amount of anesthetic solution along with it.

The use of injectable antihistamines, such as diphenhydramine (Benadryl), as weak local anesthetics has also been described previously (Chap. 9, Sec. 1). These agents may also be combined with hyaluronidase to enhance their effectiveness.

TEST QUESTIONS

1. Drugs associated with local anesthetic activity include all of the following EXCEPT:
   (a) cocaine
   (b) benzoic acid esters
   (c) lidocaine
   (d) procainamide
   (e) quinidine
   (f) diphenhydramine
   (g) chlorpromazine
   (h) mepivacaine
   (i) prilocaine

2. All of the following are para-aminobenzoic acid esters (PABA) EXCEPT:
    (a) procaine
    (b) chloroprocaine
    (c) lidocaine
    (d) propoxycaine
    (e) tetracaine
    (f) none of the above
3. All of the following are non-ester anilide derivatives of xylidine or toluidine EXCEPT:
    (a) procaine
    (b) lidocaine
    (c) mepivacaine
    (d) prilocaine
4. The advantage of adding a vasoconstrictor to a local anesthetic solution for injection purposes is to:
    (a) retard systemic absorption, thus decreasing toxicity
    (b) increase visibility by reducing hemorrhage
    (c) permit smaller volumes of solution to be used
    (d) prolong the duration of anesthesia
    (e) all of the above
    (f) none of the above
5. A disadvantage of adding a vasoconstrictor to a local anesthetic solution for injection purpose would be that:
    (a) local postoperative ischemia can develop
    (b) there are unwanted hyperglycemic effects
    (c) tachycardia may result from mild CNS stimulation
    (d) there are unwanted cardiovascular effects
    (e) all of the above
    (f) none of the above
6. The usual local anesthetic solutions stocked in a dental office and available in a 1.8 cc dental cartridge include all of the following EXCEPT:
    (a) procaine-propoxycaine with Levophed 1:30,000
    (b) ethyl aminobenzoate with epinephrine 1:100,000
    (c) lidocaine 2 per cent plain
    (d) lidocaine 2 per cent with epinephrine 1:50,000
    (e) lidocaine 2 per cent with epinephrine 1:100,000
    (f) mepivacaine 3 per cent plain
    (g) mepivacaine 2 per cent with Neo-Cobefrin 1:20,000
    (h) prilocaine 4 per cent plain
    (i) prilocaine 4 per cent with epinephrine 1:200,000
7. All of the following are topical local anesthetics EXCEPT:
    (a) mepivacaine
    (b) ethyl aminobenzoate
    (c) cocaine
    (d) tetracaine
    (e) lidocaine
    (f) none of the above
8. When the dental operator is unable to obtain profound local anesthesia with supra-periosteal or block injections the only alternative to performing painful dentistry is to:
    (a) add hyaluronidase to the solution and repeat the injections
    (b) administer a general anesthetic at a future appointment
    (c) administer parenteral sedation or relative analgesia at a future appointment
    (d) administer an extraoral injection to block the entire jaw
    (e) any of the above
    (f) none of the above

9. Local complications during administration of injectable local anesthetics most commonly involve:
   (a) broken needles
   (b) trismus
   (c) tissue desquamation
   (d) bacterial contamination
   (e) soft tissue trauma during the postoperative period
   (f) all of the above

10. Hyaluronidase is most effective when used with local anesthetic solutions that contain no vasoconstrictor because:
    (a) the vasoconstrictor reduces diffusion of the mixture
    (b) the vasoconstrictor increases the loss of enzyme activity
    (c) hyaluronidase increases absorption of the anesthetic, and such polypharmacy would be difficult to justify
    (d) all of the above

11. An antisialagogue is a drug that reduces:
    (a) thyroid function
    (b) salivary flow
    (c) anxiety
    (d) essential tremor

10

GENERAL ANESTHESIA, PARENTERAL SEDATION, AND RELATIVE ANALGESIA

SECTION 1: GENERAL ANESTHESIA

Pre-Anesthetic Medication

Agents that have been developed for the purpose of pre-anesthetic medication include (1) antihistamines (Chap. 5, Sec. 4), (2) belladonna alkaloids (Chap. 6, Sec. 2), (3) barbiturates (Chap. 7, Sec. 1), (4) non-barbiturate sedative-hypnotics (Chap. 7, Sec. 1), (5) tranquilizers (Chap. 7, Sec. 2), and (6) narcotic analgesics (Chap. 8, Sec. 1). The pre-operative use of these agents is most common in ambulatory outpatients and inpatients and in non-ambulatory inpatients who are in hospitals and about to undergo general anesthesia, but ambulatory office patients receiving either local or general anesthesia may also be treated with these agents and represent the group of patients most often encountered by the dental hygienist.

Routine medical orders for the adult hospitalized dental patient may include (1) complete blood count (CBC) and measurement of bleeding time and partial thromboplastin time (PTT), (2) urinalysis, (3) history and physical exam by the house physician, (4) a regular diet during the day and a liquid diet for supper, (5) flurazepam (Dalmane) 30 mg h.s., (6) tetracycline 250 mg q.6h. beginning today, (7) diphenhydramine (Benadryl) 50 mg h.s., (8) n.P.O. (nothing by mouth) p.m. or a.m., and (9) either meperidine (Demerol), atropine, and hydroxyzine (Vistaril) or meperidine (Demerol), atropine, and promethazine (Phenergan) I.M. one hour pre-operatively. Medical orders for children are often identical to those for adults except for the omission of flurazepam, tetracycline, and diphenhydramine; the addition of erythromycin pediatric suspension q.6h. beginning today; and substitution of a barbiturate, antihistamine, and scopolamine combination (Pedo-Sol) for the meperidine-atropine injection. There are many variations of these medical orders, depending on the nature of the operation and the opinions of the dental surgeon and anesthesiologist.

The most frequently prescribed pre-operative medications for ambulatory office patients include (1) pentobarbital (Nembutal) 100 mg with Mepergan Fortis (meperidine 50 mg, promethazine 25 mg), (2) diazepam (Valium) 5 mg, (3) secobarbital (Seconal) elixir, (4) promethazine (Phenergan Syrup or Phenergan Syrup Fortis), and (5) Pedo-Sol elixir (butabarbital, chlorpheniramine maleate, and scopolamine).

Stages of Anesthesia

When diethyl ether was first used as an inhalation anesthetic, a series of stages of anesthesia were observed during the induction phase (Fig. 10–1). The description of

Stage	Description	Respiration	Pupil Size	Corneal Reflex	Pupil Light Reflex	Muscle Tonus
I Analgesia	Loss of pain perception; vol-untary motor activity	Normal thoracic and abdominal components	Normal	Present	Present	Normal
II Delirium (excitement)	Involuntary mo-tor activity; increased blood pressure and heart rate	Shivering accompanying respiratory movements	Dilated	Present	Present	Motor activity and increased tonus
Surgical Anesthesia III — Plane I	Used for thorac-ic, head, and neck surgery; normal blood pressure and pulse	Full, slow, and deep respiratory movements	Normal	Present	Present	Slight muscle relaxation
Plane II	Used for abdom-inal surgery; normal blood pressure and heart rate	Slower and decreased ampli-tude of respiratory movements	Dilated	Present / Absent	Present	Moderate relaxation
Plane III	Seldom used; blood pressure low; artificial res-piration required	Abdominal with delayed thoracic component at a slow rate	Dilated	Absent	Present / Absent	Marked relaxation
Plane IV	Few, uses if any, in surgery; very low blood pres-sure and heart rate	Abdominal with little or absent thoracic compo-nent at a slow rate	Dilated (widely)	Absent	Absent	Marked flaccidity
IV Medullary paralysis	Not used; reflexes absent; skin cold; sphincters relaxed	Respiratory arrest	Dilated (very widely)	Absent	Absent	Extreme relaxation; flaccidity

Figure 10–1. Symptoms occurring at progressive stages with the induction of general anesthesia (Guedel Table).

events occurring during the various stages is meaningful in determining the status of the patient at any given time during anesthesia. The intravenous anesthetics (Chap. 10, Sec. 1) produce induction so rapidly that the line between one stage of anesthesia and the next is often crossed very suddenly, whereas the inhalation anesthetics (Chap. 10, Sec. 1) allow a more slow induction and have stages of anesthesia that are more readily apparent.

Stage I (analgesia) is characterized by a loss of pain perception, with decreased voluntary activity, and it is the stage a patient remains in during the relative analgesia sequence that results from using nitrous oxide oxygen (Chap. 10, Sec. 3) or intravenous sedation. Protective reflexes are operational during this time, and the patient is capable of responding to questions. As the patient drifts into the deeper planes of stage I, the eyelids often droop to a half-open position (ptosis, Verrill's sign), and the administration of local anesthesia is best tolerated by apprehensive patients during this time.

Entry into stage II is indicated by the appearance of a dilated pupil, fasciculations, increased blood pressure, and increased pulse rate (excitement, delirium). Patients entering this stage while under the influence of intravenous sedation or nitrous oxide oxygen are too deeply sedated, and appropriate measures should be taken to avoid further sedation. The patient loses consciousness in this stage.

Plate I of stage III (surgical anesthesia) begins with a return of a normal blood pressure, pulse rate, and pupil size and is distinguishable from stage I only by the appearance of unconsciousness, of slow and deep respirations, and of slight muscle relaxation. Therefore, the properly sedated patient (stage I) and the overly sedated patient (plane I of stage III) will both exhibit normal-sized pupils. It is during the first plane of stage III that all dentistry under general anesthesia is carried out.

As planes II, III, and IV of stage III are progressively entered, the musculature continues to relax, the respirations become slower, with decreased amplitude, and the pupils continue to dilate. The corneal reflex is lost at the end of plane II, and the pupil light reflex is lost at the end of plane III.

Stage IV (medullary paralysis) is characterized by widely dilated pupils, respiratory arrest, extreme muscle flaccidity, and absent reflexes. This stage is never used, and every precaution is taken to prevent the patient from entering it.

Basal anesthesia, or basal narcosis, is a state of drug-induced expression generated prior to general anesthetic administration, and it permits production of planes of surgical anesthesia with greatly reduced amounts of general anesthetic agents. It is usually produced by employing intravenous anesthetics (Chap. 10, Sec. 1), and it does not involve raising the pain threshold.

Analgesia, or relative analgesia, is a state of consciousness (stage I of anesthesia) characterized by drug-induced loss of pain perception and elevation of the pain threshold that can be produced to varying degrees by oral pre-medication with narcotic analgesics, I.M. sedation, I.V. sedation, inhalation sedation using nitrous oxide oxygen, or by physical means, such as acupuncture, hypnosis, or hyperstimulation. The term parenteral sedation includes I.M., I.V., and inhalation sedation only.

The term general anesthesia implies that the patient is unconscious and therefore includes stages II, III, and IV only; although stage I is considered a stage of anesthesia, it is more accurately termed a stage of analgesia prior to general anesthesia.

Basic Gas Laws

The **gas laws** that describe the behavior of ideal gases are only approximations but are useful in understanding the physical properties of gases important to the dental profession, such as oxygen and nitrous oxide.

Dalton's law of partial pressures states that the pressure exerted on the walls of a vessel by a mixture of gases that do not react with each other is the sum of the pressures that each gas would exert if it were present alone. Expressed in symbols, this law is as follows:

$$p_t = p_1 + p_2 + \ldots + p_n$$

p_t = total pressure
p_1 = pressure of gas 1
p_2 = pressure of gas 2
p_n = pressure of last gas in gaseous mixture

Newly filled size M tanks of oxygen contain oxygen gas under a pressure of 2000 lbs, whereas newly filled size M tanks of nitrous oxide contain nitrous oxide gas and liquid nitrous oxide at a pressure of 755 lbs. Separate lines from these two types of tanks travel to the wall jacks in the dental operating room, where the flowmeter is attached that allows the gases to mix. The line pressures are reduced at the flowmeter, and the volume of each gas in the mixture can be regulated. If the pressure at the flow valve is adjusted to 120 mm mercury when one quarter of the molecules are nitrous oxide, the pressure of nitrous oxide is 30 mm mercury, and the pressure of oxygen would be 90 mm mercury.

Boyle's law states that if the temperature of a gas is kept constant, the volume of a given mass of a gas is inversely proportional to the pressure exerted by it. Expressed in symbols, this law is as follows:

$$p_1 \times v_1 = p_2 \times v_2$$

p_1 = initial pressure
v_1 = initial volume
p_2 = final pressure
v_2 = final volume

Because a large quantity of oxygen and nitrous oxide is compressed into the small volumes of the size M tanks stored in dental offices, considerable pressure is exerted by the respective gases on the walls of the tanks; as the pressure is relieved at the flowmeters, the compressed gases occupy a larger volume and circulate through the tubing and nasal mask.

Graham's law of diffusion states that the relative rates of diffusion of two gases are inversely proportional to the square roots of their densities (or molecular weights, since densities are proportional to molecular weights). Expressed in symbols, this law is as follows:

$$\frac{R_1}{R_2} = \sqrt{\frac{d_2}{d_1}} = \sqrt{\frac{mw_2}{mw_1}}$$

R_1 = diffusion rate of gas 1
R_2 = diffusion rate of gas 2
d_1 = density of gas 1
d_2 = density of gas 2
mw_1 = molecular weight of gas 1
mw_2 = molecular weight of gas 2

Since the molecular weight of oxygen is 32 and that of nitrous oxide is 44, the ratio of diffusion of oxygen to that of nitrous oxide is 1.18; therefore, oxygen diffuses through the tubing and nasal mask 1.18 times faster than does nitrous oxide.

The deviations from accuracy in the gas laws are small when they are applied to very small molecules, such as oxygen, but are fairly large for more readily condensable gases, such as nitrous oxide, and increase rapidly as liquefying conditions are approached. This is partially explained by the attraction of the nucleus of one molecule for the electron cloud of another molecule, an attraction that tends to decrease the volume of a gas more than expected as the pressure is increased or as the temperature is decreased. Because of its smaller molecular size, oxygen boils at $-183°$ C, whereas nitrous oxide boils at the higher temperature of $-88.5°$ C.

Intravenous Anesthetics

The intravenous anesthetics include the ultrashort-acting barbiturates thiopental sodium (Pentothal), thiamylal sodium (Surital), and methohexital sodium (Brevital) (Chap. 7, Sec. 1) and the non-barbiturates ketamine and Innovar (fentanyl citrate and droperidol) (Chap. 7, Sec. 2; Chap. 8, Sec. 1).

Thiopental sodium (Pentothal) is an ultrashort-acting barbiturate that produces hypnosis between 30 and 40 seconds after I.V. injection and that induces anesthesia, but not analgesia. Since individual response to this drug is so varied, there is no fixed dosage, and sedative doses may result in surgical anesthesia (stage III) in sensitive patients. The safe upper limit of dosage for basal narcosis in a child or adult in good health is 20 mg/lb, which is decreased as needed in the elderly or debilitated. A total dose between 1 and 1.5 grams for children weighing 75 lbs or more or between 3 and 4 grams for adults weighing 200 lbs or more should not be exceeded. This drug is administered only I.V. or rectally and is available in injection form as a 2 or 2.5 per cent solution in 250, 400, and 500 mg syringes, in 0.5, 1, 5, and 10 gram multi-dose vials, in 1, 2.5, and 5 gram kits, and as a rectal suspension containing 400 mg/gram of suspension in a 2 gram syringe with applicator. Thiopental sodium builds up in adipose tissue in a concentration between 6 and 12 times that of the plasma concentration, which results in prolonged anesthesia as the drug is released from its storage sites. The dosage used during I.V. sedation is slowly titrated based on the patient's response, age, and body weight.

Thiamylal sodium (Surital) is another ultrashort-acting barbiturate in which dosage is individualized based on patient response. It is marketed as a 1, 5, or 10 gram "steri-vial" to which is added a solvent (sterile water for injection) for dilution. A 2.5 per cent solution is recommended for induction and should be injected I.V. at a rate of 1 cc/ 5 sec, to total injection of between 3 and 6 cc.

Methohexital sodium (Brevital) is also another ultrashort-acting barbiturate in which dosage is individualized. It is available for injection as 500 mg vials, as 2.5 and 5 gram vials, and in 2.5 and 5 gram ampoules to which is added sterile water for proper dilution. Between 5 and 12 cc of a 1 per cent solution of the drug will provide anesthesia for between 5 and 7 minutes, and this volume should be injected at a rate of 1 cc/5 sec. Recovery from methohexital sodium is more rapid than recovery is from thiopental sodium after equal doses, and for this reason methohexital sodium is gaining popularity for use during I.V. sedation for dental procedures when a more rapid recovery is desirable.

Ketamine (Ketaject, Ketalar) is a general anesthetic that produces anesthesia, analgesia, and cardiovascular and respiratory stimulation and that has no effect on pharyngeal-laryngeal reflexes. The drug has a wide margin of safety, and the usual dose for induction is between 1 and 4.5 mg/kg I.V. or between 6.5 and 13 mg/kg I.M. Because the pharyngeal and laryngeal reflexes remain active after administration, ketamine should be combined with succinylcholine chloride (Anectine) (Chap. 6, Sec. 2) rather than used as the sole anesthetic agent for dental procedures. It is physiologically compatible with all drugs used in anesthesia, and is available in injection form in concentrations of 10, 50, and 100 mg/cc.

The use of Innovar as anesthetic pre-medication, in induction of anesthesia, or in maintenance of anesthesia has been described previously (Chap. 7, Sec. 2; Chap. 8, Sec. 1). It is marketed in injection form containing 0.05 mg fentanyl citrate (Sublimaze) and 2.5 mg droperidol (Inapsine) per cc, in 2 and 5 cc ampoules.

Inhalation Anesthetics

The inhalation anesthetics most frequently used in dental and maxillofacial surgery include the gases nitrous oxide, cyclopropane, and ethylene and the volatile liquids halothane, methoxyflurane, and enflurane; other volatile liquids of less clinical importance that have been used for this purpose include diethyl ether, vinyl ether, ethyl vinyl ether, ethyl chloride, trichloroethylene, and fluroxene.

The most commonly used anesthetic gas is **nitrous oxide**. A dental office is a potential explosion hazard due to the presence of radiosurge units, x-ray equipment, and carpeting that can generate static electricity; therefore, the ideal general anesthetic gas for use in a dental office is non-flammable, weak, non-irritating, and practically odorless, as well as providing prompt induction and emergence. Nitrous oxide fulfills all these criteria. When administered at a satisfactory flow rate at a concentration up to 65 per cent in oxygen, this gas provides analgesia and sedation without loss of consciousness; when given in higher concentrations up to a safe maximum of 80 per cent in oxygen, light anesthesia with poor muscle relaxation results. If it is combined with pre-anesthetic medication, a general anesthetic state may result with concentrations lower than 65 per cent. A morphine index of 1.0 correlates with a concentration of 20 per cent in oxygen (Chap. 8, Sec. 1). Nitrous oxide is supplied in blue cylinders, whereas oxygen is supplied in green cylinders. The chief danger of using nitrous oxide is hypoxia (Chap. 10, Sec. 3), but as long as this complication is guarded against, the gas is extremely safe for dentists to administer without the assistance of an anesthesiologist. Because of its dental-practice-building potential and its relatively wide margin of safety in patients who are adequately oxygenated, more and more dentists are using nitrous oxide as an easy answer to their sedation problems when their training and experience in all types of sedation (oral, I.M., I.V., and inhalation) is minimal.

Cyclopropane may also be used for relative analgesia and general anesthesia. Unlike nitrous oxide, it produces full skeletal muscle relaxation in anesthetic doses of between 7 and 23 per cent in oxygen. It is not practical for dental analgesia because it is explosive, expensive, and potent and because it occasionally produces laryngospasm and cardiac arrhythmias. Nausea, vomiting, and headache are commonly seen during recovery. This gas is supplied in orange cylinders.

Ethylene may be used for relative analgesia or general anesthesia also but must be used in a high concentration (80 per cent) in oxygen. Like nitrous oxide, it is a poor muscle relaxant, and hypoxia is the primary danger in its use. Use of ethylene in dentistry is limited because it is flammable and has a disagreeable odor. It is supplied in red cylinders.

Halothane (Fluothane) may be administered with either oxygen or a mixture of oxygen and nitrous oxide for induction of general anesthesia. It produces moderate muscle relaxation, bronchodilation, and depression of laryngeal and pharyngeal reflexes, and it makes the myocardial conduction system sensitive to epinephrine and norepinephrine, which can lead to arrhythmias when these agents are combined with the use of the gas. (Chap. 11, Sec. 1). The induction dose varies from patient to patient; usually a patient is maintained on a concentration between 0.5 and 1.5 per cent, unless he begins to float back up into stage II, in which case a concentration of 4 per cent is administered and gradually reduced to about 1 per cent. Hypotension and respiratory depression may occur during halothane use, and it is non-flammable.

Methoxyflurane (Penthrane) may also be used alone or in combination with nitrous oxide for analgesia or general anesthesia. A concentration between 0.3 and 0.8 per cent is used for analgesia, up to 3 per cent may be used for induction, and between 0.1 and 0.4 per cent is usually adequate for maintenance when administered in a gas flow consisting of 50 per cent nitrous oxide in oxygen. This gas is a poor muscle relaxant in safe doses and may provide continued analgesia in the immediate postoperative period, reducing the need for narcotic analgesics. Like halothane, it is non-flammable, and it sensitizes the myocardial conduction system to epinephrine and norepinephrine.

Enflurane (Ethrane) is a general anesthetic that produces moderate muscle relaxation, and it is non-explosive. Induction occurs with a concentration between 3.5 and 4.5 per cent in between seven and ten minutes, surgical anesthesia levels can be reached with concentrations between 1.5 and 3 per cent, and maintenance concentrations should not exceed 3 per cent. Enflurane reduces ventilation of the lungs as the concentration is increased but may provoke a sigh response similar to that seen with diethyl ether. It closely resembles halothane in clinical characteristics and is associated with rapid emergence and recovery.

Acupuncture Anesthesia

Chinese physicians practice medicine not only according to the Western philosophy of treatment of disease with drugs and supportive therapy but also by means of a drugless healing art called **acupuncture,** which is not associated with iatrogenic diseases or drug-related adverse effects. According to traditional Chinese belief, the life energy of the body, ch'i, flows through the body along a network of 12 organ meridians and 2 midline meridians; along these meridians at certain places, called acupuncture points, this energy can be influenced by manipulation, and an excess or deficiency of this energy produces pain or disease.

In 1973 the Norwegian medical delegation to the People's Republic of China witnessed approximately 30 major operations involving acupuncture in surgery. It was demonstrated that (1) acupuncture was almost always given in combination with large doses of analgesics and sedative-hypnotics (phenobarbital 100 mg night before and meperidine 1 mg/kg I.M. 30 minutes before, supplemented with local anesthesia with procaine), (2) acupuncture is not as frequently used as the news media suggest (declining to 5 per cent in 1974 from a previous 60 per cent in 1967), and pain relief was not obtained according to Western criteria in as much as 82 per cent of instances of use.

There is no evidence to support the traditional Chinese meridian or channel theory, and these meridians are unrelated to any known lymphatic, circulatory, or nervous systems. The main acupuncture points are located within the dermatome of the diseased organ and are usually near the nerve branches. Theories of the mechanism of acupuncture based on neurophysiological and psychophysiological data seem to be more tenable. The meridian theory is no longer followed by Chinese researchers or physicians.

Hyperstimulation of the skin innervated by spinal nerves gives rise to afferent fiber activity, and the effects of acupuncture, as well as of transcutaneous peripheral nerve stimulation, are due to afferent nervous impulses (Chap. 10, Sec. 3). There is a modulation of sensory input in the substantia gelatinosa of the spinal cord that was first demonstrated by Melzack and Wall in 1965 (gate control theory). It was shown that the cells of the substantia gelatinosa exert an inhibitory effect on afferent fiber terminals entering the spinal cord, an effect which is increased by activity in large diameter fibers and decreased by activity in small diameter (pain) fibers. Therefore, any sudden volley of large diameter fiber impulses would inhibit the central transmission of pain impulses along small diameter fibers by closing the gate to conscious pain perception. There is a connection between these observations and the mechanism of acupuncture.

Chinese anesthesiologists produce anesthesia with local or general anesthetics about 90 per cent of the time, with general anesthesia used relatively infrequently. Chinese patients prefer to be awake during surgery because sleep and coma are popularly equated with a departure of the soul from the body, and the possible benefits of general anesthesia in ensuring vagal blockade, ventilation of the lungs, and muscular relaxation are not explained to patients. The Chinese patient generally submits to acupuncture in the belief that he will benefit from reduced side-effects and that if the pain becomes too great an adequate local and general anesthetic back-up is available.

Acupuncture "anesthesia" produces neither anesthesia nor analgesia in the conventional sense, and local anesthesia is an important part of the technique. Patients are premedicated with barbiturates, analgesics, and an anticholinergic agent, such as scopolamine 0.3 mg Sub-Q. The anesthesia classification system used in Shanghai includes four grades of effectiveness: (1) grade I allows for slight pain during the procedure and the use of local anesthetics and intravenous meperidine; (2) grade II permits occasional light groans for pain and local anesthetics, intravenous meperidine, and changes in vital signs (Chap. 12, Sec. 1); (3) grade III permits obvious pain sensation and the use of local anesthetics, intravenous meperidine, and changes in vital signs; and (4) grade IV is characterized by marked pain and changes in vital signs, because of which it is necessary to shift to drug anesthesia to accomplish the operation. Grades I, II, and III are considered effective in China; in the United States it is likely that only those patients of Grade I who experience no pain at all would be considered effectively managed.

Acupuncture analgesia produces a small but reliable increase in pain threshold, which can be reversed by naloxone. It is unlikely that this effect is related to hypnosis or the placebo effect because hypnotically induced analgesia is not reversed by naloxone and does not outlast the treatment period, as does acupuncture analgesia, and placebos fail to alter pain thresholds. It is believed that acupuncture analgesia activates a pain inhibitory system, such as that proposed by Melzack and Wall, which can also be activated by electrical stimulation of the mesencephalic central grey area or by administration of narcotic analgesics.

Acupuncture has been shown to be a harmless therapeutic modality for chronic pain when patients are carefully screened by physicians using Western diagnostic methods and strict sterile techniques.

Diseases Limiting the Choice of Anesthesia

Common diseases in which a local rather than a general anesthetic is indicated for dental treatment include (1) respiratory diseases, such as asthma, emphysema, bronchiectasis, or acute respiratory infections; (2) liver disease, such as cirrhosis; and (3) diabetes mellitus. Patients who have a history of these diseases and who undergo general anesthesia will be more difficult to ventilate, will have more difficulty detoxifying from the effects of the anesthetic, or will have their disease aggravated by the hyperglycemic effects of anesthesia.

Common diseases in which a general rather than a local anesthetic is indicated for dental treatment include (1) hyper- and hypothyroidism, (2) adrenal cortical insufficiency (Addison's disease), (3) cardiac arrhythmias, and (4) hypertensive cardiovascular disease. Patients who have a history of these diseases and undergo a local anesthetic injection may be more uncooperative, may have their condition aggravated by the endogenous release of epinephrine secondary to anticipation of injections, or may not be able to react satisfactorily to stressful situations.

Complications

The most frequent complications associated with the use of general anesthetics include (1) diffusion anoxia, or insufficient atmospheric oxygen, (2) inadequate pulmonary ventilation, (3) inadequate oxygen transport to the tissues, (4) increased oxygen demand, (5) lung abscess, and (6) aspiration pneumonia.

It is extremely dangerous to allow patients to inhale pure nitrous oxide undiluted with oxygen or to suddenly breathe room air containing only 21 per cent oxygen after nitrous oxide oxygen analgesia. Nitrous oxide is a gas that is carried in the blood plasma in physical solution, rapidly crossing back and forth across the respiratory membrane (pulmonary capillaries, interstitial cells, and pulmonary alveoli) to establish an equilibrium. When the nitrous oxide in the inspired air is reduced, the nitrous oxide rapidly rushing into the pulmonary alveoli will dilute the oxygen and carbon dioxide already present, resulting in hypoxia and a decreased respiratory drive. To avoid diffusion anoxia and possible brain or kidney damage, patients are allowed to breathe 100 per cent oxygen at the end of the analgesic sequence until the nitrous oxide is eliminated (Chap. 10, Sec. 3).

Inadequate pulmonary ventilation in patients can be prevented by using a source of 100 per cent oxygen under positive pressure until the primary condition is brought under control. Conditions that contribute to insufficient ventilation include drug-induced respiratory depression, mechanical obstruction of the air passages, and interference with the respiratory muscles by convulsive seizures or paralysis. Inadequate oxygen transport in severely anemic patients or in those who are profoundly hypotensive can also be prevented by using 100 per cent oxygen. Oxygen consumption by the body is increased with hyperthyroidism and fever (a 7 per cent increase in metabolic rate per 1° F increase in body temperature). If an increased oxygen demand is expected, a source of 100 per cent oxygen under positive pressure will also prevent complications.

Lung abscess has been known to occur following dental extractions under general anesthesia, and the causative agent was presumed to be either a piece of bone, a tooth structure, or a septic piece of calculus that was aspirated into the trachea during oral surgery. The use of a sufficiently large gauze throat pack will discourage aspiration of such particles. Aspiration pneumonia results from the vomiting of gastric juice during anesthesia and aspiration of it into the trachea; this is usually preventable by ordering that nothing be taken by mouth for eight hours before surgery and that the diet be liquid for supper the night before to ensure an empty stomach.

SECTION 2: PARENTERAL SEDATION

Intramuscular Sedation

Although oral pre-medication is widely used for those patients who approach their dental treatment with various degrees of apprehension or dread, the results are variable from patient to patient using a standardized drug dosage. This form of sedation has high patient acceptance but requires a protracted time period for adequate sedation to begin and may fail in the severely anxious patient, in the obstructive child, or in the patient in pain.

The onset of intramuscular sedation is more rapid than in oral and provides more predictable results; however, patient acceptance is lower, and the cost is usually greater. This form of sedation best lends itself to use as a pre-anesthetic medication prior to general anesthesia in hospitalized patients (Chap. 10, Sec. 1).

I.M. sedation is not as reliable, predictable, or effective as I.V. sedation, except in the case of ketamine administration (Chap. 10, Sec. 1). Use of I.M. sedation in office dental patients is usually restricted to those requiring local anesthesia in which I.V. sedation, inhalation sedation, and general anesthesia is unsuitable.

Venipuncture Technique

The veins usually employed in venipuncture to establish an intravenous route of administration for I.V. sedation are located in the proximal forearm and the dorsum of the hand. The most suitable veins in the proximal forearm include (1) the median antebrachial vein, (2) the cephalic vein, (3) the median cephalic vein, and (4) the accessory cephalic vein (Fig. 10–2).

In the cubital fossa the brachial artery is slightly deeper than the median basilic vein, and only a fascial layer is between the two vessels; therefore, the median basilic vein, although it may be very superficial and inviting, is generally avoided in order to prevent puncturing of the brachial artery. If two equally inviting veins can be chosen from either the medial or the lateral side of the forearm, it is best to choose the vein on the lateral side.

Some patients may present with deep veins or veins that "roll," which makes successful venipuncture more difficult. A few light slaps with the hand on the ventral side of the forearm will result in superficial venospasm, which makes visualization of the superficial veins easier. A rubber tube tourniquet may be wrapped around the upper arm to obstruct venous return in the forearm, or a sphygmomanometer cuff can be inflated to a level between the systolic and diastolic pressures to obstruct venous return and yet ensure adequate arterial blood flow and rapid determination of blood pressure.

When a vein has been chosen, it should be entered by holding the bevel of the needle up, disinfecting the skin overlying the area with an alcohol sponge, and entering the vein by burying the needle within it at only a slight angle with respect to the skin. A short section of the needle shank should be visible outside the puncture area. A flashback bulb should be present on the Venoset tubing to enable the operator to press the bulb

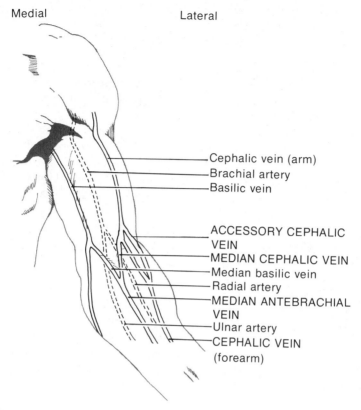

Medial   Lateral

Cephalic vein (arm)
Brachial artery
Basilic vein

ACCESSORY CEPHALIC VEIN
MEDIAN CEPHALIC VEIN
Median basilic vein
Radial artery
MEDIAN ANTEBRACHIAL VEIN
Ulnar artery
CEPHALIC VEIN (forearm)

Figure 10–2. Superficial veins of the proximal forearm suitable for venipuncture (in capital letters).

and withdraw venous blood back into the tubing to check for proper needle placement. The patient's elbow should be immobilized by means of tying the forearm to an intravenous armboard with restraints. The hub of the needle is taped to the skin with adhesive tape, and the clamp on the tubing is adjusted to allow a suitable flow of intravenous fluids.

Veins that "roll" may cause the needle to "ride the vein" for a short distance before penetrating and thus cause greater discomfort to the patient. This problem can be minimized by pressing the thumb down on the skin adjacent to the vein and pushing lightly in the direction of the vein to hold it still. Some operators prefer to puncture the skin adjacent to these veins rather than that directly over them and to make the needle enter the side of the vein rather than the top.

Intravenous Sedation

Intravenous sedation should be considered for apprehensive patients requiring local anesthesia for dental procedures in which inhalation sedation is contraindicated. It is not ideally suited for very young children, obese patients, or others in whom venipuncture would be extremely difficult; such patients should receive either I.M. sedation, general anesthesia, or relative analgesia through various non–drug-related measures. Intravenous sedation is contraindicated in pregnant patients, in patients who are vulnerable to hypoxia (those with anemia, asthma, or emphysema), in patients who are hypoglycemic or who are taking insulin (diabetes mellitus), and in those who are easy to overdose owing to a decreased response to drugs (as in epilepsy). The advantages of using this method of sedation include drug response that is predictable, controllable, and efficient; short postoperative recovery; and lower mortality than with general anesthesia; however, a recovery area is needed, a patient escort must be arranged, and a full comprehension of the indications, restrictions, and complications of its use are essential.

At a separate appointment the procedure should be discussed with the patient or the parents, or both. Early morning appointments are generally best because the patient must have nothing by mouth for eight hours prior to sedation. The patient's pulse rate and base line blood pressure, rate and depth of respiration, Verrill's sign, verbal responses, and eyelash reflex are monitored. When narcotics are used, pupil size is unreliable sign, because narcotics cause pupils to constrict.

The most frequent complications with intravenous sedation include hematoma, venospasm, infiltration, intra-arterial injection, phlebothrombosis, and certain drug-related difficulties (laryngospasm, respiratory depression, and drug interactions). These problems can be avoided by making sure the needle enters the vein, by injecting slowly with barbotage (withdrawing blood into the syringe barrel to dilute the contents prior to injection), by having an adequate medical history taken, and by being prepared to manage emergency situations. Infiltrations are best managed with procaine injection into the surrounding tissue to produce vasodilation. Laryngospasm secondary to debris impacted at the glottal opening is treated by means of pharyngeal suction and 100 per cent oxygen, ventilating the patient hard two or three times; should this fail to break the laryngospasm, the patient is given succinylcholine chloride (Anectine) 10 mg I.V., and respiration is supported until the muscles repolarize.

The following techniques are the most commonly used for intravenous sedation, but there are many variations:

1. Diazepam alone—diazepam between 5 and 20 mg, supplemented with local anesthesia.

2. Diazepam with supplemental methohexital (Foreman technique)—diazepam between 3 and 20 mg, then methohexital 1 per cent, between 1 and 5 cc, supplemented with local anesthesia.

3. Intravenous amnesia technique of Shane—alphaprodine between 6 and 36 mg, hydroxyzine between 25 and 50 mg, and atropine between 0.3 and 0.6 mg in a mixture, then methohexital 1 per cent as needed, supplemented with local anesthesia.

4. Intravenous pre-medication (Jorgensen technique)—pentobarbital between 10 and 100 mg, then meperidine 25 mg and scopolamine 0.32 mg in a mixture, supplemented with local anesthesia.

5. Intermittent Brevital anesthesia (minimal increment technique of Drummond-Jackson)—methohexital between 80 and 100 mg, then one half the initial dose, injected every 15 seconds until sleep begins. Increments are given as needed. Local anesthesia is NOT used.

6. Twilight sedation technique of Berns—secobarbital between 25 and 50 mg, then meperidine between 25 and 50 mg, then methohexital 1 per cent, 3 cc, supplemented with local anesthesia.

7. Vistaril-Demerol technique of Abramson—meperidine 50 mg and hydroxyzine 50 mg in a mixture, supplemented with local anesthesia.

8. Microdose techniques of Goldstein and Dragon—alphaprodine 40 mg, levallorphan 1 mg, promethazine 25 mg, and sterile water 2 cc in a mixture; 5 cc in a syringe, injected 1 cc at a time, first initially, then 2 minutes later, then 15 minutes later, then 0.5 cc every 15 minutes, supplemented with local anesthesia.

9. Drip Brevital technique of Howard and Friedman—methohexital 0.1 per cent drip started, then methohexital 1 per cent, between 6 and 12 cc, supplemented with local anesthesia. If the patient proves resistant, give potentiators: diazepam between 5 and 10 mg or alphaprodine between 10 and 15 mg.

10. Neuroleptanalgesia with Innovar—Innovar 2 cc, then methohexital 1 per cent, supplemented with local anesthesia.

11. Nembutal-Demerol, or Nem-Dem, technique of Lehrman—pentobarbital between 50 and 100 mg, then meperidine between 25 and 100 mg, supplemented with local anesthesia.

Laborit referred to his lytic cocktail as "artificial hibernation," and it consisted of meperidine 25 mg, promethazine 6.25 mg, and chlorpromazine 6.25 mg per cc. It was discovered that it was not compatible with homeostasis in that it resulted in severe circulatory depression and profound lowering of the temperature. The preferred extension of Laborit's concept is neuroleptanalgesia with Innovar.

Intravenous and inhalation techniques may be combined, as in the chemanesia-analgesia method of Monheim, which is a modified Jorgensen technique with gases added. It consists of pentobarbital or secobarbital between 50 and 100 mg; then meperidine 50 mg and hydroxyzine 50 mg in a mixture, with a dose between 12 and 50 mg; then nitrous oxide and oxygen in a 1:1 ratio, supplemented with local anesthesia and maintenance of the patient on gases in a ratio of 25:75. However, it is best to keep the procedure as simple as possible, with as few drugs as needed to accomplish anxiety control.

The author prefers a modified Foreman technique in which a mixture of alphaprodine 30 mg, levallorphan 0.5 mg, and atropine 0.6 mg may be interposed between administration of diazepam and methohexital.

SECTION 3: RELATIVE ANALGESIA

Nitrous Oxide Analgesia

Patients who are going to experience nitrous oxide oxygen sedation for the first time should be given an explanation of the sequence of events that will occur and the subjective sensations they will feel during the analgesic sequence. This discussion should emphasize that the gas will be used as a "vapor tranquilizer" to disconnect the patient from his surroundings while he is fully awake, rather than to induce sleep. The patient should be told that it is a pleasant procedure, extremely safe, and that many patients request it a second time after using it. He should also be told that his mouth will not be covered and that the small nasal mask will not give him the feeling that he is being smothered, that during sedation his speech may be slower than normal or slurred, that a warmth may spread over his body and his extremities may feel heavy or tingle, and that he may dream that he is somewhere else.

Since some patients experience euphoria during nitrous oxide anesthesia (laughing gas), inhalation sedation with nitrous oxide oxygen should not be considered in patients who are emotionally unstable or who currently have a respiratory disease (Chap. 10, Sec. 1).

The expiratory valve of older nasal masks has been replaced by a scavenger hose connecting the nasal mask to suction to prevent expired gases from escaping into the air and thus chronically exposing dental personnel to those gases, which could contribute to lung disease (Chap. 3, Sec. 1). After the scavenging hose is connected to the suction and the plastic stopcock on the hose is opened a small amount to adjust the vacuum to a proper level, the round key, usually in the possession of the doctor, is used to turn on the flowmeter. A short whistling noise is heard as the line gases enter the flowmeter and as oxygen escapes through the nasal tubing at a minimum flow rate of 2 liters/minute. Modern flowmeters are manufactured to allow a flow of at least 2 liters oxygen/minute. even with the flow valve turned off as a fail-safe measure taken to avoid hypoxia. This whistling noise may alarm the patient unless he is warned that the machinery will make a little noise when it is turned on.

The flow of oxygen is then adjusted to a rate between 8 and 10 liters/minute, and the mask is placed over the patient's nose, with a 2 inch $\times$ 2 inch square of gauze over the philtrum of the upper lip as needed for cushioning. The patient is then asked to hold the mask on his nose in a comfortable position with both hands while the slack is taken up in the tubing under the headrest ("tightening the pigtails"). Since room air is 78 per cent nitrogen and 21 per cent oxygen, the patient is given 100 per cent oxygen at this time to allow most of the nitrogen to be expired and to richly oxygenate the blood.

After the patient breathes 100 per cent oxygen at a flow rate of between 8 and 10 liters/minute for between 4 and 5 minutes, the flow rate is reduced to 4.5 liters/minute, and nitrous oxide is introduced at a flow rate of 1.5 liters/minute; this produces a mixture of 25 per cent nitrous oxide in oxygen delivered at a flow rate of 6 liters/minute, which equals the respiratory minute volume for the average male (tidal volume $\times$ respiratory rate) (Fig. 10–3). The beginning percentage of nitrous oxide is always adjusted to a level of 25 per cent, but the flow rates should be slightly increased for athletes or decreased for females, small adults, or children.

If the patient does not report subjective sensations of nitrous oxide concentration, the oxygen is reduced to 4 liters/minute and the nitrous oxide is increased to 2 liters/minute, producing a 33 per cent concentration; a constant flow rate of 6 liters/minute maintained. The concentration of the gas can be increased 0.5 liters approximately every 60 seconds until a safe maximum of 65 per cent is reached, but most patients usually respond to concentrations between 33 and 50 per cent.

As the dental procedure is nearing completion, the patient should be gradually "backed down" the concentration scale by reducing the flow rate of nitrous oxide and increasing the flow rate of oxygen. After the patient has breathed a concentration of 25 per cent nitrous oxide for approximately 60 seconds, the oxygen is turned up to between 5 and 8 liters/minute, and the nitrous oxide is turned off. One hundred per cent oxygen must be administered during this time to avoid diffusion anoxia (Chap. 10, Sec. 1), and it should be continued for a full five minutes before dismissing the patient. The nasal mask is then disinfected for future use.

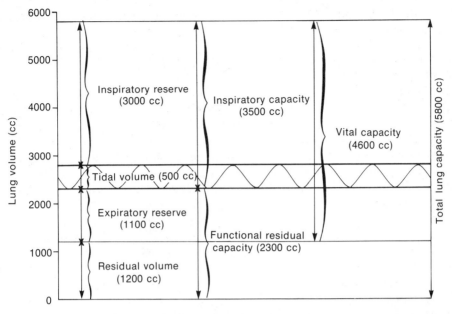

Figure 10–3. Pulmonary volumes and capacities.

Hypnotically Induced Analgesia

Surgical procedures ranging from dental extractions to appendectomies, thyroidectomies, caesarian sections, and open heart surgery have been painlessly carried out using hypnosis as the sole anesthetic agent (hypnoanesthesia). It is estimated that over 90 per cent of the population show an increase in pain threshold with appropriate hypnotic suggestions.

The induction of hypnosis is remarkably simple, and the hypnotist instructs the patient to focus his attention, to think about his eyes growing heavy, and to drift off as if to sleep. No drug is given and nothing dramatic is done, but moments later a suitable individual when questioned will respond that he is becoming insensible to pain. There are no clear-cut changes in the patient's electroencephalogram (EEG); he responds to the hypnotist's voice and may show every evidence that he is wide awake.

Patients who have had hypnoanesthesia during surgery often continue to assert its effectiveness long after the surgery and require little postoperative analgesia, if any. The increase in pain threshold resulting from hypnoanesthesia cannot be reversed by naloxone as with acupuncture anesthesia (Chap. 10, Sec. 1) and is independent in mechanism from the placebo effect, which fails to alter pain thresholds.

Hypnosis is helpful in a high proportion of dental patients in that the patient becomes less anxious and is easier to manage, and the method allows the administration of local anesthetics without pre-medication (hypnotically induced analgesia). Posthypnotic suggestion has also been used to render certain patients more responsive to the wearing of removable dentures. Since hypnosis is safe, non-habit forming, easily applied, and associated with no adverse effects, it should be considered before invasive or mutilating procedures that have been used to control chronic pain in the past. Although no current explanation accounts for hypnotically induced analgesia (rapid induction analgesia, RIA), it has been used as an effective analgesic that can be used instead of chemical analgesia or anesthesia and that is effective in virtually every instance.

Hyperstimulation Analgesia

Renewed interest in artificial stimulation of the peripheral nerves began after the publication of the gate theory of Melzack and Wall in 1965 (Chap. 10, Sec. 1), and this has led to two important applications for the control of dental pain: (1) transcutaneous electrical stimulation (TES) and (2) audioanalgesia.

The first electrical stimulators having electrodes applied to the skin or mucous membrane became available in 1970. Today a modern transcutaneous neural stimulator is powered by three 1.5 volt batteries, and it generates square wave impulses between 50 and 300 μsec in duration with a frequency between 10 and 100 Hz; the electrodes can be applied to the infraorbital area or to any other area of the face, and the elevation in the pain threshold that results during or after stimulation using a single electrode is the same on the ipsilateral and contralateral sides. This indicates that the effect is not confined to the first synapse but occurs at higher levels. Permanent stimulation using implanted electrodes has been shown to relieve intractable pain of benign origin in about 33 per cent of cases.

When earphones are placed on a patient's head and soft music is played, with a random mixture of frequencies ranging from 50 to 45,000 Hz (white sound) the pain threshold may also be raised (audioanalgesia). This method also makes inaudible any undesirable sounds that may excite the apprehensive patient, such as the whine of the airotor handpiece.

TEST QUESTIONS

1. Agents used for the purpose of pre-anesthetic medication include all of the following EXCEPT:
   (a) antihistamines
   (b) belladonna alkaloids
   (c) barbiturates
   (d) non-barbiturate sedatives
   (e) tranquilizers
   (f) narcotic analgesics
   (g) antibiotics

2. Routine medical orders for the adult hospitalized dental patient about to undergo general anesthesia may include any of the following EXCEPT:
   (a) complete blood count (CBC)
   (b) measurement of partial thromboplastin time (PTT) and bleeding time
   (c) urinalysis
   (d) history and physical exam by the house physician
   (e) a regular diet during the day and a liquid diet for supper
   (f) flurazepam 30 mg h.s.
   (g) diphenhydramine 50 mg h.s.
   (h) tetracycline 250 mg q.6h. beginning today
   (i) n.P.O. p.m. or a.m.
   (j) succinylcholine chloride 50 mg I.V. one hour pre-operatively
   (k) meperidine 50 mg, atropine 0.6 mg, promethazine 25 mg in a mixture given I.M. one hour pre-operatively

3. The stage of anesthesia characterized by initial loss of pain perception, decreased voluntary activity, and "Verrill's sign" is:
   (a) Stage I
   (b) Stage II
   (c) Stage III, Plane I
   (d) Stage III, Plane II
   (e) Stage III, Plane III
   (f) Stage III, Plane IV
   (g) Stage IV

4. All of the following are inhalation anesthetics EXCEPT:
   (a) halothane
   (b) thiopental sodium
   (c) thiamylal sodium
   (d) methohexital sodium
   (e) ketamine
   (f) Innovar

5. All of the following inhalation anesthetics are volatile liquids EXCEPT:
   (a) halothane
   (b) nitrous oxide
   (c) methoxyflurane
   (d) enflurane

6. The chief danger in using nitrous oxide is:
   (a) cardiac arrhythmias
   (b) laryngospasm
   (c) hypoxia
   (d) explosiveness

7. Inhalation anesthetics that sensitize the myocardium to epinephrine and norepinephrine are:
   (a) nitrous oxide
   (b) halothane
   (c) methoxyflurane
   (d) enflurane
   (e) both a and b
   (f) both b and c
   (g) both c and d
   (h) all of the above

8. Acupuncture analgesia produces a small but reliable increase in pain threshold that can be reversed by:
   (a) naloxone
   (b) oxymorphone
   (c) oxycodone
   (d) meprobamate

9. Local anesthesia is preferable to general anesthesia for dental patients who have a history of any of the following diseases EXCEPT:
   (a) asthma
   (b) emphysema
   (c) bronchiectasis
   (d) acute respiratory infections
   (e) cardiac arrhythmia
   (f) chronic liver disease
   (g) diabetes mellitus

10. General anesthesia is preferable to local anesthesia for dental patients who have a history of any of the following diseases EXCEPT:
    (a) hyperthyroidism
    (b) hypothyroidism
    (c) Addison's disease
    (d) cardiac arrhythmia
    (e) hypertensive cardiovascular disease
    (f) diabetes mellitus

11. At the end of a nitrous oxide oxygen analgesia sequence the patient is given 100 per cent oxygen to prevent:
    (a) neuroleptanalgesia
    (b) fasciculations
    (c) diffusion anoxia
    (d) nitrogen narcosis

12. When a modern nitrous oxide oxygen flowmeter is closed the oxygen flow rate is automatically maintained at a minimum of:
    (a) 1 liter/min
    (b) 2 liters/min
    (c) 3 liters/min
    (d) 4 liters/min

13. All of the following general anesthetics are flammable EXCEPT:
    - (a) nitrous oxide
    - (b) halothane
    - (c) methoxyflurane
    - (d) enflurane
    - (e) cyclopropane
    - (f) ethylene
    - (g) a, b, c, and d
    - (h) b, c, d, and e
    - (i) c, d, e, and f
    - (j) all of the above (i.e., none are flammable)

14. The most frequent complications associated with general anesthetics include all of the following EXCEPT:
    - (a) muscle relaxation
    - (b) diffusion anoxia
    - (c) decreased pulmonary ventilation
    - (d) inadequate oxygen transport
    - (e) lung abscess
    - (f) aspiration pneumonia
    - (g) increased oxygen demand

15. I.M. sedation is not as reliable, predictable, or as effective as I.V. sedation, except for use in the administration of:
    - (a) ketamine
    - (b) Innovar
    - (c) thiopental sodium
    - (d) methohexital sodium

16. The most suitable veins for I.V. administration of drugs for dental sedation are located in any of the following areas EXCEPT:
    - (a) the dorsum of the hand
    - (b) the cephalic vein (arm)
    - (c) the cephalic vein (forearm)
    - (d) the median cephalic vein
    - (e) the accessory cephalic vein
    - (f) the median antebrachial vein

17. I.V. sedation is not suitable for dental patients having a current history of any of the following EXCEPT:
    - (a) pregnancy
    - (b) obesity
    - (c) anemia
    - (d) emphysema
    - (e) asthma
    - (f) hypoglycemia
    - (g) diabetes mellitus
    - (h) epilepsy
    - (i) hypertension

18. The most unreliable means of monitoring a dental patient during I.V. sedation is:
    - (a) pulse rate
    - (b) blood pressure
    - (c) pupil size
    - (d) respiratory excursions
    - (e) Verrill's sign
    - (f) verbal responses
    - (g) eyelash reflex

19. Drug-related complications associated with I.V. sedation include all of the following EXCEPT:
    - (a) larynogospasm
    - (b) respiratory depression
    - (c) adverse interactions
    - (d) infiltrations

20. Most dental patients respond to nitrous oxide oxygen sedation in concentrations ranging from:
    - (a) 25 to 33 per cent
    - (b) 33 to 50 per cent
    - (c) 50 to 67 per cent
    - (d) 67 to 80 per cent

21. Relative analgesia is produced by certain non–drug-related measures that may include any of the following EXCEPT:
    - (a) acupuncture
    - (b) hypnosis
    - (c) oral premedication
    - (d) hyperstimulation

11

DRUG INTERACTIONS AND ABUSE

SECTION 1: DRUG INTERACTIONS

Alcohol

Ethyl alcohol is a sedative-hypnotic agent found in many commercial beverages that can be easily obtained by ambulatory patients under treatment with drugs. It depresses the CNS, and its effects in combination with other agents may be unpredictable or lethal.

Potentially lethal combinations result when alcohol is used with other sedative-hypnotics, such as barbiturates and chloral hydrate, narcotics, coronary vasodilators, muscle relaxants, and tricyclic antidepressants. Alcohol also potentiates many other agents, such as the major and minor tranquilizers, diuretics, antihistamines, tetracyclines, and certain non-narcotic analgesics and antihypertensive agents. It may induce severe hypoglycemia in diabetic patients receiving insulin or oral antidiabetic drugs, but small amounts of alcohol have been used in the diet to decrease insulin requirements, with the rationale that alcohol provides energy without requiring insulin for its metabolism. Sulfonamides potentiate the toxic effects of alcohol by inhibiting oxidation of acetaldehyde. Alcohol may increase the possibility of gastric hemorrhage in patients taking salicylates and may inhibit the anticonvulsant action of phenytoin. It also interferes with absorption of vitamin B_{12} and has an unpredictable effect on coumarin anticoagulants; it may adversely affect the liver and make patients more sensitive to anticoagulants, or it may inhibit the action of the drugs themselves. Patients taking anticoagulants should restrict their intake of alcohol.

The effects of alcohol are antagonized by CNS stimulants, such as caffeine or amphetamines.

Patients under treatment with "sleeping pills," "nerve pills," "pain pills," "angina pils," "water pills," "blood pressure pills," or insulin or "diabetes pills" should be ordered not to drink anything alcoholic while under treatment.

Tobacco

The active ingredient in tobacco (nicotine) has been correlated with lung cancer, with adverse effects on blood coagulation factors, with increased blood levels of endogenous corticosteroids, with elevated blood sugar, and with dietary changes. Tobacco consumption is frequently an attempt to correct an underlying metabolic defect (hypoglycemia), and when the metabolic defect does not exist there is no need for tobacco or food consumption to raise blood sugar suddenly (Chap. 3, Sec. 1).

Heavy smokers who consume 11 or more cigarettes daily have a lower dietary intake of B vitamins, vitamin C, vitamin E, and total protein compared to non-smokers. The smoker's intake of refined carbohydrates is statistically higher than that of a non-smoker, which enhances the smoker's susceptibility to chronic degenerative diseases. Smoking-related losses of vitamin B_{12} appear to be due to reaction of B_{12} with the cyanide in inhaled tobacco smoke, whereas losses of vitamin B_6 appear to involve a reaction of the vitamin with carbon monoxide in the smoke. Decreased plasma levels of vitamin C due to smoking are well established, but the exact mechanism has not been identified.

Smoking has significant implications for drug therapy in that (1) for certain drugs, smokers need different doses of a different frequency of administration than non-smokers, (2) when smokers stop or reduce their smoking their drug regimen may need adjustment, and (3) smokers may have different reactions to certain drugs than do non-smoking patients, with fewer or more numerous adverse effects.

The half-life of theophylline (the time required for one half a dose of theophylline to be removed from the body) is reduced from about seven hours in non-smokers to about four hours in smokers. Therefore, to achieve the same effects that occur in a non-smoker with this drug, smokers either need to have more frequent administration of theophylline or to have the dose increased by between 50 and 100 per cent.

Smokers metabolize 40 per cent more pentazocine per unit time than do non-smokers, necessitating larger and more frequent doses for analgesia used than with non-smokers. Smoking is also correlated with lower plasma levels of phenacetin and higher rates of "ineffective" responses to propoxyphene.

Patients taking anticoagulants for thrombosis or for other clotting problems should be advised to quit smoking because smoking reduces clotting time by potentiating platelet aggregation.

Smoking is also known to inhibit the action of barbiturates and to produce an increase in blood pressure when combined with propanolol.

Antibiotics

The penicillins are inhibited in their mechanism of action by erythromycin and the tetracyclines and are potentiated by the salicylates, chymotrypsin, and large doses of sulfonamides. The penicillins themselves are known to inhibit heparin and to potentiate the coumarin anticoagulants.

Erythromycin tends to inhibit the bactericidal activity of the penicillins but to potentiate their activity against resistant strains of *Staphylococcus aureus*. The antibacterial effects of erythromycin and lincomycin are antagonistic.

Tetracyclines are potentiated by alcohol, chymotrypsin, and citric acid, and oral absorption of them is inhibited by food. They should be administered one hour before meals or two hours after. These drugs also interfere with the intestinal synthesis of vitamin K by microorganisms and therefore potentiate coumarin anticoagulants. They antagonize the bactericidal effects of the penicillins, which is particularly intense with methicillin. Oral absorption is inhibited by complexing agents, such as antacids, dairy products, or dietary supplements containing calcium or iron. Administration of parenteral tetracycline combined with methoxyflurane anesthesia may seriously impair renal function, which can be fatal.

Lincomycin antagonizes the antibacterial action of erythromycin and is inhibited by kaolin-containing antidiarrheal medicines (Kaopectate) and by cyclamates. It has also been shown to have neuromuscular blocking properties that may enhance other neuromuscular blocking agents. These interactions are also shared by clindamycin.

The cephalosporins act synergistically with certain penicillins (ampicillin and benzyl penicillin) and aminoglycosides (kanamycin and streptomycin), but they are incompatible in parenteral mixtures with erythromycin, tetracyclines, or alkaline earth metals (calcium, magnesium, or strontium).

Sulfonamides are inhibited by local anesthetics that have a para-aminobenzoic acid (PABA) nucleus and are potentiated by salicylates and promethazine. They will themselves potentiate the actions of alcohol, coumarin anticoagulants, insulin, oral antidiabetic agents, phenytoin, methotrexate, and (in large doses) penicillins. Sulfonamides increase the excretion of vitamin C, and vitamin C increases excretion of sulfonamides.

Aminoglycosides should not be combined with other neuromuscular blocking agents or general anesthetics owing to the risk of muscular paralysis; such paralysis may be reversed by neostigmine administration. Potent diuretics enhance aminoglycoside toxicity.

Insulin

The hypoglycemic effect of insulin is potentiated by alcohol, salicylates, sulfonamides, antineoplastic agents, MAO inhibitors, beta-blocking agents, and coumarin anticoagulants. Amphetamines increase the metabolic rate and when combined with insulin may induce lower blood glucose levels than would the same amount of insulin alone. Insulin potentiates the action of oral antidiabetic agents.

The effects of insulin are antagonized by epinephrine, glucagon, corticosteroids, furosemide, thiazides, thyroid preparations, and general anesthesia.

Corticosteroids

Although the corticosteroids will potentiate the action of sedative-hypnotics, the corticosteroids are inhibited by barbiturates, chloral hydrate, and diphenhydramine. Nicotine (smoking) increases plasma steroid levels. When corticosteroids are combined with meperidine, antihistamines, tricyclic antidepressants, adrenergic stimulants, or cholinergic blockers, the intraocular pressure will increase, which is hazardous in patients with glaucoma. The corticosteroids antagonize insulin, cholinergic stimulants, anticholinesterases, and coumarin anticoagulants and may produce severe and often fatal hypotension with general anesthetics unless the dose of corticosteroids is increased preoperatively. These drugs may also produce hypokalemia, especially when combined with diuretics, which could enhance digitalis toxicity.

The salicylates may produce their anti-inflammatory effects by displacing corticosteroids from their plasma protein binding sites.

Vitamins

Vitamin B complex increases prothrombin time and when administered in combination with coumarin anticoagulants may lead to hemorrhage. Riboflavin tends to decompose tetracyclines, phenytoin decreases folate levels, and alcohol causes malabsorption of cobalamine.

Vitamin C decreases prothrombin time and antagonizes coumarin anticoagulants, and it enhances iron absorption in "mega" doses and potentiates sulfonamides, salicylates, and barbiturates. It increases the excretion of atropine and quinidine. Administration of atropine, sulfonamides, salicylates, and barbiturates increases the excretion of vitamin C.

Cholestyramine inhibits the absorption of fat-soluble vitamins (A, D group, E group, and K group). Vitamin K inhibits coumarin anticoagulants by encouraging formation of prothrombin and factors VII, IX, and X. Many antibiotics depress the synthesis of vitamin K by intestinal microorganisms and tend to potentiate coumarin anticoagulants.

Analgesics

All narcotic analgesics (morphine, codeine, synthetic opiates, and opioids) potentiate alcohol, sedative-hypnotics, tranquilizers, antihistamines, muscle relaxants, and other narcotic analgesics. They increase the possibility of orthostatic hypotension in patients taking thiazide diuretics. Beta-blocking agents, such as propanolol, behave as CNS depressants synergistically in the presence of morphine.

The salicylates potentiate the actions of penicillins, sulfonamides, corticosteroids, insulin, phenytoin, methotrexate, and (in large doses) coumarin anticoagulants. The action of salicylates is potentiated by furosemide and vitamin C (which decreases salicylate excretion). Salicylates inhibit vitamin C (by increasing ascorbate excretion) and are themselves inhibited by reserpine and phenobarbital. Beta-blocking agents abolish the anti-inflammatory effects of salicylates. The administration of salicylates in combination with tricyclic antidepressants or methotrexate may be fatal.

Propoxyphene is potentiated by alcohol, tranquilizers, and sedative-hypnotics and ranks second only to barbiturates as the leading prescription drug associated with fatalities. Lethal overstimulation of the CNS leading to convulsions and death may be produced when caffeine or amphetamines are used to treat propoxyphene overdosage.

Anticoagulants

Heparin sodium potentiates thyroxine and coumarin anticoagulants and is itself potentiated by salicylates (which inhibit platelet adhesiveness) and hyaluronidase (which stimulates heparin absorption). The actions of heparin sodium are inhibited by penicillins, tetracyclines, nicotine (smoking), digitalis, hydroxyzine, phenothiazines, protamine sulfate, and (in large doses) antihistamines.

The coumarin and indandione anticoagulants potentiate insulin and may be inhibited by certain of the benzodiazepine tranquilizers. These anticoagulants are potentiated by a wide variety of agents, including certain anesthetics, anticonvulsants, salicylates, antineoplastic agents, erythromycin, tetracyclines, sulfonamides, phenothiazines, methyldopa, chloral hydrate, trypsin-chymotrypsin preparations, diazepam, phenytoin, glucagon, heparin sodium, iodine, MAO inhibitors, morphine, mefenamic acid, hydroxyzine, and oxyphenbutazone and also by vitamin C deficiency. These drugs are also inhibited by an equally wide variety of agents, including corticosteroids, barbiturates, diuretics, xanthines, aminocaproic acid, cholestyramine, digitalis, meprobamate, diphenhydramine, vitamin C, and green leafy vegetables (vitamin K). The response to alcohol or to antihistamines used in combination with these anticoagulants is variable; i.e., the anticoagulant may be either potentiated or inhibited. Short-term reserpine therapy inhibits anticoagulants, whereas long-term reserpine therapy potentiates them.

Antihistamines

The antihistamines tend to potentiate the actions of epinephrine, norepinephrine, tricyclic antidepressants, alcohol, anticonvulsants, analgesics, organic nitrates and nitrites, thiopental sodium, and anticholinergic agents. Xerostomia secondary to chronic use of antihistamines with anticholinergic agents may lead to dental caries and premature loss of teeth. Antihistamines tend to inhibit the actions of acetylcholine and cholinesterase inhibitors, anticoagulants, hydrocortisone and other corticosteroids, phenytoin, and of course, histamine itself.

The actions of antihistamines are inhibited by beta-blocking agents. Administration of MAO inhibitors combined with antihistamines is contraindicated because MAO inhibitors slow the metabolism of the norepinephrine released by antihistamines and potentiate the cardiovascular effects of norepinephrine and the anticholinergic effects of the antihistamines. Since the phenothiazines block the accumulation of norepinephrine at storage sites, free norepinephrine would increase in concentration and would be potentiated by MAO inhibitors. The sedative effects of the antihistamines are inhibited by caffeine and amphetamines.

Sedative-hypnotics and tranquilizers are both potentiated by antihistamines, but continued use of either combination may lead to mutual inhibition, tolerance, and habituation. Antihistamines given pre-operatively increase the depth and duration of barbiturate narcosis.

Sedative-Hypnotics

Some of the sedative-hypnotics are known as enzyme inducers (barbiturates and chloral hydrate), and they increase the rate of metabolism of other drugs; when the drug metabolites are less active than the drug, enzyme induction inhibits drug action, whereas when the drug metabolites are more active than the drug, enzyme induction potentiates the drug action. Tolerance results when a drug induces its own metabolizing enzymes. The interactions of most sedative-hypnotics, except ethyl alcohol, which is treated separately (Chap. 11, Sec. 1), involve the enzyme inducers.

The enzyme inducers potentiate all narcotic analgesics and chlorpromazine; they also potentiate alcohol, MAO inhibitors, and tricyclic antidepressants, which are contraindicated for use in combination with them. An enzyme inducer antagonizes itself and other enzyme inducers and inhibits the action of benzodiazepines, meprobamate, phenothiazines, and corticosteroids. It also inhibits the oral anticoagulants, except chloral hydrate, which potentiates it.

The enzyme inducers are inhibited by phenytoin and are potentiated by alcohol, corticosteroids, and MAO inhibitors.

Tranquilizers

The phenothiazines potentiate alcohol; anticholinergic agents; antihistamines; muscle relaxants; CNS depressants, such as narcotics (morphine, meperidine) and general anesthetics (thiopental sodium); aspirin; insulin; quinidine; and antihypertensive agents, which may lead to hypotensive episodes; treatment of such episodes with epinephrine could lead to "epinephrine reversal," aggravating the hypotension (Chap. 11, Sec. 1). Phenothiazines inhibit heparin sodium and the CNS-stimulating properties of amphetamines, but they potentiate the sedative effects of the barbiturates and benzodiazepines.

Phenothiazines are potentiated by alcohol, antidepressants (MAO inhibitors and dibenzazepines), benzodiazepines, and atropine. The potentiation of phenothiazines by anticholesterases can be reversed by anticholinergics, although anticholinergics potentiate phenothiazines themselves. The hypotension induced by phenothiazines can be reversed by norepinephrine or phenylephrine, and phenothiazines are inhibited by long-term barbiturate therapy. Their alpha-blocking activity can be increased by beta-blocking agents, and they may lower the convulsive threshold, necessitating higher doses of anticonvulsants for control of seizures.

Both the major and minor tranquilizers potentiate alcohol and anticholinergic agents and are potentiated by antidepressants. Chlordiazepoxide potentiates phenytoin. The spectrum of interactions for other tranquilizers is similar to that of the phenothiazines except for those involving alpha-blocking activity.

Tricyclic Antidepressants

The dibenzazepines (tricyclic antidepressants) potentiate the actions of epinephrine, norepinephrine, narcotics, amphetamines, belladonna alkaloids and other anticholinergic agents, antihistamines, barbiturates, benzodiazepines, organic nitrates and nitrites, and centrally acting muscle relaxants. Lethal potentiation occurs when they are combined with salicylates, alcohol, phenothiazines, or MAO inhibitors. Although the dibenzazepines potentiate anticonvulsants, they tend to lower the seizure threshold in epileptic patients, necessitating higher doses of anticonvulsants for seizure control. Tricyclic antidepressants inhibit certain antihypertensive agents (reserpine and guanethidine), cholinesterase inhibitors, and mephentermine sulfate and inhibit oral absorption of oxyphenbutazone.

The actions of tricyclic antidepressants are potentiated by narcotics and beta-blocking agents. The associated cardiovascular depression can be reversed with isoproterenol, and the actions of nortriptyline are inhibited by hydrocortisone.

Monoamine Oxidase Inhibitors

The MAO inhibitors potentiate a wide variety of agents, including amphetamines, sympathomimetic vasoconstrictors (alpha stimulants), anticholinergic agents, antihistamines, antihypertensives, anticoagulants, diuretics, coronary vasodilators, muscle relaxants, phenothiazines, minor tranquilizers, atropine, caffeine, cocaine, and doxapram, as well as themselves. Lethal interactions result when they are given with insulin or tricyclic antidepressants. They also potentiate CNS depressants (alcohol, barbiturates, chloral hydrate, codeine, morphine, meperidine, and general anesthetics).

MAO inhibitors are potentiated by narcotics and beta-blocking agents and are inhibited by phenobarbital and phenothiazines. Chlorpromazine potentiates the hypotensive effect of pargyline.

Muscle Relaxants

The propanediol (meprobamate) and dibenzazepine (diazepam) centrally acting muscle relaxants potentiate CNS depressants and MAO inhibitors. They are potentiated by phenothiazines and are inhibited by barbiturates and diphenhydramine.

The anticholinergic (promethazine) muscle relaxants may induce mental confusion, anxiety, or tremors when combined with propoxyphene.

The competitive (d-tubocurarine) peripherally acting muscle relaxants are potentiated by general anesthetics, MAO inhibitors, quinidine, and excess carbon dioxide. They are inhibited by epinephrine, norepinephrine, and anticholinesterases.

The depolarizing (succinylcholine chloride) peripherally acting muscle relaxants potentiate fluorine anesthetics (halothane, methoxyflurane, and enflurane), anticholinesterases, phenothiazines, and acetylcholine. They are potentiated by MAO inhibitors, local anesthetics, procainamide, quinidine, diuretics, and anticholinesterases. When they are administered in combination with methotrimeprazine, severe hypotension may result.

Antiemetics

The interactions of the phenothiazine tranquilizers are shared by the antiemetics chlorpromazine, promethazine, and prochlorperazine.

The interactions of the antihistamines are shared by the antiemetics dimenhydrinate, diphenhydramine, and hydroxyzine.

Trimethobenzamide is relatively free of interactions with other agents.

Excessive pre-medication with antiemetics prior to local anesthesia in the elderly patient or in the young child may lead to excessive CNS depression.

CNS Stimulants and Depressants

Analeptics (caffeine and amphetamines) should not be given to patients suffering from overdosage of narcotics, propoxyphene, or antihistamines because they may initiate fatal convulsions.

Anticonvulsants (barbiturates, phenytoin, and diazepam) tend to inhibit hydrocortisone and are potentiated by anticoagulants, narcotics, MAO inhibitors, and phenytoin. Barbiturates, especially phenobarbital, inhibit anticonvulsants and themselves by enzyme induction. Reserpine and phenothiazines lower the convulsive threshold and may necessitate an increase in anticonvulsant dosage.

Cardiovascular and Autonomic Agents

The organic nitrates and nitrites used as coronary vasodilators potentiate the actions of antihypertensives, anticholinergics (antihistamines and tricyclic antidepressants), and meperidine and its derivatives and are potentiated by alcohol and beta-blocking agents. They tend to inhibit the actions of histamine, epinephrine, and norepinephrine and are inhibited by cholinergic agents.

The xanthines tend to inhibit the actions of the coumarin anticoagulants.

The digitalis glycosides also inhibit the oral anticoagulants and are potentiated by phenytoin, procainamide, quinidine, and propanolol. Their actions are inhibited by triamterene, and their toxicity is enhanced by thyroid preparations, diuretics, insulin, reserpine, and isoproterenol.

The thiazide diuretics increase insulin requirements and potentiate alpha- and beta-blocking agents, antihypertensives, digitalis glycosides, tricyclic antidepressants, and competitive muscle relaxants (*d*-tubocurarine) and also potentiate the orthostatic hypotension resulting from administration of phenothiazines, narcotics, barbiturates, alcohol, and procainamide. They inhibit the action of pressor amines, such as norepinephrine.

Furosemide is a sulfonamide itself and shares the interactions characteristic of the sulfonamides (Chap. 11, Sec. 1). In addition to these interactions, it increases insulin requirements; potentiates other diuretics, competitive muscle relaxants (*d*-tubocurarine), and antihypertensives; and enhances toxicity of salicylates and digitalis. It tends to inhibit the actions of oral anticoagulants and pressor amines.

Guanethidine potentiates insulin and sympathomimetics (catecholamines and other vasopressors), and also potentiates the hypotensive effects of general anesthetics. It is potentiated by diuretics and inhibited by mephentermine and anticholinergic agents. It may be inhibited by sympathomimetics, antihistamines, antidepressants, amphetamines, or cocaine.

Methyldopa potentiates oral anticoagulants and CNS depressants (alcohol, narcotics, and general anesthetics) and is potentiated by diuretics. It may be inhibited by adrenergic stimulants or antidepressants. Adverse reactions and hypertension often result when it is administered in combination with antidepressants.

Hydralazine is potentiated by thiazide diuretics, triamterene, MAO inhibitors, and general anesthetics and is inhibited by amphetamines and sympathomimetics. It tends to inhibit the actions of epinephrine, norepinephrine, and pyridoxine (vitamin B_6).

Lidocaine potentiates procainamide and CNS depressants (alcohol, narcotics, and general anesthetics) and is potentiated by pre-anesthetic medication. It tends to inhibit sulfonamides, and its nerve-blocking activity is inhibited by pargyline. Patients sensitive to lidocaine are usually cross-sensitive to quinidine and procainamide.

Procainamide potentiates antihypertensive agents, muscle relaxants, lidocaine, quinidine, and propanolol and is potentiated by lidocaine. It tends to inhibit the actions of acetylcholine and cholinesterase inhibitors, and its hypotensive effects are inhibited by pressor agents.

Quinidine potentiates antihypertensive drugs, anticholinergic agents, anticoagulants, muscle relaxants, digitalis glycosides, procainamide, and propanolol and is potentiated by phenytoin. It inhibits the actions of acetylcholine and cholinesterase inhibitors and may lead to arrhythmias when given in combination with Rauwolfia alkaloids (reserpine).

Sympathomimetics (catecholamines, methoxamine, metaraminol, mephentermine, phenylephrine, ephedrine, amphetamines, and levonordefrin and related vasopressors) are potentiated by alcohol, antihistamines, antidepressants, guanethidine, and cocaine but are inhibited by other antihypertensive agents and by organic nitrates and nitrites. They tend to inhibit the actions of hydralazine and methyldopa and may produce arrhythmias when combined with digitalis glycosides, guanethidine, or halogenated general anesthetics (halothane, methoxyflurane, and enflurane). Mephentermine inhibits guanethidine, whereas dopamine inhibits morphine. Epinephrine is inhibited by hydralazine and, when administered in combination with alpha-blocking agents, causes a paradoxical lowering of blood pressure due to excessive $beta_2$ stimulation of skeletal muscle vessels and to a decrease in total peripheral resistance ("epinephrine reversal"). Paradoxical hypotension may also occur when other alpha-$beta_1$-$beta_2$ stimulants are combined with alpha blockers, and it may lead to other drug-related reversals.

Atropine potentiates anticholinergic agents and meperidine and is potentiated by antidepressants. It tends to inhibit the actions of acetylcholine, cholinesterase inhibitors, pilocarpine, vitamin C, and the respiratory depression of morphine. It is inhibited by reserpine and vitamin C and when given in combination with methotrimeprazine, it may lead to hypotension.

Phentolamine, an alpha blocker, antagonizes the myocardial sensitization to general anesthetics induced by sympathomimetic agents.

Propanolol, a beta blocker, potentiates organic nitrates and nitrites, digitalis glycosides, antihypertensives, quinidine, d-tubocurarine, insulin, and the CNS depression induced by morphine and general anesthetics. It tends to inhibit the actions of antihistamines, isoproterenol, and anti-inflammatory agents (salicylates, hydrocortisone, and others) and is inhibited by isoproterenol. It is potentiated by phenytoin.

Local Anesthetics

All local anesthetics potentiate CNS depressants (alcohol, narcotics, and general anesthetics) and enhance the toxicity of other local anesthetics. Epinephrine should not be used as a vasoconstrictor with local anesthesia in cardiac patients when the dose would exceed 0.2 mg of epinephrine, and it also should not be used in hyperthyroid patients or in those receiving adrenergic blocking agents.

Procaine potentiates procainamide, prolongs the action of penicillins and heparin sodium, and inhibits the antibacterial activity of sulfonamides by virtue of its PABA nucleus. It is potentiated by MAO inhibitors and inhibited by phenobarbital, and its effects are antagonistic to physostigmine.

General Anesthetics

General anesthetics potentiate antihypertensive agents, competitive muscle relaxants, and CNS depressants (alcohol, narcotics, barbiturates, and phenothiazines). They are potentiated by beta-blocking agents, alcohol, antihistamines, phenothiazines, and MAO inhibitors. When given together with doxapram or any of the catecholamines, arrhythmias or ventricular tachycardia may result; these effects are antagonized by phentolamine. Severe hypotension may occur during general anesthesia in patients on long-term steroid therapy unless the steroid dose is increased pre-operatively. General anesthetics may also enhance the actions of anticoagulants by inhibiting formation of coagulation factors.

The use of nitrous oxide with fluroxene produces an increase in central venous pressure and cardiac output.

General Rules

The following generalizations will help prevent the majority of the hazardous drug interactions that could be encountered in the practice of dentistry and dental hygiene:

1. Refrain from prescribing or dispensing any drug to patients taking antidepressants (dibenzazepines or MAO inhibitors) or anticoagulants unless a physician indicates in writing to do so. Remember that aspirin is lethal with tricyclic antidepressants.

2. Caution the patient to abstain from drinking alcohol during drug treatment.

3. Reduce and adjust the dose of pre-anesthetic medication (sedative-hypnotics, tranquilizers, and narcotics) given to patients taking antidepressants, coronary vaso-dilators, antihistamines, or muscle relaxants. If nitrous oxide is combined with pre-operative sedation, be prepared for the eventuality of a general anesthetic state.

4. Avoid local anesthesia with lidocaine in patients taking procainamide; avoid local anesthesia with epinephrine in patients taking antidepressants, phenothiazines, or quinidine.

5. Avoid pre-medication with phenothiazines in epileptic patients and pre-medication with barbiturates in patients taking digitalis glycosides.

6. Use only one antibiotic at a time to treat infections.

SECTION 2: DRUG ABUSE

Drugs Most Often Abused

The following drugs and combination products are most commonly involved in episodes of drug abuse and were grouped into Schedules by the Controlled Substances Act of 1970 (Chap. 1, Sec. 3):

1. Schedule I

    a. diacetylmorphine (heroin, H, horse, junk, smack)
    b. lysergic acid diethylamide (LSD, acid, hawk, the chief)
    c. marijuana (Cannabis, pot, grass, boo)
    d. peyote (cactus)

2. Schedule II

    a. morphine (M, Miss Emma)
    b. hydromorphone (Dilaudid)
    c. codeine
    d. Percodan
    e. meperidine (Demerol)
    f. cocaine (coke, snow, happy dust, corinne)
    g. amphetamines ("uppers")
        1. amphetamine sulfate (Benzedrine, bennies)
        2. dextroamphetamine sulfate (Dexedrine, dexies, copilots)
        3. methamphetamine hydrochloride (Methedrine, STP, crystals)
    h. barbiturates ("downers")

1. pentobarbital (Nembutal, yellow jackets)
2. secobarbital (Seconal, red birds)
3. amobarbital (Amytal, blue heavens)

3. Schedule III

a. Empirin Compound with Codeine
b. Fiorinal with Codeine
c. Phenaphen with Codeine

4. Schedule IV

a. non-narcotic analgesics
   1. propoxyphene hydrochloride (Darvon)
   2. pentazocine (Talwin)
b. barbiturates and tranquilizers ("downers")
   1. phenobarbital (Luminal, purple hearts)
   2. meprobamate (Equanil, Miltown)
   3. chlordiazepoxide (Librium)
   4. diazepam (Valium)

The student should note that nearly all the lawful drugs in this list may be prescribed or dispensed by dentists for the treatment of oral disease.

Signs of Drug Abuse

The dental hygienist often sees the new patient for the first appointment and may perform a visual and oral examination before the dentist to detect possible narcotics users. The following tips may be helpful in analyzing new patients:

1. Notice long, buttoned sleeves worn in warm weather.

2. Be suspicious of patients presenting with one arm bandaged or suspended in a harness without a plaster cast.

3. Notice small blood stains on skin or clothes or adhesive bandages on the backs of the hands.

4. When you record the blood pressure check arms for needle marks.

5. Notice a sloppy, unkempt appearance.

6. Notice excessive yawning, sneezing, nervousness, slurred speech, or slowness of response in answering questions.

7. Be suspicious of a thirsty patient who frequently licks his lips.

8. Notice constricted pupils in dim light or a nose red from scratching or rubbing.

9. Be wary of any patient who presents with a history of pain so incompatible with oral and radiographic findings that a diagnosis cannot be made.

10. Be wary of several people in succession with practically the same discomfort and symptoms.

11. Be wary of the patient just passing through town with a toothache and an

empty pill bottle who declines treatment, stalls for time, or changes the subject when you suggest that he forward his radiographs from his previous dentist.

12. Be wary of the patient with irritated mucosa at the apex of a slightly decayed tooth. The addict is clever—he may use a sharp needle to simulate an abscess.

13. Be wary of patients in pain who are allergic to most narcotics except one that worked well for them once before, which they do not pronounce well.

14. Be wary of the patient who wants an antibiotic for a toothache. He may be trying to throw off suspicion by dwelling on the antibiotic, which is often prescribed with a narcotic.

15. Be wary of the patient who telephones the dentist at odd hours with a toothache or who always prefers the last appointment of the day and arrives habitually late.

Addict Manipulation of Dental Personnel

The process of tricking a dentist into writing a prescription is referred to as "making a dentist," and the prescription drugs most obtained by this means are narcotics, certain non-narcotic analgesics, and certain tranquilizers. The United States Government Drug Abuse Warning Network (DAWN) reports that alcohol, heroin, and diazepam are the most frequently abused drugs in the United States, based on emergency room and crisis center overdosage reports from 23 major cities; diazepam was used alone in 44 per cent of the cases, and in more than half the incidences it was obtained by legal prescription. The drug addict (user) as well as the drug dealer (pusher), usually tries to obtain tranquilizers from physicians and narcotics from dentists; the younger addicts who still have their teeth to use as an excuse for obtaining a prescription tend to focus their interest on older dentists near retirement, who (presumably) are unaware of the drug abuse problem, or on younger, inexperienced dentists, who are just beginning their practices and who (presumably) will go to any length to satisfy a new patient in the hope of gaining referrals for the growth of their practices.

Organized dentistry unknowingly screens dentists for addicts and dealers who phone the local dental society by supplying them with the names of dentists who practice their own endodontics or oral surgery (such dentists are usually licensed to prescribe Schedule II drugs). By this means, several dental offices can be contacted by the drug abuser with a high degree of success; many local dental societies are now publishing descriptions of suspicious patients with pertinent oral findings so that individuals who attempt to "make the rounds" to several offices will not be successful. Dentists who suspect that a patient is angling for a prescription only should simply state, "I'm sorry, but that's a drug I don't prescribe. My advice is to contact your physician for further treatment." It won't take long for word to get around through the grapevine that this dentist does not "write;" whenever such a patient is satisfied with the treatment he receives the dentist can expect many more similar patients.

The drug dealer is more difficult to spot than the addict because (1) the dealer fails to display the signs of drug abuse (Chap. 11, Sec. 2), (2) he is less careless than the addict in his office behavior and generally thinks more clearly, and (3) family members often accompany the dealer to the office to corroborate the pain story related to the dentist. The street sale of restricted drugs is extremely lucrative, but when drugs are dispensed at the request of a lawful prescriber charges cannot be brought against a dealer without proof of sale to a third party; this is almost impossible without the testimony of an eye-witness or a signed confession. Furthermore, the dealer knows that the addicted customers cannot betray the relationship to the police without risking the agony of withdrawal, and dealers won't sell to anyone but their usual customers for fear of selling to undercover narcotics agents.

Dentists and dental hygienists can do their part to limit the illegal sale of drugs by communicating information about suspicious patients to their local dental societies, which can then notify local medical societies, hospital emergency rooms, pharmacies, and the police, as well as other dentists. The single factor that permits the existence of drug dealers—the factor that is essential for the survival of such parasites—is the present state of non-communication among members of the dental, medical, and pharmaceutical professions.

Drugs Most Often Stolen

The majority of stolen drugs as reported on Drug Enforcement Administration Form 106 are routinely prescribed by dentists and include the following drugs and combination products:

1. Analgesics

   a. morphine
   b. Empirin Compound with Codeine
   c. Fiorinal with Codeine
   d. hydromorphone (Dilaudid)
   e. Percodan
   f. meperidine (Demerol)

2. Amphetamines

   a. dextroamphetamine sulfate (Dexedrine)
   b. methamphetamine hydrochloride (Methedrine)

3. Barbiturates

   a. pentobarbital (Nembutal)
   b. secobarbital (Seconal)
   c. amobarbital (Amytal)

4. Tranquilizers

   a. chlordiazepoxide (Librium)
   b. diazepam (Valium)
   c. amitriptyline hydrochloride (Elavil)

Office Drug Security

Most addicts and drug pushers can write a prescription as well as any doctor, and they pay large sums of money for the street sale of prescription pads, as well as for the drugs themselves. If such a drug abuser sees where a dentist stores emergency drugs, he may return at night to steal whatever can be readily sold. Approximately $500 to $1000 in cash or proceeds from the sale of stolen goods are required each day to keep an addict supplied with drugs, depending on his habit, and he can act despicably to obtain what he wants. One blank script with the doctor's personal BNDD number (DEA number) is worth $50 to $75 on the streets.

With these facts in mind, one should practice the following general office policies:

1. Prescription pads should be kept in the doctor's personal possession during office hours and locked in a safe or locked cabinet after hours. They should not be left out in plain view of patients seated in the dental chair.

2. Prescription blanks should not have the doctor's DEA number printed on them; this should be filled in by the doctor as needed.

3. The doctor should avoid carelessness in writing prescriptions so that a prescription once written cannot be altered to dispense a larger dose than intended.

4. Office drugs should be kept out of sight and in small quantities. The office staff should be instructed not to discuss the amounts or location of such drugs with any patient or with persons outside the office.

TEST QUESTIONS

1. Unless prior clearance is obtained in writing from the patient's physician, no drug should be prescribed or dispensed to any dental patient taking:
   (a) anticoagulants
   (b) antidepressants
   (c) salicylates
   (d) both a and b
   (e) both b and c
   (f) all of the above

2. Patients should be cautioned to abstain from alcohol consumption while under drug treatment of any kind because:
   (a) alcohol is easily obtained by ambulatory patients
   (b) unpredictable or lethal effects may result from mixing alcohol with many drugs
   (c) alcohol potentiates many other agents
   (d) all of the above

3. A reduction in dose of pre-anesthetic medication is indicated for those patients taking:
   (a) antidepressants
   (b) coronary vasodilators
   (c) antihistamines
   (d) muscle relaxants
   (e) all of the above
   (f) none of the above

4. When nitrous oxide oxygen sedation is combined with pre-anesthetic medication the operator should be prepared for the eventuality of a:
   (a) hypotensive episode
   (b) general anesthetic state
   (c) convulsive seizure
   (d) ventricular tachycardia

5. Patients taking procainamide should NOT be given lidocaine for local anesthesia. This is to prevent:
   (a) ventricular tachycardia
   (b) severe hypotension
   (c) both a and b
   (d) neither a nor b

6. Patients taking quinidine should NOT be given local anesthesia using epinephrine as a vasoconstrictor. This is to prevent:
   (a) ventricular fibrillation
   (b) congestive heart failure
   (c) bacterial endocarditis
   (d) all of the above

7. Epinephrine reversal may result when local anesthesia with epinephrine is given in combination with any drug that:
   (a) stimulates alpha receptors
   (b) stimulates beta receptors
   (c) blocks alpha receptors
   (d) blocks beta receptors

8. Patients taking digitalis glycosides should not receive pre-medication with barbiturates because:
   (a) barbiturates could decrease the effects of these drugs
   (b) severe hypotension may result
   (c) a general anesthetic state may result
   (d) all of the above

9. Epileptic patients should NOT receive pre-medication with phenothiazines unless the dosage of anticonvulsant is increased, because the phenothiazines:
   (a) inhibit the action of anticon- vulsants
   (b) lower the convulsive threshold
   (c) both a and b
   (d) neither a nor b

10. Patients taking tricyclic antidepressants may have a fatal interaction occur if the dental hygienist recommends taking:
    (a) aspirin
    (b) alcohol
    (c) phenothiazines
    (d) MAO inhibitors
    (e) any of the above

11. Epinephrine for use as a vasoconstrictor in local anesthetic solutions should NOT be administered to patients who are taking:
    (a) phenothiazines
    (b) tricyclic antidepressants
    (c) MAO inhibitors
    (d) alpha-blocking agents
    (e) quinidine
    (f) any of the above

12. Dental caries and premature loss of teeth may occur secondary to xerostomia resulting from chronic use of:
    (a) antihistamines
    (b) anticholinergic agents
    (c) belladonna alkaloids
    (d) any of the above

13. Administration of any enzyme inducer, such as chloral hydrate or a barbiturate, may result in:
    (a) inhibition of other drugs
    (b) potentiation of other drugs
    (c) tolerance
    (d) any of the above

14. Cardiac arrhythmias may result when epinephrine is used for hemostasis or gingival retraction during general anesthesia using:
    (a) halothane and methoxyflurane
    (b) nitrous oxide and enflurane
    (c) both a and b
    (d) neither a nor b

15. The antibacterial activity of the sulfonamides may be inhibited by administration of local anesthesia using:
    (a) procaine-propoxycaine
    (b) lidocaine
    (c) mepivacaine
    (d) prilocaine

16. All of the following could be signs of drug abuse EXCEPT:
    (a) long sleeves in warm weather
    (b) an arm bandaged or suspended in a harness without a cast
    (c) a sloppy unkempt appearance
    (d) persistent thirst or licking of lips
    (e) constricted pupils in bright light
    (f) a nose red from scratching or rubbing

17. Office rules to follow to discourage the drug dealer who is posing as a dental patient
    are to:
    (a) keep prescription pads out of sight and locked up at night
    (b) avoid printing the dentist's DEA number on the prescription blanks
    (c) avoid carelessness in writing the subscription so that once written it cannot be
        altered to dispense a larger dose
    (d) keep emergency drugs out of sight and in small quantity
    (e) avoid discussing the amounts or location of office drugs with persons outside
        the office
    (f) all of the above

12

EMERGENCIES

SECTION 1: DIAGNOSIS AND MANAGEMENT OF PATIENTS

Vital Signs

The patient's vital signs, or "vitals," are (1) blood pressure, (2) pulse rate, (3) respiratory rate, and (4) temperature. These measurements give an immediate evaluation of the medical status of the patient and are monitored during the postoperative period following major surgery and during acute emergencies.

Blood pressure maintenance is a function of five variables, four of which are under autonomic control and have been previously described (Chap. 6, Sec. 2). The mercury manometer is used as the standard of reference, and blood pressure (BP) is measured in units of mm mercury (Hg), signifying the force per unit of vessel area that would support a column of mercury a certain number of millimeters in height. The pumping action of the heart is intermittent, and the blood pressure normally alternates between a systolic pressure of 120 mm mercury and a diastolic pressure of 80 mm mercury; systole refers to the phase of the cardiac cycle characterized by contraction, whereas diastole refers to the period of relaxation. Blood pressure is recorded as a quotient, with the systolic pressure in the numerator and the diastolic pressure in the denominator, i.e., 120/80. The mean blood pressure is the sum of the diastolic pressure and one third the difference of the systolic and diastolic pressures, i.e., 93 mm mercury. The average blood pressure is the sum of the diastolic pressure and one half the difference of the systolic and diastolic pressures, i.e., 100 mm mercury. Blood pressure readings should be taken at the time of hospital admission, on the evening prior to major surgery, on the morning of surgery, q.4h. for four days postoperatively after major surgery and prior to office dental surgery, and readings should also be taken in all new dental patients and in recall patients.

The pulse rate at rest is between 60 and 100 beats/minute, with a mean value of 72 beats/minute. The pulse is most commonly palpated on the ventrolateral side of the wrist (radial pulse) or just medial to the sternocleidomastoid muscle in the neck (carotid pulse). The pulse pressure felt with the fingers is the difference of the systolic and diastolic pressures, i.e., 40 mm mercury. The velocity of transmission of the pressure pulse down the aorta (between 3 and 5 meters/sec), down the large arteries (between 7 and 10 meters/sec), and down the small arteries (between 15 and 35 meters/sec) is much greater than the velocity of blood flow, which is only 33 cm/sec in the aorta and which decreases to 1/1000 in the capillaries (0.3 mm/sec). Therefore, the pressure pulse arrives at the palpated arteries between 15 and 100 times faster than does the blood ejected from the left ventricle. The patient is said to be in sinus rhythm when the pulse rate is within normal limits, in sinus bradycardia when the pulse rate is less than 60/minute, and in sinus tachycardia when the pulse rate is greater than 100/minute with no electrocardiogram indications of arrhythmia. Sinus bradycardia may be seen in athletes conditioned by exercise or in patients experiencing drug-induced respiratory depression; sinus tachycardia may be seen in patients who are nervous, in patients who are in syncope or other forms of shock, or in patients in febrile states (a 1° F increase in body temperature increases pulse rate 10 beats/minute). Marey's law states that under rest conditions, blood pressure is inversely proportional to pulse rate; therefore, sinus tachycardia is the logical sequel to a fall in blood pressure and occurs to maintain tissue perfusion. Under conditions of exercise, Marey's law does not hold; i.e., blood pressure is proportional to pulse rate. The absence of a pulse in a living subject indicates cardiogenic shock (Chap. 6, Sec. 1) and ventricular fibrillation, a condition of disorderly spread of excitation through the myocardium that, left untreated, results in death. Although blood pressure in children is less than that in an adult, the pulse rate for young children may be between 100 and 120 beats/minute.

The normal respiratory rate is 12 ventilations/minute in adults but this value is also higher for young children. The rate may rise to between 40 and 50 breaths/minute during exercise in which the tidal volume can become as great as the vital capacity (Fig. 10–3). The respiratory minute volume (tidal volume × respiratory rate) can be increased by as much as 25-fold for short periods of time, but it is normally 6 liters/minute for the average male.

Body temperature is measured by means of a mercury dry-bulb thermometer inserted rectally or sublingually, and the normal reading is 37° C or 98.6° F. If the temperature is elevated (99° F and above) the patient is febrile; if it is not, he is afebrile. The temperature of febrile patients should be taken q.4h. until it remains at a normal level for two consecutive readings. Rectal readings should be employed with those patients who cannot or will not cooperate with sublingual placement of the thermometer, such as infants and very young children, the very old or senile, or unconscious patients. Febrile patients should never be spoken of as "having a temperature"; all patients have a temperature, even dead ones.

Indirect Blood Pressure Determination

Since it is impractical to insert a cannula directly into an artery and measure intra-arterial blood pressure, an indirect approach using the palpatory (radial) and auscultatory methods is employed. An inflatable bag or bladder inside a cloth cuff is wrapped around the patient's upper arm directly over the brachial artery. The cuff must completely encircle the upper arm, and if the arm is obese, the standard-sized cuff (14 X 52 cm with a balloon 12.5 X 23 cm) may give falsely high pressure readings. The standard cuff is appropriate for an arm circumference up to 30 cm; for arms over 30 cm in circumference, a cuff 17 X 54 cm with a balloon 15 X 38 cm should be used. This oversized cuff not only will accommodate larger arms but also will not introduce errors into the readings for persons with normal-sized arms. An extremely oversized cuff 21 X 82 cm with a balloon 19 X 39 cm can be used on the leg of grossly obese persons.

An aneroid (bellows) sphygmomanometer is calibrated against a mercury manometer and may be used in place of a mercury column. After the cuff is properly placed with the label over the ventral surface of the arm the valve leading to the squeeze bulb is closed by turning it clockwise until it locks, and the cuff is then inflated by pumping the bulb to a pressure between 10 and 20 mm mercury above the value necessary to stop blood flow in the brachial artery. This value is determined by palpating for the disappearance of the radial pulse coincident with inflating the cuff. The bag (bladder) pressure is then gradually reduced by opening the valve on the squeeze bulb with a slight counter-clockwise turn to allow the balloon to deflate at a rate of between 2 and 4 mm mercury/second. If the cuff is deflated too rapidly, errors will appear in the readings. The systolic pressure is noted on the aneroid at the palpation of the first beat of the radial pulse (palpatory or radial method).

The stethoscope is placed in the ears with the diaphragm on the skin overlying the cubital fossa, distal to the compressed brachial artery, and the cuff is inflated above the systolic pressure again. As the cuff pressure is again deflated to equal the systolic pressure the sounds originally described by Korotkoff are produced; as the pressure is slowly decreased in the cuff, the sounds change in phase, character, and magnitude. There are four types of Korotkoff sounds: (1) phase I, a rhythmic tapping coincident with the heartbeat that gradually increases in intensity; (2) phase II, a period in which the tapping sounds change to a murmur or swishing sound; (3) phase III, a period in which the sounds are crisper and of greater intensity than in phase I; and (4) phase IV, marked by abrupt muffling and decreasing intensity, as if the sounds were fading out. Phase V is the point at which the sounds disappear altogether. The phases are separated by a pressure interval approximately equal to 13 mm mercury (Fig. 12-1). The systolic pressure is defined as the pressure reading at the onset of phase I, and the diastolic pressure, as the reading at the onset of phase IV (auscultatory method).

In some individuals phase IV persists to zero, which may indicate aortic insufficiency or may be normal for that person; it may also indicate excessive pressure over the stethoscope diaphragm. The point of onset of phase V is called the second diastolic pressure, and recording in these instances should include systolic, diastolic, and the end point, i.e., 120/80/30 and 120/80/0.

Sometimes, particularly in hypertensive patients, the Korotkoff sounds disappear during the last part of phase I or during the onset of phase II, a phenomenon which is termed the "auscultation gap." It may cover a range of 40 mm mercury before the sounds return at a lower pressure. Unless the operator first palpates for the disappearance of the radial pulse as the cuff pressure is lowered, it is possible to seriously underestimate the

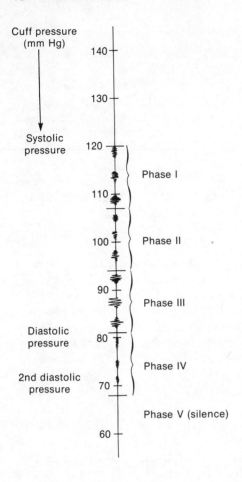

Figure 12–1. Phases of the Korotkoff sounds (BP = 120/80/68)

systolic pressure or to overestimate the diastolic pressure, if an auscultation gap is noted.

When all the sounds have been heard, the cuff should be rapidly and completely deflated to allow the release of blood trapped in the veins before further determinations are made. Venous return can be improved by holding the patient's arm above the head for about 20 seconds.

Diagnosis of Abnormal Blood Pressure

Any patient whose systolic pressure is equal to or greater than 160 or whose diastolic pressure is equal to or greater than 95 is considered to be hypertensive and should have repeated measurements performed by his physician, dentist, or a community screening program. The hypotensive patient whose systolic pressure is equal to or less than 80 or whose diastolic pressure is equal to or less than 65 should also have repeated measurements. The lower limit of hypertension is therefore 160/95, the upper limit of hypotension is 80/65, and the normotensive range is from 80 to 160 systolic/65 to 95 diastolic.

Drug treatment is indicated for hypertensive patients whose diastolic pressures are equal to or greater than 105, and sustained elevations above 130 should be considered a medical emergency. Extreme pain may cause extremely elevated pressures, and if the diastolic pressure is above 110 there is increased incidence of cerebrovascular accident (stroke) secondary to dental procedures performed without sedation or antihypertensive drugs. If dental treatment cannot be delayed, the severity of the dental problem must be weighed against the possible danger of the level of the blood pressure and the time involved in obtaining medical help if it should be needed during a stressful dental procedure.

Essential hypertension is high blood pressure that cannot be attributed to any known cause; most patients with high blood pressure have essential hypertension. However, hypertension may be caused by many diseases, such as renal disease, adrenal disease such as Cushing's syndrome, pheochromocytoma, diabetes mellitus, toxemia of pregnancy, and hypo- or hyper-thyroidism, and it may also be caused by use of oral contraceptives.

The phenothiazine tranquilizers and certain antihypertensive drugs, such as reserpine, guanethidine, and methyldopa, often cause orthostatic (postural) hypotension; therefore, abrupt changes from the supine position to the sitting or standing position at the end of a dental appointment should be avoided. Such patients should be gradually raised from the supine position and allowed to stand and should be questioned about feeling weak or dizzy before allowing them to leave. Another person should accompany the patient home if symptoms of hypotension persist.

Vasovagal Syncope

Certain immediate steps should be taken during the majority of office emergencies after the dentist makes a tentative diagnosis of the patient's condition:

STEP 1: Recline the patient to a head down (Trendelenburg) position to improve venous return and cardiac output.

STEP 2: Check for a patent airway, making sure it is open.

STEP 3: Administer 100 per cent oxygen (O_2) under positive pressure at a flow rate equal to the patient's respiratory minute volume (6 liters/min for an adult male).

STEP 4: Be prepared to send for medical help, support respiration, and support circulation. This involves teamwork with other auxiliaries and availability of emergency drugs and equipment.

These steps will be performed for all office emergencies except (1) acute asthmatic attack, when the patient is kept sitting erect because of respiratory difficulty; (2) convulsive seizure, when the patient is reclined to a comfortable position and restrained; (3) acute hyperventilation syndrome, when oxygen is NOT given; and (4) subluxation, when none of the above STEPS is applicable (Chap. 12, Sec. 1).

Vasovagal syncope is a form of neurogenic shock (Chap. 6, Sec. 1) characterized by faintness, dizziness, nausea, pallor, cold perspiration, hypotension, sinus tachycardia, dilated pupils, and possible loss of consciousness. It is the most common dental emergency and is sometimes precipitated in the patient by anticipation of injections, extractions, or other dental procedures the patient may approach with dread. If fainting occurs complete STEPS 1 through 4, then:

STEP 5: Loosen the patient's collar.

STEP 6:   Check the carotid pulse.

STEP 7:   Break one or two ampoules of aromatic spirits of ammonia ("smelling salts") under the patient's nose to encourage breathing through reflex stimulation.

STEP 8:   Check BP—if systolic pressure is above 80 mm continue oxygen and monitor BP; if systolic is 80 mm or below give alpha stimulants, such as phenylephrine (Neo-Synephrine) 5 mg INTRAMUSCULARLY, mephentermine (Wyamine) 30 mg INTRAVENOUSLY, or methoxamine (Vasoxyl) 5 mg INTRAVENOUSLY. Repeat in 20 minutes as needed for treatment of hypotension (Chap. 6, Sec. 2).

Allergic Reactions with Urticaria

Allergic reactions with urticaria are most commonly precipitated in dentistry by administration of penicillins or local anesthetic solutions, many of which contain antibacterial preservatives, such as methylparaben or propylparaben, or antioxidants, such as ethylenediaminetetraacetic acid (EDTA), sodium bisulfite, or sodium thiosulfate, that tend to inhibit decomposition of vasoconstrictors. Patients who have had an allergic response to administration of a local anesthetic solution may be allergic to the preservatives in the solution rather than to the anesthetic drug itself. Allergy to epinephrine and norepinephrine solutions without preservatives is non-existent.

If an allergic reaction is delayed and is limited to the skin (skin eruptions, urticaria, or mild angioneurotic edema) an antihistamine should be prescribed in maintenance doses (Chap. 5, Sec. 4), and the patient should be referred to an allergist. If further dental treatment cannot be delayed, the patient should remain on antihistamine therapy prior to any appointments in which local anesthesia will be used, or general anesthesia can be used instead of local. Further injections of local anesthetic solutions should be attempted only with the consent of the patient's physician, because subsequent allergic reactions may be serious or fatal.

If the allergic reaction is immediate and severe with involvement of the tracheobronchial tree (congestion, edema, respiratory depression) complete STEPS 1 through 4, then:

STEP 5:   Give epinephrine 1:1000, 0.5 cc SUBCUTANEOUSLY.

STEP 6:   Check the carotid pulse.

STEP 7:   Support respiration by breathing for the patient as needed, using mouth-to-mouth breathing, a mechanical resuscitator, or a bag and mask. Be sure the chest moves, whichever method is chosen.

Watch the patient carefully. If the previous measures have not relieved the condition, proceed to STEP 8:

STEP 8:   Give diphenhydramine hydrochloride (Benadryl) 50 mg slowly, INTRAVENOUSLY. Leave needle in vein for STEP 9.

STEP 9:   Start INTRAVENOUS glucose 5 per cent drip to establish a means for rapid drug administration.

STEP 10: Give hydrocortisone sodium succinate (Solu-Cortef) 100 mg slowly, INTRAVENOUSLY, through the tubing of the glucose drip. The drug is supplied in a Mix-O-Vial that supplies 100 mg in 1.8 cc of distilled water when mixed.

If the allergic reaction is immediate and severe with involvement of the cardiovascular system (pallor, hypotension, sinus tachycardia), complete STEPS 1 through 4 and STEPS 5 through 7, then:

STEP 8: Initiate cardiopulmonary resuscitation (CPR) if a carotid pulse cannot be detected (Chap. 12, Sec. 2).

Watch the patient carefully. If the patient's condition does not improve proceed to STEP 9:

STEP 9: Give epinephrine 1:1000, 0.5 cc slowly, INTRAVENOUSLY. Leave needle in vein for STEP 10.

STEP 10: Start INTRAVENOUS glucose 5 per cent drip to establish a means for rapid drug administration.

STEP 11: Give hydrocortisone sodium succinate (Solu-Cortef) 100 mg slowly, INTRAVENOUSLY, through the tubing of the glucose drip. The drug is supplied in a Mix-O-Vial that supplies 100 mg in 1.8 cc of distilled water when mixed.

Anaphylactoid Reactions

An anaphylactoid reaction is an allergic reaction that is characterized by an abrupt respiratory and cardiovascular depression with the signs and symptoms of both (urticaria, weakness, sweating, dyspnea, cyanosis, hypotension, unconsciousness, and cardiogenic shock) (Chap. 1, Sec. 2). It usually occurs during the first few minutes following injections and is often fatal, even when treated vigorously. When such a reaction is suspected, there is no time to debate the diagnosis or plan the treatment—the dentist and his staff must act almost by reflex if the patient's life is to be saved.

The STEPS involved in the treatment of this condition are identical to those followed in treatment of a severe allergic reaction but are executed in a different order. Complete STEPS 1 through 4, then:

STEP 5: Give epinephrine 1:1000, 0.5 cc SUBCUTANEOUSLY.

STEP 6: Give epinephrine 1:1000, 0.5 cc slowly, INTRAVENOUSLY. Leave needle in vein for STEP 7.

STEP 7: Start INTRAVENOUS glucose 5 per cent drip to establish a means for rapid drug administration.

STEP 8: Support respiration by breathing for the patient as needed, using mouth-to-mouth breathing, a mechanical resuscitator, or a bag and mask. Be sure the chest moves, whichever method is chosen.

STEP 9: Check the carotid pulse.

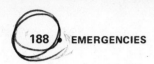

STEP 10: Initiate cardiopulmonary resuscitation (CPR) if a carotid pulse cannot be detected (Chap. 12, Sec. 2).

STEP 11: Give hydrocortisone sodium succinate (Solu-Cortef) 100 mg slowly, INTRAVENOUSLY, through the tubing of the glucose drip. The drug is supplied in a Mix-O-Vial that supplies 100 mg in 1.8 cc of distilled water when mixed.

Continue STEP 10 until adequate medical help arrives or until a spontaneous carotid pulse returns; when the carotid pulse returns, proceed to STEP 12:

STEP 12: Continue to support respiration and check BP—if the systolic pressure is above 80 mm continue oxygen administration and monitor BP; if systolic is between 60 and 80 mm, give epinephrine 1:1000, 0.5 cc INTRA-MUSCULARLY; if systolic is 60 mm or less, give epinephrine 1:1000, 0.5 cc slowly, INTRAVENOUSLY.

STEP 13: Give diphenhydramine hydrochloride (Benadryl) 50 mg INTRAMUSCU-LARLY to minimize any further action of released histamine.

Angina Pectoris

The patient who experiences an attack of angina pectoris is not having a heart attack but rather is experiencing a vague squeezing pain in the center of the chest that may radiate into the shoulders, arms, or jaws. The attacks are usually frequent and last no more than 15 minutes. Inadequate coronary blood flow is blamed for the painful attacks, and relief is generally obtained with adequate rest and administration of a coronary vasodilator (Chap. 6, Sec. 1), which improves myocardial oxygenation. Hypotension, nausea, and sweating are absent, and fatalities are uncommon. Many attacks are induced by emotional episodes. If such mild to moderate chest pain occurs in a patient in the dental office, complete STEPS 1 through 4, then:

STEP 5: Give glyceryl trinitrate (nitroglycerin) 0.6 mg, SUBLINGUALLY, and repeat, up to three doses. Relief should be expected in between 2 and 4 minutes. If the pain is more severe, break one or two ampoules of amyl nitrite under the patient's nose and expect relief of his pain in 45 seconds.

STEP 6: Give reassurance to the patient and allow him to rest; if pain is not relieved, suspect a myocardial infarction and give treatment accordingly.

Myocardial Infarction

An infarct is a blockade of an end artery that feeds all or part of an internal organ, and it results in partial or complete ischemia of the tissue area supplied by the end artery. When this occurs in the myocardium (usually from a thromboembolism), the patient experiences a crushing substernal pain that may also radiate into the shoulders, arms, or jaws, and he also suffers from cyanosis, sweating, nausea, hypotension, and dyspnea, and his skin may appear pale or ashen gray. In contrast to the pain of angina (Chap. 12, Sec. 1), the pain of myocardial infarction is agonizing, infrequent, and usually prolonged for several hours, and it is not necessarily induced by emotion. If such a heart attack occurs in a dental patient, complete STEPS 1 through 4, then:

STEP 5: Loosen the patient's collar.

STEP 6: Check the carotid pulse—if pulse is 60 or below give atropine sulfate 0.6 mg, INTRAVENOUSLY. Initiate cardiopulmonary resuscitation (CPR) if a carotid pulse cannot be detected (Chap. 12, Sec. 2). Leave needle in vein for STEP 7.

STEP 7: Start INTRAVENOUS glucose 5 per cent drip to establish a means for rapid drug administration.

STEP 8: Support respiration by breathing for the patient as needed, using mouth-to-mouth breathing, a mechanical resuscitator, or a bag and mask. Be sure the chest moves, whichever method is chosen.

STEP 9: Check BP—if systolic pressure is above 80 mm continue administration of oxygen and monitor BP; if systolic is between 60 and 80 mm, give mephentermine (Wyamine) 15 mg, INTRAVENOUSLY; if systolic is between 40 and 60 mm or below give 60 mg, INTRAVENOUSLY.

STEP 10: Give hydrocortisone sodium succinate (Solu-Cortef) 100 mg slowly, INTRAVENOUSLY, through the tubing of the glucose drip. The drug is supplied in a Mix-O-Vial that supplies 100 mg in 1.8 cc of distilled water when mixed.

STEP 11: Give analgesics—meperidine (Demerol) 50 mg, INTRAVENOUSLY or morphine sulfate 5 mg, INTRAVENOUSLY.

Toxic Reaction to Local Anesthetic

A toxic reaction to a drug is defined as the symptoms manifested as a result of excessive administration or overdosage (Chap. 1, Sec. 2), and it usually results from inadvertent intravascular injection of a local anesthetic solution or from the administration of too large a dose at one time. The body can detoxify up to 20 mg of local anesthetic per minute when it is injected intravenously, without reaction; therefore, if more than 1 cc per minute of a 2 per cent solution is given I.V., a toxic reaction may result. There are 36 mg lidocaine in each 1.8 cc carpule of a 2 per cent solution, and the maximum dose should not exceed 300 mg; therefore, if more than eight carpules are administered to an adult at one time, a toxic reaction may also result. This complication can be prevented by (1) using a minimal volume of solution with a vasoconstrictor, (2) aspirating before injecting, (3) injecting slowly, (4) watching the patient carefully during injection and discontinuing injection if toxic symptoms appear, and (5) determining the nature of any illness the patient may have before beginning treatment.

The early signs of a toxic reaction involve stimulation of the CNS, the respiratory center, and the cardiovascular system, resulting in visual disturbances, restlessness, confusion, feeling a lump in the throat, rapid breathing, and increased pulse rate and blood pressure. The later signs of toxicity include depression of the CNS, the respiratory center, and the cardiovascular system, resulting in stupor, convulsions caused by cerebral anoxia, unconsciousness, cyanosis, respiratory failure, hypotension, sinus tachycardia, and peripheral vascular collapse. The signs of depression may begin without a prior period of stimulation. If a toxic reaction begins in a dental patient, complete STEPS 1 through 4, then begin treatment for myocardial infarction:

STEP 5: Loosen the patient's collar.

STEP 6: Check the carotid pulse—if the pulse is 60 or below, give atropine sulfate 0.6 mg, INTRAVENOUSLY. Initiate cardiopulmonary resuscitation (CPR) if a carotid pulse cannot be detected (Chap. 12, Sec. 2). Leave needle in vein for STEP 7.

STEP 7: Start INTRAVENOUS glucose 5 per cent drip to establish a means for rapid drug administration.

STEP 8: Support respiration by breathing for the patient as needed, using mouth-to-mouth breathing, a mechanical resuscitator, or a bag and mask. Be sure the chest moves, whichever method is chosen.

STEP 9: Check BP—if systolic pressure is above 80 mm continue administration of oxygen and monitor BP; if systolic is between 60 and 80 mm, give mephentermine (Wyamine) 15 mg, INTRAVENOUSLY; if systolic is between 40 and 60 mm, give 30 mg, INTRAVENOUSLY; if systolic is 40 mm or below, give 60 mg, INTRAVENOUSLY.

STEP 10: If convulsions are sustained, DO NOT give a barbiturate, which could mask convulsions. Give succinylcholine chloride (Anectine) 50 mg, INTRAVENOUSLY, and repeat STEP 8, using bag and mask.

Insulin Shock

Insulin "shock," a complication of insulin administration for treatment of pancreatic diabetes (diabetes mellitus), is more correctly termed "insulin intoxication," since it is not directly associated with a progressive deterioration of the circulation, as are other forms of shock (Chap. 4, Sec. 2; Chap. 6, Sec. 1). The condition is precipitated by fasting immediately after insulin administration or by inadvertent insulin overdosage, resulting in an abrupt fall in blood glucose; symptoms reflect the release of endogenous adrenalin and include pallor, sinus tachycardia, profuse sweating, trembling extremities, headache, nausea and vomiting, disorientation, and in severe cases, convulsions and loss of consciousness. The diabetic dental patient who remembers to take his morning insulin but who is in a hurry to get to the dentist and fails to eat breakfast may develop insulin shock after arriving at the office. This potentially serious complication can be prevented by obtaining an adequate medical history and by questioning the patient at each appointment about (1) whether the diabetes is controlled or uncontrolled, (2) what the patient ate at his last meal, (3) how long ago he ate it, and (4) when he took his last dose of insulin or antidiabetic drugs.

Non-diabetic patients may also display milder hypoglycemic episodes when subjected to stress from dental procedures performed after a meal high in sugar, caffeine, or refined carbohydrates (Chap. 4, Sec. 2) or after prolonged fasting. In these patients the symptoms are identical to insulin shock but are much less severe.

Treatment consists of raising the blood glucose level; complete STEPS 1 through 4, then:

STEP 5: If the patient is conscious, give lemon-lime soda or other sweetened drink orally through a straw with the patient's head turned to the side. If the patient becomes unconscious, start INTRAVENOUS glucose 5 per cent drip and allow it to run completely open.

STEP 6:   Support respiration by breathing for the patient as needed, using mouth-to-mouth breathing, a mechanical resuscitator, or a bag and mask. Be sure the chest moves, whichever method is chosen.

If unconsciousness or respiratory failure persists, proceed to STEP 7:

STEP 7:   Give epinephrine 1:1000, 0.5 cc SUBCUTANEOUSLY.

Diabetic Coma

Uncontrolled pancreatic diabetes (diabetes mellitus) results in ketoacidosis (buildup of unmetabolized ketone bodies in the bloodstream) with symptoms of polydipsia, polyuria, glycosuria, weakness, disturbed vision, dry mouth and dry mucous membranes, flushed skin, acetone breath odor, hunger for air, nausea and vomiting, hypotension, and sinus tachycardia. Dental treatment of patients who present with any of these symptoms should be delayed until the possibility of diabetes mellitus is ruled out; serious oral infections should be treated initially with antibiotic therapy rather than by surgery. Although infections increase insulin requirements, surgery performed on infected tissue in a patient with uncontrolled diabetes may result in spreading the infection through a larger surgical wound and increasing, rather than decreasing, the insulin demand. A diabetic (ketoacidotic) coma and unconsciousness is the inevitable result of uncontrolled diabetes, and it can occur in a dental office as well as anywhere else. Treatment consists of giving insulin and I.V. fluids to lower the blood glucose level and to correct dehydration; complete STEPS 1 through 4, then:

STEP 5:   Check the carotid pulse—if pulse is 60 or below give atropine sulfate 0.6 mg, INTRAVENOUSLY. Initiate cardiopulmonary resuscitation (CPR) if a carotid pulse cannot be detected (Chap. 12, Sec. 2). Leave needle in vein for STEP 6.

STEP 6:   Start INTRAVENOUS saline (0.9 per cent NaCl) drip and allow it to run completely open.

STEP 7:   Support respiration by breathing for the patient as needed, using mouth-to-mouth breathing, a mechanical resuscitator, or a bag and mask. Be sure the chest moves, whichever method is chosen.

STEP 8:   Check BP—if systolic pressure is above 80 mm continue administration of oxygen and monitor BP; if systolic is between 60 and 80 mm give mephentermine (Wyamine) 15 mg, INTRAVENOUSLY; if systolic is between 40 and 60 mm give 30 mg, INTRAVENOUSLY; if systolic is 40 mm or below give 60 mg, INTRAVENOUSLY.

Watch the patient carefully; at the earliest opportunity proceed to STEP 9:

STEP 9:   Give regular insulin 40 units, INTRAVENOUSLY, under medical supervision.

Acute Asthmatic Attack

Bronchial asthma is a disorder characterized by dyspnea secondary to narrowing of the lumens of the smaller bronchi and bronchioles, and it results in the symptoms of wheezing, prolonged expiration, bronchiolar congestion, and in severe cases, in chest distention and cyanosis. It usually results from infections of the respiratory tract (intrinsic asthma) or from allergy to external antigens (extrinsic asthma), such as ingested foods or drugs. Patients who have a history of asthma will usually be taking beta$_2$ stimulants as needed (Chap. 6, Sec. 2). If this should occur, proceed to STEP 1:

STEP 1: Keep the patient upright—DO NOT recline the patient to a head-down (Trendelenburg) position.

Complete STEPS 2 through 4, then proceed to STEP 5:

STEP 5: Give epinephrine 1:1000, 0.5 cc SUBCUTANEOUSLY. Repeat in 15 minutes as needed.

STEP 6: Give aminophylline 250 mg, slowly, INTRAVENOUSLY. Do not exceed 100 mg/minute and watch for hypotension. Leave needle in vein for STEP 7.

STEP 7: Start INTRAVENOUS glucose 5 per cent drip to establish a means for rapid drug administration.

STEP 8: If the patient is hysterical, give diazepam (Valium) 10 mg slowly, INTRAVENOUSLY. Do not exceed 5 mg/minute.

Convulsive Seizure

Epilepsy is an intermittent disorder of the CNS characterized by organized discharge of cerebral neurons (Chap. 7, Sec. 3). The incidence of epilepsy in the United States is approximately 2 per cent, and in about 90 per cent of the cases a convulsive seizure occurs (grand mal). The seizure usually begins with tonic contraction of muscles, twitching and turning of head and eyes, loss of consciousness, cyanosis, and oozing of saliva and possibly blood from the mouth (if the tongue is bitten). If a convulsive seizure should occur, proceed to STEP 1:

STEP 1: Recline the patient to a comfortable position and restrain him by tying restraints around arms and legs—DO NOT recline the patient to a head down (Trendelenburg) position.

Complete STEPS 2 through 4, then proceed to STEP 5:

STEP 5: Place a dry towel horizontally between upper and lower posterior teeth to prevent tongue-biting.

STEP 6: Give diazepam (Valium) 10 mg slowly, INTRAVENOUSLY. Do not exceed 5 mg/minute. Leave needle in vein for STEP 7.

STEP 7: Start INTRAVENOUS glucose 5 per cent drip to establish a means for rapid drug administration.

Watch the patient carefully; if the convulsion is sustained proceed to STEP 8:

STEP 8: Give pentobarbital (Nembutal) 100 mg slowly, INTRAVENOUSLY.

When the convulsion stops, allow the patient to sleep or remain quiet. If the face is flushed or cyanotic the patient may have had a cerebrovascular accident (CVA, stroke); if this is noted proceed to STEP 9:

STEP 9: Support respiration by breathing for the patient as needed, using mouth-to-mouth breathing, a mechanical resuscitator, or a bag and mask. Be sure the chest moves, whichever method is chosen. Continue administration of oxygen until medical supervision arrives.

Acute Hyperventilation Syndrome

Hysterical overbreathing leads to excessive loss of carbon dioxide (CO_2) in the expired air, increased blood pH (–log of hydrogen ion concentration), reduced carbon dioxide combining power, and cerebral vasoconstriction, which may produce cerebral hypoxia. It may follow direct stimulation of the respiratory system; as in fever states, CNS lesions, salicylism, or psychogenic hyperventilation; reflex stimulation of peripheral chemo-receptors; or stimulation of stretch receptors by space-occupying lesions in the abdomen or thorax, as occur in cirrhosis, congestive heart failure, or pneumonitis. If acute hyper-ventilation occurs, complete STEPS 1 and 2, and proceed to STEP 3:

STEP 3: Limit carbon dioxide loss by having the patient rebreathe into a paper bag or oxygen facemask with low oxygen flow (1 liter/min). Have the patient count to ten out loud between breaths. DO NOT administer oxygen at a flow rate equal to the patient's respiratory minute volume (6 liters/min for an adult male).

Complete STEP 4, and proceed to STEP 5:

STEP 5: If patient is uncooperative or hysterical, give diazepam (Valium) 10 mg slowly, INTRAVENOUSLY. Do not exceed 5 mg/min.

Subluxation

When the mandible is depressed from the centric occlusion position of maximal inter-cuspation of the teeth, the mandibular condyles undergo a simple rotational movement when the mandible first begins to open without changing their respective positions in the glenoid fossae of the right and left temporal bones. As the mouth opens more widely, the mandibular condyles continue rotating and begin to translate down the articular eminences anterior to the glenoid fossae, with their forward advance halted by the eminentia themselves. Subluxation is a condition characterized by condyles riding anteriorly over the heights of the articular eminentia and being trapped anterior to their normal positions. This is painful and frightening for the patient not only because he has opened his mouth too wide and is unable to close it but also because his muscles of mastication (masseter, temporalis, medial pterygoid, and lateral pterygoid muscles) are usually in spasm. Forceful superior movements of the mandible will not only fail to reposition the dislocated temporomandibular joint but may succeed in fracturing the necks of the mandibular condyles or the condyles themselves.

If this should ever occur in a dental patient, proceed to STEP 1:

STEP 1: Keep the patient upright—DO NOT recline the patient to a head-down (Trendelenburg) position.

STEP 2:   Wrap your thumbs in a dry towel and place them on the occlusal surfaces of the lower posterior teeth with the index fingers beneath the inferior border of the mandible. Press downward with your thumbs and attempt to guide the mandible back into its posterior position. Remove your thumbs quickly when you begin to feel clamping on them.

If manual efforts fail to reposition the dislocated mandible, proceed to STEP 3:

STEP 3:   Give diazepam (Valium) 10 mg slowly, INTRAVENOUSLY. Do not exceed 5 mg/minute. Wait 10 minutes and repeat STEP 2.

If manual efforts fail to reposition the dislocated mandible again, proceed to STEP 4:

STEP 4:   Repeat STEP 3.

If the jaw muscles are unusually sore and painful when the mandible is repositioned, proceed to STEP 5:

STEP 5:   Give diazepam (Valium) 10 mg orally, q.4h. as needed for muscle pain, and advise the patient to use a warm water shower on both sides of the jaw and head. Stabilize the jaws with a Barton bandage.

SECTION 2: CARDIOPULMONARY RESUSCITATION

Methods of Administration

Serious life-threatening emergencies (severe allergic reactions, anaphylactoid reactions, toxic reactions, or myocardial infarctions) may progress into cardiogenic shock (Chap. 6, Sec. 1) and may result in brain death if not reversed within between 4 and 6 minutes following cardiac and respiratory arrest. Prior to brain death, the kidneys are damaged to varying degrees by circulatory failure depending on the degree of anoxia, and when this occurs drastic measures must be taken to (1) get air into the lungs and (2) compress the heart between the sternum and the vertebral column to circulate the blood. Although external cardiac compressions are only 40 per cent effective in circulating blood the chances of preventing brain death with cardiopulmonary resuscitation (CPR) long enough to get the patient to intensive care alive are better than 50:50.

Air inhaled into the lungs contains 21 per cent oxygen, whereas air exhaled from the lungs contains 16 per cent oxygen; since the normal tidal volume is 500 cc for the average adult, the volume of exhaled air from the rescuer that is needed to provide adequate tissue perfusion of oxygen in the victim is 719 cc. Therefore, the rescuer should overestimate the amount of exhaled air needed to provide adequate alveolar ventilation by giving about 1000 cc with each breath.

When a cardiac arrest is witnessed, a precordial thump may be used within the first 15 seconds of shutdown to shock the heart into beating rhythmically. The rescuer makes a fist and taps on the sternum with the same firmness as if affectionately "popping" someone on the shoulder—the ribcage should not be crushed with the blow. It is not the pressure but the shock of the stimulus that is often successful in restoring the heartbeat. A precordial thump is of no value unless performed within the first 15 seconds following a witnessed cardiac arrest.

Vomiting occurs during the first 2 to 7 minutes in 50 per cent of the cases treated with CPR. If such patients are not immediately intubated with an inflatable endotracheal tube that blocks the esophagus, the patient may aspirate vomitus into the trachea and die. If vomitus begins to ooze from the patient's mouth as the chest wall is compressed, there is no hope in saving the victim because his lungs, trachea, and pharynx are blocked, and air is unable to enter. When patients are extubated, there is a 100 per cent chance of vomiting, but a trained physician can remove vomitus on extubating without causing aspiration into the trachea. Unless vomitus is oozing from the mouth of the patient as the chest is compressed, CPR should not be stopped for any reason until medical supervision arrives and the patient is pronounced dead.

The STEPS involved in performance of CPR for a single rescuer are as follows:

STEP 1: Establish unresponsiveness (between 4 and 10 sec). Shake the shoulder and shout, "Are you OK?"

STEP 2: Open airway, establish breathlessness (between 3 and 5 sec), and give four quick ventilations (between 3 and 5 sec). Extend the patient's neck and look, listen, and feel for ventilations with ear to mouth and hand on chest. Maximum elapsed time should be 20 seconds.

STEP 3: Check the carotid pulse, establish pulselessness (between 5 and 10 sec). If a pulse is present, ventilate 12 times/min; if there is no pulse, proceed to STEP 4. Maximum elapsed time should be 30 seconds.

STEP 4: Begin four cycles of 15 chest compressions: two ventilations with a rate of 80/min (80 sec total time for this). Measure the width of three fingers superiorly from the tip of the xiphoid process of the sternum and compress the center of the body of the sternum to a depth of $1\frac{1}{2}$ to 2 inches. The compressions must be made vertically, with rigid arms and no bouncing; let your body weight provide the force to prevent fatigue. Maximum elapsed time should be 110 seconds.

STEP 5: Check the carotid pulse, establish spontaneous breathing (5 sec). Repeat STEPS 4 and 5 until the pulse reappears. Maximum elapsed time should be 115 seconds.

When two rescuers are available, the STEPS are identical except the chest compressions and lung ventilations are given in a ratio of 5:1 instead of 15:2. One rescuer performs chest compressions while the other ventilates on the contralateral side. Inflations are performed between the fifth and sixth chest compressions, and compressions are given at a rate of 60/minute.

Infants are resuscitated in the same manner as adults with the following exceptions:

1. The baby's neck need not be extended to open the airway.

2. The best position is with the arm under the body with the hand supporting the baby's head.

3. Four quick ventilations are performed by giving small puffs of air over both the mouth and nose.

4. Check the precordial pulse (over the left nipple) instead of the carotid pulse. *(?) (Brachial)*

5. The xiphoid process cannot be found readily. Begin chest compressions with two fingers over the mid-sternum and compress sternum $\frac{1}{2}$ to $\frac{3}{4}$ inches at a rate of 100/min. Ventilate at a rate of 20/minute.

Drug-Related Treatment

The portion of the myocardium having the most rapid depolarization, the part where the cardiac muscle cell membranes are most permeable to sodium ions, is in the wall of the right atrium at the sinoatrial node (SA node, pacemaker). The normal spread of excitation begins at the SA node and travels through the myocardium to the atrioventricular node (AV node), near the interventricular septum, which sends a wave of excitation through the bundle of His in the septum to the Purkinje's fibers scattered through the ventricular walls. This results in atrial contraction followed by ventricular contraction. When this automatic process is interrupted by arrhythmias, such as ventricular fibrillation, a direct current countershock can be applied across the chest to cause all portions of the heart to depolarize at the same time; when the current is removed, the SA node, having the greatest rhythmicity, should then take over and direct an orderly spread of excitation. A Life-Pack-5 is a defibrillator that is in use by many paramedics and that delivers a countershock of 400 watt-seconds over its paddles; it also contains a "scope" (EKG), three electrode leads, and a recorder. The defibrillator paddles can give a reading on the scope and recorder without having the leads (electrodes) attached to the extremities. The limitation of defibrillating is that cardiac standstill cannot be converted to sinus rhythm or to anything else without first having an arrhythmia to convert. Cardiotonic drugs are used to stimulate the myocardium in the hope of producing either sinus rhythm or an arrhythmia that can be converted by means of countershock.

The fastest acting cardiotonic drug used in cardiogenic shock is epinephrine (Adrenalin Chloride) (Chap. 6, Sec. 2). If CPR has been continued for five minutes without producing a spontaneous pulse, continue CPR and proceed to STEP 1:

STEP 1: Give epinephrine 1:1000, 1 cc INTRAVENOUSLY. Leave needle in vein for STEP 2.

STEP 2: Start INTRAVENOUS glucose 5 per cent drip to establish a means for rapid drug administration.

STEP 3: Give sodium bicarbonate 7.5 per cent, 50 cc INTRAVENOUSLY to counteract metabolic acidosis.

STEP 4: Give hydrocortisone sodium succinate (Solu-Cortef) 100 mg, INTRAVENOUSLY.

SECTION 3: ASPIRATION AND OBSTRUCTED AIRWAY

Heimlich Maneuver

The lodging of food or impaction of foreign bodies at the glottal opening of the larynx produces a choking spasm which may result in laryngospasm, and within four minutes, in death. In dentistry this may happen during (1) use of wax try-ins for removable dentures, (2) use of small casting try-ins, (3) crown or bridge removal, (4) pin placement, (5) canal débridement using hand files without rubber dam or gyromatic angles, and (6) subgingival débridement and prophylaxis, if loose cervical fillings become dislodged, rubber cups are lost from prophylaxis angles, or the blades of scaling instruments break off in the mouth. The operator should instruct the patient to hold still and should then apply suction to the oropharynx to remove any foreign bodies at the moment it is realized that a foreign body is present floating in the saliva. If no foreign bodies were taken up in the suction and none can be located in the mouth, the dentist should inform the patient that a foreign body entered the mouth and was not retrieved, and he should order chest radiographs to be taken. If the findings are negative on examination of the chest radiographs, the foreign body should pass through and into the stool in about three days.

If a patient is lying supine in the dental chair and begins to choke, proceed to STEP 1:

STEP 1: Identify complete airway obstruction by asking the patient, "Can you speak?" (between 2 and 3 sec).

STEP 2: Turn the patient on his side and deliver four blows to the back rapidly and forcibly on the spine between the shoulder blades; support the patient's chest with the other hand (between 3 and 5 sec). Maximum elapsed time should be 8 seconds.

STEP 3: Have the patient sit up and wrap your arms around his waist from behind. Place a fist, thumb side down, between the belt and ribcage and grasp your fist with your other hand. Deliver eight abdominal thrusts by pressing your fist suddenly backward and upward (between 8 and 10 sec). Maximum elapsed time should be 18 seconds. This expels a portion of the expiratory reserve volume from the lungs (Fig. 10–3). (Heimlich maneuver).

If the patient loses consciousness, proceed to STEP 4:

STEP 4: Place the patient in a supine position, extend the head to open the airway, and attempt to ventilate by giving four quick ventilations (between 10 and 12 sec). Maximum elapsed time should be 30 seconds.

STEP 5: Repeat STEP 2.

STEP 6: Turn the patient supine and position yourself with your knees close to the patient's hips. Place the heel of one hand between the belt and ribcage with the other hand on top. Deliver eight abdominal thrusts by pressing into the abdomen quickly and upward (between 10 and 12 sec). Maximum elapsed time should be 47 seconds.

STEP 7: Check for a foreign body in the mouth by turning the head to the side, open the mouth, and sweep deeply into the mouth with a hooked finger (between 6 and 8 sec). Maximum elapsed time should be 55 seconds.

STEP 8: Repeat STEP 4.

STEP 9: Repeat STEPS 2, 6, 7, and 4 in rapid sequence until patient regains consciousness and returns to normal breathing (between 21 and 31 sec per sequence). If after one sequence the patient's airway is still obstructed, perform a tracheostomy (Chap. 12, Sec. 3).

Tracheostomy

If the patient's airway continues to be obstructed by a foreign body believed to be at the level of the vocal cords, superior to the cricothyroid membrane, and if death from inadequate alveolar ventilation appears imminent, the dentist should perform a tracheostomy (tracheotomy), even if he has never performed one before. There is no time to prepare the patient psychologically for the procedure, and the operator should proceed directly to STEP 1:

STEP 1: Extend the head and palpate the neck for the inferior border of the thyroid cartilage. Give the skin below the thyroid cartilage an alcohol sponge wipedown and inject lidocaine 2 per cent with epinephrine 1:100,000, 0.5 cc SUBCUTANEOUSLY into the midline area between the thyroid cartilage and the sternum. Proceed immediately to STEP 2.

STEP 2: Insert a 10 or 12 gauge tracheostomy needle through the skin halfway between the inferior border of the thyroid cartilage and the superior border of the sternum to a depth of about 1 cm. Remove the mucus and blood by suction and stabilize the needle with adhesive tape or by tying it to the back of the neck. DO NOT force the needle against a resistance or puncture the posterior wall of the trachea. If considerable hemorrhage occurs, lightly clamp a hemostat above and below the point of puncture (Fig. 12–2).

STEP 3: Keep the lumen of the tracheostomy needle well suctioned and free of blood and mucus. Reassure the patient that everything will be all right but that he will temporarily lose his voice. Keep a pad and pencil handy for patient communication until medical supervision arrives.

When the trachea is first opened a loud, violent inspiration occurs, followed by the escape of a large amount of blood and mucus. In some patients the two anterior jugular veins are replaced by a median vein that divides in the suprasternal space of Burns into right and left branches running horizontally to join the external jugular veins; accidental severing of this median vein during tracheostomy will give rise to additional hemorrhage

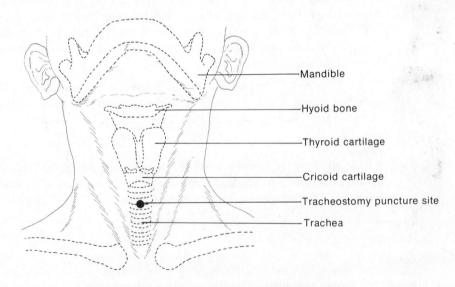

Mandible

Hyoid bone

Thyroid cartilage

Cricoid cartilage

Tracheostomy puncture site

Trachea

Figure 12–2. Anatomical landmarks for tracheostomy.

The isthmus of the thyroid gland is usually caudal to the first two or three tracheal cartilaginous rings, and this area is most suitable for puncturing the trachea because no blood vessels of appreciable size are usually present; caudal to the thyroid gland large veins are likely to be present and the trachea is much deeper with respect to skin surface.

TEST QUESTIONS

1. The term "vital signs" includes all of the following EXCEPT:
   (a) blood pressure   (d) temperature
   (b) pulse rate   (e) blood glucose level
   (c) respiratory rate
2. Indirect blood pressure determination is best made by using the palpatory (radial) method before the auscultatory method to totally prevent underestimation of the:
   (a) systolic pressure   (c) pulse pressure
   (b) diastolic pressure   (d) auscultation gap
3. Blood pressure determination of 162/96 for a 25 year old patient would classify the patient as:
   (a) normotensive   (c) hypertensive
   (b) hypotensive   (d) none of the above
4. Blood pressure determination of 158/94 for a 70 year old patient would classify the patient as:
   (a) normotensive   (c) hypertensive
   (b) hypotensive   (d) none of the above
5. Blood pressure determination of 96/60 for a 10 year old patient would classify the patient as:
   (a) normotensive   (c) hypertensive
   (b) hypotensive   (d) none of the above
6. Blood pressure determination of 96/60 for a 25 year old patient would classify the patient as:
   (a) normotensive   (c) hypertensive
   (b) hypotensive   (d) none of the above
7. When a diagnosis of vasovagal syncope is made, all of the following drugs should be readied for administration EXCEPT:
   (a) aromatic spirits of ammonia
   (b) alpha stimulants (phenylephrine, mephentermine, methoxamine)
   (c) oxygen
   (d) epinephrine 1:1000
8. When a diagnosis of allergic reaction with urticaria is made, all of the following drugs should be readied for administration EXCEPT:
   (a) epinephrine 1:1000
   (b) diphenhydramine hydrochloride
   (c) hydrocortisone sodium succinate
   (d) oxygen
   (e) atropine sulfate

9. When a diagnosis of anaphylactoid reaction is made, all of the following drugs should be readied for administration EXCEPT:
   (a) epinephrine 1:1000
   (b) diphenhydramine hydrochloride
   (c) hydrocortisone sodium succinate
   (d) oxygen
   (e) atropine sulfate

10. When a diagnosis of angina pectoris is made, all of the following drugs should be readied for administration EXCEPT:
    (a) nitroglycerin
    (b) oxygen
    (c) amyl nitrite
    (d) atropine sulfate

11. When a diagnosis of myocardial infarction is made, all of the following drugs should be readied for administration EXCEPT:
    (a) atropine sulfate
    (b) mephentermine
    (c) hydrocortisone sodium succinate
    (d) meperidne
    (e) oxygen
    (f) nitroglycerin

12. When a toxic reaction to a local anesthetic injection occurs, all of the following drugs should be readied for administration EXCEPT:
    (a) atropine sulfate
    (b) mephentermine
    (c) succinylcholine chloride
    (d) oxygen
    (e) meperidine

13. When severe insulin shock is diagnosed, all of the following drugs should be readied for administration EXCEPT:
    (a) sugar solution
    (b) oxygen
    (c) epinephrine 1:1000
    (d) atropine sulfate

14. When diabetic coma is diagnosed, all of the following drugs should be readied for administration EXCEPT:
    (a) atropine sulfate
    (b) sugar solution
    (c) oxygen
    (d) mephentermine
    (e) insulin

15. When an acute asthmatic attack is diagnosed, all of the following drugs should be readied for administration EXCEPT:
    (a) oxygen
    (b) epinephrine 1:1000
    (c) aminophylline
    (d) diazepam
    (e) atropine sulfate

16. When a convulsive seizure is diagnosed, all of the following drugs should be readied for administration EXCEPT:
    (a) oxygen
    (b) diazepam
    (c) pentobarbital
    (d) mephentermine

17. When acute hyperventilation syndrome is diagnosed, all of the following drugs should be readied for administration EXCEPT:
    (a) oxygen
    (b) diazepam
    (c) pentobarbital
    (d) both a and b
    (e) both a and c
    (f) both b and c

18. When manual efforts fail to reposition a dislocated temporomandibular joint the treatment of choice includes I.V. injection of:
    (a) diazepam
    (b) naloxone
    (c) succinylcholine chloride
    (d) pentobarbital

19. When cardiac arrest occurs, all of the following drugs should be readied for adminis-
    tration EXCEPT:
    (a) epinephrine 1:1000
    (b) oxygen
    (c) sodium bicarbonate
    (d) hydrocortisone sodium succinate
    (e) meperidine

13

PHARMACOLOGICAL MANAGEMENT OF PATIENTS WITH SYSTEMIC OR ORAL DISEASE

SECTION 1: PHARMACOLOGICAL CONSIDERATIONS IN PATIENTS WITH SYSTEMIC DISEASE

Medical-Dental History

The dental hygienist is concerned with the treatment of certain oral conditions diagnosed by the dentist. Although these conditions are diagnosed based on the information obtained from the clinical oral examination, the radiographic examination, and the patient's history, the single most important factor in the establishing of a diagnosis is the history. The medical-dental history form (Fig. 13–1) should contain (1) both primary and permanent tooth grids for charting existing dental work, evidence of pathologic conditions seen clinically, and evidence seen radiographically; (2) space for patient biographical data; (3) space for recording medical information, including blood pressure and pulse rate; (4) space for recording special clinical observations, such as the presence of tori, tooth mobility, hyperactive gag reflex, and so forth; and (5) space for the patient's signature attesting to the truthfulness of his statements. Such a record is not only necessary to effectively plan a patient's treatment but is also evidence that the medical status of the patient was investigated by questioning according to accepted standards before treatment was begun.

Some practitioners feel that only a member of the office staff or only the dentist should take the patient's medical history; others feel that it is permissible for the patient to fill out his own form. In either case, the dentist or dental hygienist should check to be sure that all the questions have been answered and that the patient has verified the truth of the answers with his signature. A responsible adult should be asked to complete the history form for patients under the age of 18.

The dental hygienist should bear in mind that any dental operator who so much as probes a new patient for periodontal pocket measurements without taking an updated medical history is guilty of negligence and that accepting a properly filled out history form that makes an inadequate survey of a patient's physical condition is also negligence.

Precautions During Pregnancy

Since the effects of many drugs on the developing human embryo or fetus are not known, and apprehension resulting from dental procedures has been the cause of spontaneous abortions, certain precautions should be taken with pregnant patients.

When pregnancy is suspected or confirmed, the patient's obstetrician should be consulted as to whether or not dental treatment should be attempted during the pregnancy. The dentist should describe the pertinent oral findings to the physician and should ask his or her advice concerning emergency treatment, if this should be necessary. All dental procedures except emergencies and routine oral examination and prophylaxis should be delayed if possible until the pregnancy is concluded. No diagnostic radiographs should be taken, but in dire emergencies they are permissible if a lead-lined apron is placed across the patient's abdomen and pelvis to protect the uterine environment. When local anesthesia has been administered the physician should be notified of the preoperative diagnosis and the services rendered.

The hormonal changes of pregnancy often cause changes in the eating habits, the oral hygiene habits, and the resistance of the patient's gingival tissues to infection. Pregnant women should have a periodic oral examination during each trimester, and a dental prophylaxis is permitted by the physician. Appointments should be short and pleasant, with treatment as conservative as possible. A dietary fluoride supplement taken daily is advisable during the second and third trimester (Chap. 3, Sec. 2).

PERSONAL HISTORY

LAST NAME _____ FIRST NAME _____

ADDRESS _____

CITY _____ STATE _____ zip code _____

| 1 | 2 | 3 | 4 | 5 | 6 | 7 | 8 | 9 | 10 | 11 | 12 | 13 | 14 | 15 | 16 |

Calculus deposit?____ Slight?____ Moderate?____ Excessive?____

| 32 | 31 | 30 | 29 | 28 | 27 | 26 | 25 | 24 | 23 | 22 | 21 | 20 | 19 | 18 | 17 |

HOW LONG?

Age _____ Date of Birth _____ Phone _____ Spouse or Parent _____

Married___ Single___ No. of children _____ Occupation _____

Widowed___ Divorced___ Employer _____ How long? _____

Ref. by _____ Employers address _____ Phone _____

Prev. address _____ How long? _____ Spouse employed by _____ Phone _____

Nearest relative _____ Address _____

Address _____ Spouse occupation _____

Phone _____

MEDICAL HISTORY   B/P _____ P.R. _____

Date _____

When were your teeth x-rayed last?
When was your last Phys.Exam?
Physician _____ Phone _____
Address _____
Is your general health good?
Are you now going treated by a Phys.?
if yes, nature of illness
Have you ever recieved x-ray or
radio-active isotope treatments?
By whom? _____ When? _____
Are you at present taking any
medicine?
If yes, What?
Are you on a diet? Why?
Are you allergic to penicillin?
other drugs or food?
if yes, What?
Has a Physician ever told you that
you have heart trouble?
high blood pressure?
rheumatic heart?
low blood pressure?
rheumatic fever?
hepatitis?
liver disease?
T.B.?
nervous condition?
diabetes?
Are you pregnant?
if yes, how many months?
Do you ever have chest pains?
if yes, where?
Are you short of breath on exertion?
Do you have a cough?
if yes, is it productive?

YES NO

Have you ever been seriously ill?
Have you ever had a major operation?
if yes, what?
Have you ever been hospitalized?
if yes, what for?
Are you considered a nervous person?
Do you bruise easily?
Have you ever had excessive bleeding?
following tooth extraction?
following cuts?
Do your gums bleed? When?
Are your teeth sensitive? to heat?
cold, or sweets?
Do you clench your teeth while
concentrating?
Do you grind your teeth during sleep?
or awake?
Is one tooth ever sore? loose?
Do you wake in the morning with
tired jaws?
Have you lost many teeth?
Why?
Have they ever been replaced by,
fixed bridge?___ removable partial?
or dentures?
How do you feel about your teeth?
How do you feel about dentures?
NOTES

YES NO

The above information is true and
correct to the best of my knowledge.

Signature: _____

CLINICAL NOTES

Figure 13–1. Patient history form.

Management of Patients with Cardiac Disease

The patient who presents with a history of a cardiovascular disorder will usually be well informed about it, and the disorders most commonly will involve (1) heart "murmur," (2) congenital heart disease, (3) rheumatic valvular heart disease, (4) coronary artery disease (angina pectoris, myocardial infarction), (5) cardiac arrhythmia, (6) congestive heart failure, or (7) hypertension.

The majority of heart "murmurs" are functional in nature; i.e., they are harmless extra sounds made during the cardiac cycle that cause no clinical disability; pre-medication of these patients for dental procedures is not necessary. Organic "murmurs" result from serious cardiac pathologic conditions, such as valvular incompetence, patent ductus arteriosus, or patent foramen ovale; pre-medication with an antibiotic of patients having organic murmurs for dental procedures is desirable to aid in the prevention of bacterial endocarditis, a condition secondary to bacteremia (Chap. 13, Sec. 1), and characterized by growth of bacterial colonies on defective valve leaflets or on endo-cardial surfaces. Patients having a history of congenital heart disease or rheumatic valvular heart disease should also be pre-medicated with an antibiotic.

No dental treatment should be planned for any patient within the three months following a heart attack (myocardial infarction), except for treatment of dire emergencies with appropriate sedation. Patients taking coronary vasodilators for treatment of angina pectoris will often carry their medication with them, but the dentist should stock his own nitroglycerin tablets and amyl nitrite "pearls" in the event that the patient forgets to bring them and has an attack.

Patients who have cardiac arrhythmias will usually be taking either quinidine, procainamide hydrochloride, or propanolol in maintenance doses. If the patient is taking quinidine, and local anesthesia is to be used, administration of epinephrine as a vaso-constrictor should be avoided because an accidental I.V. injection could produce ven-tricular fibrillation; it is best to avoid vasoconstrictors altogether with this type of patient. Local anesthesia with lidocaine should be avoided in those patients taking procainamide hydrochloride because an accidental I.V. injection may produce ventricular tachycardia and severe hypotension.

Patients who have a history of congestive heart failure and who are taking digitalis glycosides should not be pre-medicated with barbiturates, which may decrease the effect of these drugs; however, patients who are hypertensive or who have coronary heart disease will profit greatly from barbiturate pre-medication.

Prevention of Bacterial Endocarditis

Patients having a history of rheumatic fever, rheumatic valvular heart disease, con-genital heart disease, or organic heart murmur usually have damaged or abnormal heart valves or endocardium. The transitory bacteremia resulting from routine subgingival débridement and dental prophylaxis may result in the growth of bacterial vegetations on scarred endocardial surfaces or valve leaflets, which if large enough could break off and travel to a vital organ to become impacted in an end artery as an infarct. Prevention of this complication consists of pre-medication with an antibiotic; patients unwilling to comply with pre-medication either should not be treated at all or should sign a release form stating that they do not hold anyone in the office responsible for complications that may develop as a result of their failure to comply with the dentist's orders. Actually, all dentists are morally and ethically obligated not to treat such patients at all, and the dental hygienist should adhere to the same philosophy, because bacterial endocarditis may even occur despite preventive measures.

It is not possible to predict which patients with structural heart disease or which specific dental procedure will cause an infection, but patients with prosthetic heart valves are more likely to develop bacterial endocarditis than are other patients. Certain dental procedures, such as extractions or subgingival débridement, are more likely to initiate bacteremia than are other procedures, but there have been no controlled clinical trials in humans, and recommendations for antibiotic prophylaxis are based upon experiments in animal models.

Even without dental procedures, poor oral hygiene or ulcers caused by ill-fitting dentures may be a source of bacteremia, and patients at high risk should maintain a high level of oral health. There are no data to suggest that shedding of deciduous teeth is a significant cause of bacteremia, but devices that provide water under pressure to clean between teeth, and dental floss should be used with caution in patients with poor oral hygiene and cardiac defects because they have been shown to produce bacteremia. There are insufficient data at present to make a recommendation about use of these aids in patients susceptible to endocarditis.

The most common organism implicated in bacterial endocarditis following dental procedures is the alpha-hemolytic streptococcus (e.g., *Streptococcus viridans*); antibiotic prophylaxis should be specific for this organism, and parenteral administration should be favored when practical. For all dental procedures likely to result in gingival bleeding, antibiotic administration according to either regimen A or B may be used in patients having the cardiac disorders: (1) most congenital heart diseases, (2) rheumatic valvular heart disease, (3) other acquired valvular heart disease, (4) idiopathic hypertrophic subaortic stenosis, and (5) mitral valve prolapse. Patients with prosthetic heart valves should be treated according to Regimen B only.

In unusual circumstances or in the case of delayed healing, additional doses of antibiotic may be necessary, even though the bacteremia rarely persists longer than 15 minutes after the dental procedure is terminated. In some patients receiving continuous oral penicillin for prevention of rheumatic fever, alpha-hemolytic streptococci relatively resistant to penicillin are sometimes found in the oral cavity. In these cases it is likely that use of regimen A would be sufficient, but the dental surgeon may choose one of the suggestions in Regimen B or oral erythromycin.

Regimens A and B are the following:

REGIMEN A: PENICILLIN

1. Parenteral and oral combined

Adults: Aqueous crystalline penicillin G, 1,000,000 units I.M. mixed with procaine penicillin G, 600,000 units I.M., between 30 and 60 minutes pre-operatively. Begin penicillin V 500 mg orally q.6h. for eight doses.

Children: Aqueous crystalline penicillin G, 30,000 units/kg I.M. mixed with procaine penicillin G, 600,000 units I.M., between 30 and 60 minutes pre-operatively. For children under 60 lbs, begin penicillin V 250 mg orally q.6h. for eight doses.

2. Oral

Adults: Penicillin V 2.0 gm orally between 30 and 60 minutes pre-operatively, then 500 mg orally q.6h. for eight doses.

Children: Same as above. For children under 60 lbs, give 1.0 gm orally between 30 and 60 minutes pre-operatively, then 250 mg orally q.6h. for eight doses.

For patients allergic to penicillin:

3. Parenteral and oral combined (See regimen B.)

4. Oral

Adults: Erythromycin 1.0 gm orally between 90 and 120 minutes pre-operatively, then 500 mg q.6h. for eight doses.

Children: Erythromycin 20 mg/kg orally between 90 and 120 minutes pre-operatively, then 10 mg/kg q.6h. for eight doses.

REGIMEN B: PENICILLIN PLUS STREPTOMYCIN

Adults: Aqueous crystalline penicillin G, 1,000,000 units I.M. mixed with procaine penicillin G, 600,000 units I.M., plus streptomycin, 1.0 gm I.M. between 30 and 60 minutes pre-operatively; then give penicillin V 500 mg orally q.6h. for eight doses.

Children: Aqueous crystalline penicillin G, 30,000 units I.M. mixed with procaine penicillin G, 600,000 units I.M., plus streptomycin 20 mg/kg I.M. Timing of doses is same as above. For children of less than 60 lbs, give penicillin V 250 mg q.6h. for eight doses.

For patients allergic to penicillin:

Adults: Vancomycin 1.0 gm I.V. given for between 30 and 60 minutes via I.V. infusion, then erythromycin 500 mg orally q.6h. for eight doses.

Children: Vancomycin 20 mg/kg I.V. given for between 30 and 60 minutes via I.V. infusion, not to exceed a total dose of 44 mg/kg for 24 hours. Timing of doses is the same as above. Erythromycin dosage is 10 mg/kg q.6h. for eight doses.

Management of Hypertensive Patients

Arterial hypertension is a sustained elevation of the systolic or diastolic blood pressures or both (Chap. 12, Sec. 1) and is termed either primary (essential) or secondary. Essential hypertension is not linked to a single etiology, whereas secondary hypertension is due to some recognizable cause, such as renal disease, an adrenal disorder, or hyperthyroidism. Certain tranquilizers and antihypertensive drugs, such as ganglionic blocking agents, hydralazine, guanethidine, methyldopa, reserpine, and phenothiazines, may produce orthostatic hypotension (a fall in blood pressure in response to sitting upright from a reclining position); hypertensive patients taking such medication should be raised gradually from the supine operating position and observed for signs of dizziness before being allowed to stand up at the end of a dental appointment. The use of antisialagogues, such as atropine or methantheline bromide, should be avoided in hypertensive patients, since they may produce tachycardia. The use of vasoconstrictors for hemostasis or gingival retraction should be avoided in cases of hypertension, but local anesthesia with vasoconstrictors is preferable to general anesthesia, provided that the total dose of epinephrine does not exceed 0.2 mg.

Pre-operative sedation should be considered for potentially stressful dental procedures even in patients whose hypertension is adequately controlled, and for all dental procedures performed on hypertensive patients who are particularly apprehensive.

Management of Patients with Liver Disease

The patient with a history of liver disease (alcoholic liver disease, fatty liver, fibrosis, or cirrhosis) other than hepatitis is often unable to metabolize and detoxify drugs as rapidly as is normal, and drug intoxication may occur; this may be prevented by reducing the daily dose administered to such patients or by combining potentially toxic agents with synergists to allow a lower than average dose to be more effective. Local anesthetics should be administered with vasoconstrictors to delay systemic absorption and reduce toxicity.

Protective surgical gloves should be worn by the operator during examination and treatment of patients who have had hepatitis, even if recovery occurred many years ago (Chap. 5, Sec. 3; Chap. 9, Sec. 2).

Management of Patients with Lung Disease

Patients with a history of chronic lung disease (asthma, pleurisy, cystic fibrosis, or chronic obstructive pulmonary disease) are obviously not good candidates for inhalation sedation or general anesthesia and should have local anesthesia administered when anesthesia is needed. Dental treatment should be delayed in patients with acute infections (tracheobronchitis, pneumonia, and upper respiratory infections) until symptoms have disappeared. The operator should wear a mask over nose and mouth if treatment of a patient with a pulmonary infection cannot be delayed. If inhalation sedation or general anesthesia is used by necessity in patients who have a history of tuberculosis or chronic lung disease, hypoxia is more likely to occur secondary to reduced intra-alveolar surface area induced by scarring; such patients require an increased oxygen flow during anesthesia. The probability of allergic reactions is greater in those who have asthma, and asthmatics should be pre-medicated with an antihistamine prior to dental procedures.

Management of Nervous Patients

Patients who are nervous prior to and during dental procedures will usually admit it and should be given either oral pre-medication or parenteral sedation to alleviate emotional stress. Such patients should be accompanied to and from the office by a responsible adult and should be reassured that adequate drugs are currently available to treat virtually any possible complication or situation. Fear of pain is often nothing more than lack of knowledge, and the dental hygienist should encourage the nervous patient to ask questions about his dental treatment; apprehension is the natural uneasiness many patients have because they have not had a certain dental procedure performed in a certain manner before and therefore have no basis for comparison. Apprehsnsion can be controlled by drugs, but fear of pain is best dispelled by careful use of words, which are as important as the drugs themselves (Chap. 1, Sec. 3).

Management of Diabetic Patients

Patients who have a history of diabetes mellitus have vascular complications that result in poor circulation and reduced ability to resist infections or to heal tissue. In diabetic patients, all precautions to prevent oral infections should be exercised, since infections increase insulin requirements (Chap. 4, Sec. 1). Since epinephrine also increases insulin requirements and inhibits pancreatic insulin release, it should not be used for gingival retraction or hemostasis or as a vasoconstrictor in local anesthetic solutions administered to diabetics. Local anesthesia without a vasoconstrictor is preferred over general anesthesia (Chap. 10, Sec. 1). Prior to most dental procedures or extended appointments, the patient should be pre-medicated with a sedative to minimize the release of endogenous adrenalin.

Prior to oral surgery the patient should be pre-medicated with both a sedative and an antibiotic, and sutures may be left in place for two weeks in severe diabetics without causing excessive foreign-body reaction. Dental implants (vitreous carbon, endosteal blade-vent, osteogenic bone pins, and endodontic stabilizers, or subperiosteal) are contra-indicated except for intramucosal snap inserts. A multivitamin-mineral combination containing vitamin C, vitamin E, magnesium and zinc should be prescribed post-operatively.

Management of Cancer Patients and Cancer Chemotherapy

Cancer is a disease that touches everyone's life; one person in every four will develop cancer in a lifetime. Oral cancer accounts for about 5 per cent of all cancerous neoplasms in men and about 2 per cent in women, with five year survival rates of only 30 per cent. Since 60 per cent of all oral cancers are well advanced by the time of their discovery, and since there are 15,000 new cases occurring annually in the United States, a concerted effort is being made on the part of dentists and dental hygienists to diagnose suspected malignancies of the mouth in their early stages, when they are asymptomatic and easily treated.

The etiology or oral cancer is believed to be related to use of alcohol or tobacco, exposure to sunlight, viral activity, and nutritional deficiencies that cause normal cells to develop defective cell membranes, abnormalities of membrane transport, high densities of negative charge resulting in decreased cohesiveness, and cell division cycles prolonged from a range of 24 to 48 hours to a period about 120 hours long. These abnormal cells produce a proteolytic enzyme (plasminogen activator) that promptly produces plasmin, which in turn destroys the cell cytoskeleton (microtubules and microfilaments). Although the primary treatment for any form of cancer is surgery, various pharmacological agents are used as adjunctive therapy when the malignancy is inoperable, when surgery would be excessively mutilating, or when recurrence is likely after surgery. At the present time the chemical cure of a malignant tumor has not been achieved, but over 50 per cent of all cancers can be cured using chemotherapy combined with either surgery or radiotherapy, or with both.

Cancer chemotherapy is a traumatic psychological experience, especially for children;

the injections are usually painful, they may cause dizziness, and they may result in a temporary loss of body hair, which may grow back with a different texture or color. Agents that are currently being used include (1) antibiotics, such as bleomycin; (2) alkylating agents, such as cyclophosphamide; (3) radioactive isotopes, such as ^{60}cobalt, ^{131}iodine, ^{198}gold, or ^{32}phosphorus; (4) steroids, such as hydrocortisone or prednisone; (5) antimetabolites, such as cis-platinum, sodium fluoride, amethopterin, thiouracil, or mercaptopurine; and (6) miscellaneous agents, such as hydroxyurea. Amygdalin (vitamin B_{17}, laetrile) is a substance derived from apricot pits that has been widely promoted for the prevention and cure of cancer. At the present time in 12 states it is legal to receive laetrile treatments, but there has been no reliable evidence that laetrile is more active against any cancer than any other placebo is, and according to the FDA laetrile is of no value in human nutrition. Most of the promotional efforts to support laetrile have come from (1) the National Health Federation, which also supports antifluoridation of public drinking water, health foods, and certain medical treatments generally unaccepted by organized medicine; (2) the International Association of Cancer Victims and Friends, publishers of the Cancer News Journal, (3) the Cancer Control Society, publishers of the Cancer Control Journal; and (4) the Committee for Freedom of Choice in Cancer Therapy, which views efforts to regulate laetrile and other unproven substances as an invasion of personal privacy. The policy of organized medicine on the use of laetrile is that its effectiveness against cancer is unproven and that its use in such cases exploits the victims of cancer and their families by preying upon the emotions of the hopelessly ill for the profit of the unscrupulous. Apricot pit extracts also contain cyanides that, if ingested, can result in fatal cyanide poisoning. Although hopeful states of mind can beneficially alter the course of the disease in some patients, the dental profession should neither encourage the use of an alleged cancer remedy nor discount a placebo effect that has involved a spontaneous remission (Chap. 1, Sec. 1).

When the acidity of the saliva increases and the pH of the saliva drops to 5.5, the enamel begins to slowly dissolve. External radiation to the mouth and jaws decreases the pH of the saliva to 4.0 and produces xerostomia and an increased lactobacillus count, all of which tend to accelerate enamel breakdown. Since radiation also greatly reduces the cellular activity and reparative capacity of any tissue through which it passes, natural teeth in the path of radiation often develop radiation caries secondary to inhibition of the flow of dentinal fluid, and bone necrosis may occur when dental extractions are performed on such teeth shortly before or soon after radiotherapy. When bone necrosis occurs, the necrotic portion of jawbone must be surgically excised, creating a larger surgical wound and additional bone necrosis, and the entire jaw may eventually require surgical removal. To avoid causing osteoradionecrosis, at least three weeks healing time should elapse following dental extractions before radiotherapy is begun. In a study comparing the causes of jawbone necrosis in 304 cancer patients, the incidence of necrosis was 29 per cent in patients who had teeth removed at least three weeks before radiotherapy, compared to an incidence of 4 per cent when extractions were performed after radiotherapy. These results indicate that teeth in the path of radiation should be retained if the patient has a choice in the matter.

Radiated patients should have a recall dental visit every four months for subgingival débridement and prophylaxis, should use an ADA-recommended fluoride-containing dentifrice at least twice daily, should have a topical fluoride treatment with each recall visit, and should use a stannous fluoride topical product at home every day (Chap. 3, Sec. 2).

Management of Patients Taking Steroids

The long-term use of oral steroids interferes with the normal defense mechanism of the body and gives rise to depressed adrenocortical function; patients who have taken steroids for prolonged periods of time and who develop acute oral infections or require operative procedures may experience headache, nausea, diarrhea, irritability, paresthesias, anorexia, loss of memory, and hypotension. Acute exacerbation of these symptoms results in an adrenal crisis.

When severe infection is present or anticipated following surgery in these patients, they should be pre-medicated with an antibiotic, and the dosage of the steroid should be increased prior to dental procedures, in consultation with a physician (Chap. 4, Sec. 1). It should always be assumed that without an increase in steroid dosage these patients cannot satisfactorily react to a stressful situation.

Patients taking oral anticoagulants or having a history of Addison's disease should have their dental treatment deferred until adequate steroid levels in the patient's blood are verified.

SECTION 2: PHARMACOLOGICAL MANAGEMENT OF ORAL DISEASE

Diagnosis and Treatment of Gingivitis

Gingivitis (pyorrhea) is an inflammation of the gingival tissues and is characterized by swelling, bleeding, redness, and a change in the normal texture and contour. Although the greatest single causative factor is poor oral hygiene, other causes include defective dental restorations, malocclusions, allergic reactions, scurvy, and diabetes mellitus. Inflammatory changes in the gingiva are also associated with birth control pills and heavy metals; phenytoin may produce fibrotic changes (Chap. 7, Sec. 3). Painful, swollen, livid gums that bleed easily are suggestive of leukemia. A mild gingivitis may develop during pregnancy or puberty and is secondary to hormonal changes (Chap. 4, Sec. 1; Chap. 13, Sec. 1).

Treatment of this condition is directed at improving the systemic and local factors, beginning with subgingival débridement and prophylaxis. Severe cases may require gradual-release vitamin C supplementation, but these patients are afebrile, the disease is not contagious, and antibiotics are not required.

Diagnosis and Treatment of Necrotizing Ulcerative Gingivitis

Necrotizing ulcerative gingivitis (NUG, trench mouth, or Vincent's infection) is a non-contagious gingival infection that begins on the interdental papilla and that affects the marginal and attached gingiva by direct extension. It is caused by a fusiform bacillus and a spirochete, but it is aggravated by poor oral hygiene, stress, inadequate diet, inadequate rest, and habits such as heavy smoking (Chap. 4, Sec. 2). Usually there is no fever, but lymphadenopathy is present, and the interdental papilla show a "punched-out," cratered appearance and are covered by a greyish membrane. The diagnosis is confirmed by finding an overwhelming number of fusospirochetal forms on examination of a stained smear.

Unless high fever is present, antibiotic therapy should be avoided, but analgesics may be needed during the first 24 hours after initial débridement. Periodontal surgery may be needed to correct poor tissue topography produced by the acute phase of the disease. Usually a marked improvement is seen after the first 24 hours, after which a complete débridement can be accomplished. Study of a stained smear is essential when the tonsils or pharynx is involved, to differentiate the disease from diphtheria or staphylococcal or streptococcal pharyngitis.

Diagnosis and Treatment of Periodontitis and Periodontoclasia

The term periodontal disease denotes either periodontitis or periodontoclasia (periodontosis); periodontitis results when untreated gingivitis progresses to the point that loss of dentoalveolar bone begins, whereas periodontoclasia begins as a non-inflammatory destruction of dentoalveolar bone, which then progresses into gingival inflammation. The clinical oral findings with either type include deep pocket formation, gingival recession, tooth migration, and excessive mobility. Pain is usually absent unless an acute infection is superimposed on the chronic process. Treatment includes a combination of dental extractions, periodontal surgery, splinting of loose teeth, elimination of traumatic occlusion, and subgingival débridement and prophylaxis. Body chemistry evaluations and nutritional counseling are often helpful in preventing recurrences (Chap. 4, Sec. 2).

Antibiotics and mouthwashes are of little value in treatment of either condition. Diet supplementation with multivitamin-mineral combinations containing vitamin C, magnesium, and zinc will retard bone loss.

Functions of a Periodontal Dressing

The functions of a periodontal dressing are (1) to protect the surgical wound, (2) to control healing, (3) to control bleeding, and (4) to reduce the incidence of post-operative secondary infection. At times the dressings may also act as a temporary splint for loose teeth. They are composed primarily of zinc oxide eugenol with certain additives or modifiers to improve strength or give a better working consistency.

Periodontal dressings should not be placed over exposed bone owing to the high incidence of loss of granulation tissue when the dressings are removed. Antibiotics should not be used within the dressings because topically administered antibiotics are associated with a high incidence of allergic reactions.

Diagnosis and Treatment of Periapical Abscess

A periapical (dentoalveolar) abscess is an acute or chronic suppurative process of the periapical region of a tooth secondary to infection of the dental pulp resulting from dental caries or trauma. The condition is characterized by intense, continuous pain that is aggravated by thermal shock or occlusal forces. Left untreated, infection may spread through the fascial spaces of the face and result in cellulitis and fever. Treatment consists of either extraction or endodontic therapy of the offending tooth, which in either case removes the infected pulp from the mouth. If facial swelling becomes fluctuant it should be drained, usually by intraoral incision followed by local disinfection with a suitable antiseptic (Chap. 2, Sec. 1). A periapical abscess can be drained through an endodontic access opening, but in no case should the tooth remain open for longer than two days; the practice of allowing an open tooth to drain for several weeks after pulpectomy while the patient continues antibiotic therapy is to be condemned. If high fever persists, antibiotics and antipyretic analgesics are indicated.

A properly debrided dry canal may be closed with silver points, gutta percha points, or an antibiotic sealant. When an antibiotic sealant is used, the powder is mixed with a modified eugenol containing peanut, lavender, and rose oil to form a paste, which is spun into the canal and allowed to harden. The antibiotic properties of the paste are usually retained for about seven days after endodontic therapy is completed. The formula for the sealant powder used in the N2-RC2B method (after Sargenti) is as follows:

Zinc oxide	61.00 %
Lead tetroxide	11.00 %
Bismuth subcarbonate	9.00 %
Paraformaldehyde	6.50 %
Bismuth subnitrate	4.00 %
Titanium dioxide	4.00 %
Barium sulfate	3.00 %
Hydrocortisone	1.20 %
Prednisolone	0.21 %
Phenylmercuric borate	0.09 %

The original formula contained arsenic, which is now considered too toxic for use in humans. This paste causes no inflamation when accidentally extruded into bone, and in microscopic examinations appears well encapsulated. Slow resorption of the extruded mass is complete within five years and is not associated with signs of toxicity.

Diagnosis and Treatment of Periodontal Abscess

A periodontal (lateral, parietal) abscess is a localized purulent inflammation in the periodontal tissues secondary to direct extension of infection from a periodontal pocket, trauma, or root perforation during endodontic therapy. Acute lesions are characterized by throbbing pain, gingival tenderness upon palpation, mobility, lymphadenopathy, and fever, whereas chronic lesions are often asymptomatic. In considering a differential diagnosis between periapical and periodontal abscess, it can be said that a lesion is most likely periapical if the tooth is non-vital, whereas when the apex and lateral root surface are involved by a single lesion that can be probed from the gingival margin, the lesion is most likely periodontal in origin. A gingival abscess is confined to the marginal gingiva and usually occurs in disease-free areas, whereas a periodontal abscess usually occurs in the course of chronic periodontal disease (Chap. 13, Sec. 2). Treatment of an acute periodontal abscess consists of incision and drainage, local application of an antiseptic, and rinsing the mouth with saline every hour for one or two days, followed by a simple flap operation or gingivectomy. When fever and malaise are present, a suitable antibiotic and antipyretic analgesic are indicated.

Diagnosis and Treatment of Gingivostomatitis

Primary acute herpetic gingivostomatitis is a painful inflammatory condition of the gingiva and oral mucosa characterized by the presence of multiple shallow ulcers of varying size throughout the mouth resulting from infection with herpes simplex virus. Any disease that increases the metabolic rate or induces fever can precipitate lesions, but the history usually reveals contact with an adult having a herpes simplex infection. Although fever, malaise, and cervical lymphadenopathy are present, the disease usually subsides in seven to ten days. Antibiotics are ineffective against the virus and are contraindicated; treatment consists of antipyretic analgesics and either 2 per cent lidocaine viscous q.3h. as an oral rinse or diphenhydramine elixir q.2h. as an oral rinse as needed for pain until the lesions subside.

Recurrent aphthous stomatitis ("canker sores") are similar painful ulcerations that occur only on the movable oral mucosa and rarely, if at all, on the immovable mucosa (hard palate, attached gingiva). The lesions are characteristically yellowish and are surrounded by a bright red hyperemic zone. Severe attacks may be accompanied by malaise and fever; when fever or excessive discomfort exists, antipyretic analgesics are indicated. Triamcinolone acetonide in emollient dental paste (Kenalog in Orabase) reduces discomfort and aborts the formation of beginning lesions.

Stomatitis venenata or stomatitis medicamentosa may result from either contact allergy or absorption of drugs, respectively (Chap. 1, Sec. 2).

Diagnosis and Treatment of Candidiasis

Oral candidiasis (moniliasis, "thrush") is a fungal infection of the oral cavity caused by proliferation of *Candida albicans* and related species, and it is characterized by white curd-like patches that adhere to the oral mucosa. Removal of these white patches with a gentle stroke of a gauze square leaves red areas or bleeding points that are significant in a differential diagnosis. Candidiasis is a common complication of denture stomatitis or of therapy with broad spectrum antibiotics that can result in fungal superinfections. Treatment consists of nystatin oral suspension and adequate oral hygiene (Chap. 2, Sec. 2).

Oral candidiasis may be induced by (1) endocrine disorders (diabetes mellitus, hypothyroidism), (2) malignant diseases (leukemia, agranulocytosis), (3) malnutrition and malabsorption syndrome (alcoholism, iron deficiency anemia, pernicious anemia, postgastrectomy), (4) radiation therapy, (5) drugs depressing the defense mechanism (corticosteroids, antineoplastic agents), or (6) drugs that change the oral environment (antibiotics, diuretics, antihypertensives, phenothiazines, or antidepressants). Topical nystatin does not get into the pores of acrylic dentures, and infected dentures that are not disinfected prior to returning them to the mouth may inoculate the mouth again with *Candida*. Partially or fully edentulous patients with a diagnosis of oral candidiasis must have their dentures disinfected outside the mouth to ensure success in treatment.

Diagnosis and Treatment of Pericoronitis

Pericoronitis is an inflammation of the gingiva surrounding the crown of an incompletely erupted tooth, and it occurs most commonly in the mandibular third molar area. The lesion is painful, red, swollen, and often traumatized by contact with the opposing jaw. The patient may present with malaise, fever, cervical lymphadenopathy, and cellulitis, and occasionally the pericoronal flap may be the site of necrotizing ulcerative gingivitis (Chap. 13, Sec. 2). Surgical treatment is contraindicated on the first visit unless the flap is swollen and fluctuant, in which case an incision and drainage are performed, followed by topical application of an antiseptic. The flap should be gently elevated with a scaler, and the area should be flushed with warm water to remove underlying debris and exudate; use of a saline mouth rinse every hour and an antibiotic and antipyretic analgesic are prescribed with instructions to return in 24 hours. The next day when the acute infection subsides, either the tooth is extracted or the tissue overlying the occlusal and distal surfaces of the crown is removed down to the dentoenamel junction to remove the incubation zone responsible for the infection (operculectomy).

Diagnosis and Treatment of Alveolar Osteitis

Alveolar osteitis ("dry socket") results when the blood clot in the tooth socket is lost soon after a dental extraction, and the bony walls of the alveolus are exposed to the saliva. The incidence of alveolar osteitis is between 2 and 3 per cent and is independent of the surgeon's experience or the length of the operation, but it can be minimized by adhering to strict aseptic technique, by minimizing trauma, and by returning mucoperiosteal tissue to the correct position with sutures when indicated. When alveolar osteitis occurs, the socket should be irrigated with warm water to remove debris and exudate and lightly dried with sterile cotton sponges, and a long piece of iodoform gauze dampened with eugenol should be inserted into the socket in such a way as to cover the exposed bone on all sides. The socket is closed with a plug of zinc oxide eugenol pressed slightly below the height of the contour of the gingiva, and the patient is instructed to return in 24 hours for the socket to be repacked. During the first 24 hours the pain disappears, but the packs should be repeated every day until new granulation tissue can be seen growing on the socket walls. The patient should then be advised to place a compressed piece of sterile cotton in the socket every day to prevent food impaction until the bone completely fills in the defect. A suitable antibiotic should be prescribed for the five days after placing the first pack to minimize the risk of osteomyelitis.

Limitations of Radiographic Findings

Although the diagnosis of certain oral conditions may be made only by virtue of the findings of a clinical oral examination (e.g., gingivitis), a diagnosis cannot be made only by taking a history or only by examining radiographs. There are no radiographic findings to confirm many oral conditions, and infection of any kind cannot be diagnosed from a radiograph alone. It is preposterous for any third party, including insurance companies, to require radiographs in order to verify a dental diagnosis when only the dentist has taken the history and performed an oral examination on the patient.

Any oral lesion that produces a radiolucency on a dental radiograph may on biopsy prove to be an abscess, granuloma, cyst, or some other pathological entity; unless the lesion shows a characteristic cystic or malignant appearance in the radiograph, the patient should be told he has an "abscess," even though without a biopsy a definite diagnosis is lacking. This approach will improve communication and prevent lengthy explanations, which can delay treatment and interfere with the operator's rapport.

TEST QUESTIONS

1. The single most important factor in establishing a dental diagnosis is:
   (a) the history
   (b) the clinical oral examination
   (c) the radiographic examination
   (d) none of the above

2. Pregnant women should have a periodic oral examination and dental prophylaxis during each:
   (a) month of pregnancy
   (b) trimester of pregnancy
   (c) 8 week period of pregnancy
   (d) none of the above

3. Most patients with a history of heart murmur will require pre-medication prior to dental prophylaxis with:
   (a) a bacteriostatic antibiotic
   (b) a bactericidal antibiotic
   (c) a sedative-hypnotic
   (d) none of the above, (no pre-medication is indicated)

4. Patients with poor oral hygiene and cardiac defects should be advised to:
   (a) use dental floss with caution to avoid severe bacteremia
   (b) use oral irrigating devices with caution to avoid severe bacteremia
   (c) avoid wearing ill-fitting dentures
   (d) all of the above

5. No attempt to reduce salivary flow with drugs should be made in the hypertensive patient, to preclude the development of:
   (a) bradycardia
   (b) tachycardia
   (c) severe hypotension
   (d) all of the above

6. For the patient with a history of liver disease the best choice of a local anesthetic solution from the following possible choices is:
   (a) mepivacaine 3 per cent plain
   (b) lidocaine 2 per cent w/ep 1:100,000
   (c) prilocaine 4 per cent plain
   (d) both a or c

7. Prior to dental procedures in patients with a history of asthma, they should be pre-medicated with a(n) _(1)_ and undergo sedation using only _(2)_ .
   (a) _(1)_ antisialagogue and _(2)_ nitrous oxide oxygen
   (b) _(1)_ antisialagogue and _(2)_ non-inhalation agents
   (c) _(1)_ antihistamine and _(2)_ nitrous oxide oxygen
   (d) _(1)_ antihistamine and _(2)_ non-inhalation agents

8. The best choice of a local anesthetic solution from the following possible choices for the diabetic patient is:
   (a) mepivacaine 3 per cent plain
   (b) lidocaine w/ep 1:100,000
   (c) prilocaine 4 per cent plain
   (d) both a or c

9. All of the following have been used as cancer chemotherapeutic agents EXCEPT:
   (a) bleomycin
   (b) cyclophosphamide
   (c) cobalt-60
   (d) hydrocortisone
   (e) cis-platinum
   (f) sodium fluoride
   (g) stannous fluoride
   (h) amethopterin

10. A dental patient who presents with a history of long-term steroid therapy should have dental prophylaxis deferred until:
    (a) the dose of steroids is increased by his doctor
    (b) adequate steroid levels are verified in the patient's blood
    (c) it is verified that the patient can react satisfactorily to a stressful situation
    (d) all of the above

11 to 20. Match the oral diseases in the column on the left with the appropriate drug treatment(s) in the column on the right:

Disease

11. gingivitis
12. necrotizing ulcerative gingivitis
13. periodontal disease
14. periapical abscess
15. periodontal abscess
16. acute herpetic gingivostomatitis
17. recurrent aphthous stomatitis
18. oral candidiasis
19. pericoronitis
20. alveolar osteitis

Treatment

(a) no drugs needed
(b) analgesics
(c) antibiotics
(d) vitamin-mineral combination
(e) endodontic sealant
(f) local antiseptic
(g) local anesthetic mouth rinse
(h) topical steroid
(i) antifungal agent
(j) zinc oxide eugenol pack

ANSWERS TO TEST QUESTIONS

Chapter 1

1. e	8. d	15. c	22. a	29. a
2. c	9. f	16. e	23. d	30. c
3. f	10. e	17. e	24. e	31. d
4. d	11. b	18. d	25. b	32. a
5. b	12. d	19. c	26. c	33. c
6. a	13. e	20. d	27. e	34. b
7. e	14. b	21. b	28. f	35. d

Chapter 2

1. a	6. a	11. b	16. d	21. b
2. d	7. b	12. b	17. b	22. f
3. h	8. f	13. d	18. d	
4. b	9. a	14. e	19. d	
5. c	10. c	15. b	20. c	

Chapter 3

1. d	7. g	13. d	19. b	25. c
2. i	8. h	14. b	20. c	26. b
3. a	9. k	15. g	21. b	
4. h	10. b	16. d	22. a	
5. b	11. c	17. d	23. c	
6. c	12. c	18. c	24. d	

Chapter 4

1. b	4. b	7. c	10. e	13. f
2. d	5. d	8. b	11. d	14. c
3. a	6. f	9. c	12. b	

Chapter 5

1. d	5. a	9. c	13. c	17. a
2. d	6. d	10. b	14. b	
3. a	7. d	11. d	15. f	
4. d	8. b	12. b	16. b	

Chapter 6

1. f	7. a	13. c	19. c	25. b
2. d	8. d	14. a	20. d	26. f
3. a	9. b	15. b	21. b	27. b
4. d	10. k	16. c	22. b	28. d
5. c	11. f	17. c	23. a	
6. c	12. c	18. a	24. d	

Chapter 7

1. d	5. f	9. e	13. d	17. c
2. b	6. g	10. e	14. a	
3. h	7. c	11. a	15. e	
4. b	8. e	12. e	16. f	

Chapter 8

1. f	5. a	8. h	11. k	14. f
2. b	6. c	9. c	12. a	15. b
3. f	7. b	10. f	13. i	16. a
4. c				

Chapter 9

1. e	4. e	6. b	8. e	10. d
2. c	5. e	7. a	9. f	11. b
3. a				

Chapter 10

1. g	6. c	11. c	16. b	21. c
2. j	7. f	12. b	17. i	
3. a	8. a	13. g	18. c	
4. a	9. e	14. a	19. d	
5. b	10. f	15. a	20. b	

Chapter 11

1. d	5. c	9. b	13. d	17. f
2. d	6. a	10. e	14. a	
3. e	7. c	11. f	15. a	
4. b	8. a	12. d	16. e	

Chapter 12

1. e	5. a	9. e	13. d	17. e
2. a	6. b	10. d	14. b	18. a
3. c	7. d	11. f	15. e	19. e
4. a	8. e	12. e	16. d	

Chapter 13

1. a	5. b	9. g	13. d	17. h
2. b	6. b	10. d	14. e	18. i
3. d	7. d	11. a	15. c,f	19. b,c
4. d	8. d	12. b	16. b,g	20. c,j

BIBLIOGRAPHY

American Dental Association Council on Dental Therapeutics: Accepted Dental Therapeutics. Ed. 37. Chicago, American Dental Association, 1977.

American Heart Association: Prevention of bacterial endocarditis. J. Am. Dent. Assoc., 85:1377, 1972.

American Pharmaceutical Association: Evaluations of Drug Interactions. Ed. 2. Washington, D.C., American Pharmaceutical Association, 1976.

Aviado, D. M.: Kratz and Carr's Pharmacologic Principles of Medical Practice. Ed. 8. Baltimore, Williams & Wilkins Co., 1972.

Barber, J.: Rapid induction analgesia: A clinical report. Am. J. Clin. Hypn., 19(3):138, 1977.

Bennett, C. R.: Conscious-Sedation in Dental Practice. St. Louis, C. V. Mosby Co., 1974.

Bennett, C. R. (ed.): Monheim's General Anesthesia in Dental Practice. Ed. 4. St. Louis, C. V. Mosby Co., 1974.

Berkow, R. (ed.): The Merck Manual of Diagnosis and Therapy. Ed. 13. Rahway, N. J., Merck and Co., Inc., 1977.

Berridge, M. J., and Prince, W. T.: The role of cyclic AMP in the control of fluid secretion. In: Advances in Cyclic Nucleotide Research. Vol. 1. (Edited by P. Greengard, R. Paoletti, and G. A. Robison.) New York, Raven Press, 1972.

Bevan, J. A. (ed.): Essentials of Pharmacology: Introduction to the Principles of Drug Action. Ed. 2. New York, Harper & Row, Inc., Pubs., 1976.

Bonica, J. J., and Albe-Fessard, D. G., (eds.): Advances in Pain Research and Therapy. New York, Raven Press, 1976.

Burket, L. W.: Oral Medicine, Diagnosis and Treatment. Ed. 7. Philadelphia, J. B. Lippincott Co., 1977.

Carrier, O., Jr.: Pharmacology of the Autonomic Nervous System. Chicago, Year Book Medical Pub., 1972.

Csaky, T. Z.: Introduction to General Pharmacology. New York, Appleton-Century-Crofts, 1969.

DiPalma, J. R. (ed.): Basic Pharmacology in Medicine. New York, McGraw-Hill Book Co., 1976.

Ehrlich, A. B.: The Auxiliary's Role in the Administration of Local Anesthesia. Champaign, Ill., Colwell Co., 1974.

Everett, F. G., Hall, W. B., and Phatak, N. M.: Treatment of hypersensitive dentin. J. Oral Thera. Pharm., 2:300, 1966.

Goodman, L., and Gilman, A. (eds.): The Pharmacological Basis of Therapeutics. Ed. 5. New York, Macmillan Pub. Co. Inc., 1975.

Goth, A.: Medical Pharmacology. Ed. 8. St. Louis, C. V. Mosby Co., 1976.

Graedon, J.: The People's Pharmacy. New York, St. Martin's Press, Inc., 1976.

Guyton, A. C.: Textbook of Medical Physiology. Ed. 5. Philadelphia, W. B. Saunders Co., 1976.

Holroyd, S. V. (ed.): Clinical Pharmacology in Dental Practice. St. Louis, C. V. Mosby Co., 1974.

Irby, W. B., and Baldwin, K. H.: Emergencies and Urgent Complications in Dentistry. St. Louis, C. V. Mosby Co., 1965.

Kastrup, E. K. (ed.): Facts and Comparisons. Facts and Comparisons, Inc., St. Louis, 1979.

Langa, H.: Relative Analgesia in Dental Practice: Inhalation Analgesia with Nitrous Oxide. Ed. 2. Philadelphia, W. B. Saunders Co., 1976.

Malamed, S. F.: Handbook of Medical Emergencies in the Dental Office. St. Louis, C. V. Mosby Co., 1978.

Martin, E.: Hazards of Medication. Philadelphia, J. B. Lippincott Co., 1971.

Melzack, R., and Wall, P. D.: Pain mechanisms: A new theory. Science, 150:971, 1965.

Meyers, F. H., Jawetz, E., and Goldfien, A.: Review of Medical Pharmacology. Ed. 5. Los Altos, Calif., Lange Medical Publications, 1976.

Monheim, L. M.: Local Anesthesia and Pain Control in Dental Practice. Ed. 6. St. Louis, C. V. Mosby Co., 1978.

Physician's Desk Reference. Oradell, N. J., Medical Economics, 1977.

Pratt, W. B.: Fundamentals of Chemotherapy. New York, Oxford University Press, 1973.

Root, W. S., and Hofmann, F. G. (eds.): Physiological Pharmacology. New York, Academic Press, Inc., 1963.

Rowland, M.: Drug administration and regimens. In: Clinical Pharmacology: Basic Principles and Therapeutics. (Edited by K. L. Melmon and H. F. Morelli.) New York, Macmillan Pub. Co. Inc., 1972.

Shane, S. M. E.: Principles of Sedation, Local and General Anesthesia in Dentistry, Charles C Thomas, Springfield, Ill., 1975.

Steinman, R. R.: Pharmacologic control of dentinal fluid movement and dental caries in rats. J. Dent. Res., 47(5):720, 1968.

Sutherland, V. C.: A Synopsis of Pharmacology. Ed. 2. Philadelphia, W. B. Saunders Co., 1970.

Walton, J. G., and Thompson, J. W.: Pharmacology for the Dental Practitioner. London, British Dental Association, 1970.

Wilkins, E. M.: Clinical Practice of the Dental Hygienist. Ed. 4. Philadelphia, Lea & Febiger, 1976.

Wilkin, T. J., and Davidson, P. N.: Lecture Notes on Drugs for Dental Students. Philadelphia, J. B. Lippincott Co., 1978.

Woycheshin, F. F.: An evaluation of drugs used in gingival retraction. J. Prosthet. Dent., 14:769, 1964.

DRUG INDEX

GENERAL
INDEX

Abramson technique, 159
Accepted dental therapeutics, 2
Acromegaly, 69
Action potential, 136
Active transport, 6
Acupuncture anesthesia, 153
ADA Council on Dental Therapeutics, 2
Addison's disease, 68, 155, 211
Addition, 7
Adrenergic receptors, 93–95
Adrenocorticosteroids, 66–68, 167, 211
Affinity, 7
Agonist, 7
Allergic hypersensitivity, 11, 12, 186
Alpha receptors, 94 stimulants of, 98–100
    blockers of, 101–102, 173
Alveolar osteitis, 35, 215
AMA Drug Evaluations, 2
Aminoglycosides, 34, 167
Amphetamines, 117
Amygdalin, 210
Analeptics, 115–118, 171
Anaphylactic shock, 12, 87, 187
Anemia, 44
Angina pectoris, 47, 188, 205
Antagonist, 7
Antiarrhythmic agents, 92, 172
Antibiotics, 12, 15, 31–39, 166
Anticholinergic agents, 100
Anticholinesterases, 96
Anticoagulants, 77–79, 168
Anticonvulsants, 118, 171
Antidepressants, 114, 170
Antidiabetic agents, 63–65
Antiemetics, 109–111, 171
Antifungal agents, 38
Antihistamines, 7, 12, 83, 144, 169, 171
Antihypertensive agents, 91–93, 97, 172, 205
Antineoplastic agents, 16, 209
Antipyretics, 126–128

Antiseptic, defined, 27
Antisialogogues, 100, 144
Aspiration pneumonia, 155
Aspirin index, 126
Asthmatic attack, acute, 191
Ataractics, 108–114, 117
Atrioventricular node, 90, 196
Audioanalgesia, 162
Auscultation gap, 183
Autonomic agents, 7, 96–102
Autonomic physiology, 93–96

Barbiturates, 15, 106–108, 169
Barbiturate intoxication, 11, 107
Barbotage, 158
Belladonna alkaloids, 100
Benzodiazepines, 112, 171
Beriberi, 44
Berns technique, 158
Beta receptors, 94 stimulants of, 98–100
    blockers of, 102, 173
Bleeding time, 76
Blood coagulation, 74–77
Body chemistry evaluation, 70–72
Body surface area rule, 21
British Pharmacopeia, 2
Bureau of Narcotics and Dangerous Drugs, 16
Butyrophenones, 111

Cancer Chemotherapy, 52, 209
Candidiasis, 63
Cardiac disease, 155, 205
Cardiac glycosides, 90, 172, 205
Cardiac Output, 88
Cardiogenic shock, 87
Cardiopulmonary resuscitation, 194–196
Catecholamines, 84